RATING SCALES
AND CHECKLISTS

RATING SCALES AND CHECKLISTS

Evaluating Behavior, Personality, and Attitudes

Lewis R. Aiken

JOHN WILEY & SONS, INC.

New York • Chichester • Brisbane • Toronto • Singapore

REQUIREMENTS: An IBM, PC family computer or compatible computer, a 3.5" high-
density floppy drive, PC DOS, MS-DOS, or DR DOS Version 2.0 or later, and a printer.

Library of Congress Cataloging-in-Publication Data:

Aiken, Lewis R., 1931–
        Rating scales and checklists : evaluating behavior, personality,
    and attitudes / by Lewis A. Aiken.
            p.   cm.
        Includes bibliographical references and index.
        ISBN 0-471-12787-6 (alk. paper)
        1. Psychometrics.   2. Psychological tests.   I. Title.
        BF39.A43   1996
        155'.028'7—dc20   95-39106

Printed in the United States of America

10   9   8   7   6   5   4   3   2   1

Preface

This book is concerned primarily with rating scales and checklists—designing and constructing them, administering and scoring them, and analyzing the results. Rating scales are the most common measures of job performance and second only to teacher-made achievement tests in frequency of usage of all psychological measurement procedures. Introduced by Francis Galton during the latter part of the nineteenth century, rating scales have become popular assessment devices in many applied and research contexts.

Rating scales require the respondent to make evaluative judgments on an ordered series of categories. These categories, or different points on the continuum of the scale, are checked for different frequencies or intensities of the particular behavior or characteristic being rated. Ratings, made either by the ratee (the person being rated) or by another rater, are generally considered to be less precise than personality inventories and more superficial than projective techniques. Various types of rating scales are used in assessing a wide range of behavioral and personality characteristics, including numerical scales, graphic scales, standard scales, bipolar scales, and forced-choice scales.

A type of rating scale on which the categories are dichotomous is the checklist, a relatively simple, highly cost-effective, and fairly reliable method of describing or evaluating a person. More easily constructed than a rating scale or personality inventory, but often just as valid, a checklist can be administered as a self-report or observer-report instrument. Consisting of a set of descriptive terms, phrases, or statements pertaining to actions and thoughts that the checker may endorse (viz., check, underline, or in some other way indicate acceptance of), it can be filled out by the person being evaluated or by a parent, a teacher, a supervisor, a spouse, or a peer. In completing a checklist, the respondent is instructed to mark the words or phrases on a list that apply to the individual being evaluated. When a number of judges or checkers evaluate a person on the same items of a checklist, the person's score on each item can be set equal to the number of judges who checked it.

A type of rating scale that has been used extensively in various research and applied contexts is the attitude scale. *Attitudes,* defined as learned predispositions to respond positively or negatively to certain objects, situations, institutions, or persons, are similar to interests, opinions, beliefs, and values. Different methods can be used to measure attitudes, the most popular being an attitude scale. An attitude scale consists of a set of positive and negative statements concerning a subject of interest that are responded to on a continuum consisting of a number of categories. Most common of all attitude measurement techniques are Likert scales, although other methods (Thurstone's pair comparisons and equal-appearing intervals, Guttman's scalogram analysis, etc.) have their proponents.

This volume is a comprehensive treatment of all aspects of rating scales, checklists, and attitude scales. It consists of eight chapters, three appendixes, and separate indexes of subjects, authors, and instruments. Theoretical/psychometric aspects of scaling, as well as the mechanics of designing and evaluating various types of scales for different situations, are considered. Chapter 1 is a basic introduction to psychological science and instrumentation. Chapters 2 through 4 deal with the methodology and theory of rating scales, and Chapters 5 through 8 focus on instruments in specific applied areas. Descriptive lists of both standardized and nonstandardized rating scales, checklists, and attitude scales are also provided. The advantages and shortcomings of psychological, social, and educational measurement by means of rating scales, checklists, and attitude scales are given thorough consideration, and suggestions for evaluating and improving the psychometric characteristics of these instruments are offered. In addition to the other instructional features of the book, the Questions and Exercises at the end of each chapter should assist in making the material more practical, or "real world," in nature.

This book is designed primarily for researchers and practitioners in the behavioral and social sciences who use rating scales and checklists for diagnostic purposes and for assessing the effectiveness of interventions of various kinds. It should also prove useful as a supplementary text in research methods and assessment courses in psychology, education, and health-related areas. A DOS-formatted computer diskette containing dozens of programs concerned with the construction, analysis, and applications of checklists, rating scales, attitude scales, and other psychometric instruments accompanies the text.

The author wishes to thank the copyeditor, Nancy Land, for her invaluable assistance. I have been thinking about writing this book for many years, and I am grateful to everyone who has helped to make my aspirations and thoughts into a tangible reality.

LEWIS R. AIKEN

Contents

1

Conceptual and Historical Background

During the century or so since psychology was first designated a science, it has been variously defined as the study of (1) conscious experience, (2) the whole organism, (3) human and animal behavior, and more recently, (4) behavior and cognition. Recognizing that both behavior and cognitive processes make up the subject-matter of psychology, the fourth definition is the one that we shall follow in this book.

Like the natural sciences, psychology is objective, systematic, and self-correcting. Simpler explanations and concepts are considered preferable to more complex ones. Operational definitions, which define concepts in terms of the procedures that must be performed to demonstrate them, are favored over less objective definitions.

Simplicity is related to understanding as well as to communicability: the simpler something is, the more easily it can be understood and explained to someone else. Unfortunately, simple explanations of phenomena are not always precise and may not yield accurate predictions. Most human behavior is a complex function of nature and nurture and cannot be understood or predicted by a simple deterministic equation. For this reason, we often resort to complex statistical or probabilistic models and methods in order to predict and understand why people act in certain ways.

Whether simple or complex, the explanations or propositions of psychological science must be testable and, hence, confirmable or refutable. Furthermore, the concepts (or constructs) should be subject to classification and quantification. Quantifiable constructs should be measured as precisely as possible. The measurements must also be repeatable under similar conditions and clear in what they indicate.

SCIENTIFIC METHODS

The term *scientific method* may be reminiscent of a sequence of steps to which you were introduced in grade school. As a prescription for "science-making," the scientific method has five steps:

1. A problem arises.
2. Facts or data concerning the problem are collected.
3. A hypothesis or theory is formulated.
4. An experiment is conducted.
5. Conclusions, based on the results, are drawn.

This formal sequence is the prescription for one of the scientific methods, namely the method of experimentation. Other methods of collecting data in investigations of human behavior include controlled and uncontrolled observations, developmental studies, surveys, and correlations. The most fundamental of these is observation, where event(s) of interest are observed before being collated, correlated, or experimented upon.

Experimentation is the method of choice in science because questions can be answered and hypotheses tested more rigorously through experiments. It is the only way to establish a cause-and-effect relationship between events or variables. However, in studying human behavior and cognition, we are seldom able to manipulate and control all relevant variables. Methods other than experimentation must be used to gain insight into the factors that influence how people act and think, and the results of those influences.

Observation

When using observation, one notices events or occurrences in the environment and then records what is observed. Observations are usually *uncontrolled*; behaviors or other events are observed "on the wing"—as they occur—without arranging or contriving the situation in any way. Examples of this method includes observing and recording the aggressivity and cooperativeness of children on a playground, the skill and efficiency of employees in a production shop, and the emotional outbursts of people at a sports event.

Controlled observation, on the other hand, involves arranging a situation to determine how people react under certain constraints. For example, we may be interested in observing the interactions among participants in a preselected discussion group, and in making a record of the kinds of behavior shown by the participants. The observers in this situation would not necessarily be in the same room as the discussants. A closed-circuit television camera, inconspicuously placed for recording the scene could be connected to a monitor (screen) in another room. This arrangement minimizes the effects which the observers' presence and behavior may have on the reactions of the discussants.

Methods related to observation include the following:

- *Clinical Method.* Much of what is known about personality and social behavior has been obtained from observations made by both laymen and psychologists. These observations are typically uncontrolled, as when a clinical psychologist or psychiatrist observes a person during a diagnostic or therapeutic interview. In the *clinical method*, however, the observer may have a significant effect on the patient's behavior. The patient's reactions may also affect the behavior of the therapist in a reciprocal, interactive fashion. For this reason, making completely objective observations in clinical contexts is almost impossible.

- *Case History.* Related to the clinical method is the *case history method*, which involves obtaining and analyzing detailed information concerning the behavior and circumstances of a person during his or her lifetime that are relevant to the presenting symptoms or clinical questions. Obtaining a case history is almost always necessary in conducting an intensive clinical investigation of a patient's current condition and situation.

- *Interviews.* A *diagnostic interview* of the sort incorporated under the clinical method, or conducted for purposes of preparing a case history, is only one kind of interview. Interviews used to determine employee or student selection are more common and are more likely to be structured than unstructured, although they are typically semistructured. In a *structured interview,* the interviewer asks a series of prepared questions and records the interviewee's answers. Rather than recording everything the interviewee says, the interviewer usually makes notes and/or completes a checklist or rating scale during or immediately after the interview.

Few interviews are entirely structured: interviewees typically make comments or volunteer information that is not requested. An *unstructured interview,* however, is even more unplanned and open: the interviewer exerts some direction, but the interviewee is encouraged to open up and talk freely. More skill and experience are required to conduct an effective unstructured interview than a structured one. Also demanding a great deal of experience is a *stress interview,* in which the interviewee is subjected to intense interrogation in a police-type atmosphere to discover the truth. Although stress interviewing is not used routinely for employee selection or student admissions, it can be effective when the interviewee is highly resistant or is responding in a negative manner.

- *Developmental Studies.* Also related to the clinical and case history methods is the *developmental method,* in which a written record of the physical and behavioral development of one or more individuals over a period of years is obtained. When it is not possible to obtain accurate records of the development of the same individuals over the designated time period (the *longitudinal approach*), a *cross-sectional approach* is used. In the cross-sectional approach, conclusions about development are drawn from a study of the records documenting the characteristics and responses of different groups of people at different ages.

Surveys and Sampling

A survey consists of obtaining information concerning the opinions, practices, or possessions of a select group of individuals by means of questionnaires, telephone calls, and personal interviews. Thousands of surveys are conducted every year, mainly in applied research, but in theory-based research as well. The accuracy of survey findings depends on many factors, including the extent to which the people who are questioned are representative of the population of interest (the *target population*), the care with which the survey instrument is constructed and the surveyors are trained, and contextual factors such as time of day or year during which the survey is conducted.

Several sampling plans or procedures may be used in a survey, including random or probability sampling, quota sampling, and area sampling. Random sampling is more common in psychological investigations, whereas quota and area sampling are primarily sociological research methods. In *random sampling*, which is like drawing numbers from a hat, every individual in the target population has an equal chance of being selected. In *quota* (or *stratified*) *sampling*, the population is divided into several groups on the basis of some significant variable, such as sex or socioeconomic status, and a random sample is selected from each group. The size of the sample selected from a particular group is proportional to the number of people in the target population who are in that group. Finally, in *area* (or *cluster*) *sampling*, the target population is divided into areas or clusters on the basis of geography, and a random sample of people is selected from each area.

Whatever the situation in which observations are made, observers must be objective and not let their biases and expectations distort what they observe. One way to minimize the effects of bias and other personal factors is to immediately record what was observed, and afterward make an interpretation of the event. Electronic recording is useful in this regard, but it should be supplemented by the observer's written notes, clearly expressing impressions of what took place in the observational situation.

Correlation

The method of *correlation* is used extensively in both applied and theoretical research on human behavior, particularly when it is impossible or undesirable to conduct experiments. The degree of correlation between events and variables is concerned with the extent to which two or more things (variables) occur together, or are co-related. If it is found that variables X and Y are positively correlated, a person who makes a high score on one of the variables is likely to score high on the other variable as well. Likewise, a person who scores low on one of the variables will tend to score low on the other one. Thus, a person's standing on one variable can be predicted, within a reasonable margin of error, from his or her standing on the other variable. If two variables are negatively correlated, a person who scores high on one variable will tend to score low on the other variable.

The accuracy with which a score on one variable is predictable from a score on the other variable depends on the degree of positive or negative correlation between the two variables, as indicated by the *correlation coefficient*. This numerical index of the magnitude and direction of the linear relationship between two variables can be any numerical value from -1.00 (perfect negative relationship) to $+1.00$ (perfect positive relationship); the closer the value of the coefficient is to either $+1.00$ or -1.00, the more predictable a score on one variable is from a score on the other variable. A correlation coefficient close to .00 indicates the absence of a relationship between the two variables, and prediction of scores on one variable from scores on the other is no better than chance.

The fact that two variables are highly correlated in either a positive or negative direction does not mean that one variable has a direct effect on the other. Correlation implies prediction but not causation: changes in both the X and Y variables may be caused by a third variable, Z. For example, the relationship between alcoholism and absenteeism could conceivably be due to the fact that employees who work fewer days have more time to drink, or that both alcoholism and absenteeism are caused by stress, and not that drinking causes absenteeism.

Experiment

As noted earlier, even when two variables are highly correlated, we still may not know which variable, if either, is the cause and which is the effect. For this reason, the method of correlation, which helps us to make predictions, is limited in its ability to explain. For example, knowing that watching violent television programs is related to aggression in children does not tell us which behavior causes which. What is needed to answer such cause-and-effect questions is an experiment.

Experimental questions may be rather informal, such as, "I wonder what will happen if I say this or do this to a person?" Or they may be formulated as complex hypotheses, such as, "Job satisfaction varies as a curvilinear function of the number of positive reinforcements received." In any case, the experimenter is interested in what leads to what; that is, what effect is produced by introducing some change in a situation. To make certain that the observed effect or change in the *dependent variable* is caused by the variable that is manipulated (*independent variable*), rather than by an uncontrolled variable (*extraneous* or *confounded variable*), the experimenter takes precautions. These precautions involve holding constant, or otherwise controlling, extraneous variables. Then any changes in the dependent variable (or effect) can be attributed to changes in the independent variable, rather than being caused by some extraneous variable.

It is difficult, if not impossible, to achieve perfect control in experiments involving human behavior, but several standard procedures are employed to minimize the effects of extraneous variables. One procedure is to use a large number of subjects—the people or animals selected for the experiment. This practice is particularly important when differences among individuals in physical or psychological characteristics, other than those of primary interest to the experimenter, may influence the results. Using a large sample of subjects helps ensure that the effects of extraneous individual differences will cancel each other out, and makes the results of an experiment more generalizable to individuals other than those in the sample. The experimenter wants the results of the experiment to be generalizable—applicable to a larger target population similar to the selected sample, and not limited to the sample actually used in the experiment.

Another procedure for minimizing the effects of extraneous variables is to divide the subjects in the sample into two groups—a control group and an experimental group. This division should result in the individuals in the control group being matched, subject for subject, with those in the experimental group on all variables except the independent variable, the effects of which are being examined. Because perfect matching is impossible to achieve, the available subjects are often assigned at random to the two groups. In *random assignment,* the subjects are numbered or labeled, and the labels are randomly assigned to the two groups using a table of random numbers like those found in many elementary-level statistics books. Random assignment ensures that each subject has an equal chance of being selected for either the experimental group or the control group. This approach also increases the likelihood that the two groups are equivalent with respect to any extraneous variables that might affect the results.

MEASUREMENT AND PSYCHOMETRIC INSTRUMENTS

The value of scientific data depends on the precision with which the variables under consideration are observed and measured. The accurate measurement of these variables depends on the sophistication with which the instruments for measuring them are designed and used. Historically, science and measurement go hand in hand: Progress in science leads to new measuring devices, and the new devices lead to further scientific progress. Both science and technology are highly dependent on the development of measuring instruments and techniques. This mutually beneficial relationship can be seen not only in the history of physics and chemistry, but also in the history of biology and psychology. It is not surprising that the founding of the science of psychology during the late nineteenth century was preceded by improvements in time measurements, and by the invention of other instruments useful in the study of sensation, perception, thinking, and learning. Formulation of the first psychophysical law by Gustav Fechner, and subsequent studies in psychophysics, showed that mental events could be studied scientifically, and that they were lawful and predictable.

Psychological measurement has its beginnings in experimental psychology, though now the term *measurement* is more closely associated with *testing*. The formal history of psychological testing actually began around 1900, but long before then, teachers were using tests to evaluate the progress of their students, and psychiatrists were using crude tests to measure intelligence and personality. During the first two decades of the 20th century, a more systematic, scientific approach to the construction of psychological tests was introduced. Pioneers, such as J. M. Cattell, E. L. Thorndike, and Alfred Binet, followed closely by L. M. Terman, R. S. Woodworth, E. K. Strong, and others, showed how standardized, scientific procedures could be applied to the construction of mental tests. This approach was effective not only in measuring abilities, but also in assessing personality traits, interests, and other behavioral, cognitive, and affective processes. But how precise are these psychometric instruments in what they measure? And do they measure what they are supposed to? The second question, concerning validity, will be answered in Chapter 4. An answer to the first question, concerning precision of measurement, depends to a large extent on the particular *scale of measurement* being used.

Scales of Measurement

The term *scale* has many meanings. There is a balance scale, a decimal scale, a social scale, a taxation scale, a union scale, and a wage scale. In addition, there are bud scales, fish scales, mill scales, and even scales over one's eyes! *Scale* also refers to a graded series of tests or tasks for measuring intelligence, achievement, adjustment, and so on. Furthermore, it has come to be used, albeit rather loosely, to designate a particular psychometric instrument that purports to assess a person's standing on some variable, such as a scale of anxiety, depression, or Machiavellianism. When included in the title of a psychometric instrument, *scale* is essentially equivalent to "inventory," "questionnaire," or "test." Finally, as used in psychometrics, *scale* has traditionally referred to a measurement continuum on which objects, persons, events, or other entities can be ordered with respect to the quantity or quality of some variable. This is the sense in which the term will be employed here.

According to the pioneer psychologist E. L. Thorndike (1918), "Whatever exists at all exists in some amount." And, as echoed by W. A. McCall (1939), "Anything that exists in amount can be measured." *Measurement*, in its simplest form, involves assigning numbers to events. If measurement were limited to the function of labeling, it would serve only classification purposes. As we shall see, however, expanded application of these numbers in scientific functions makes measurement of greatest use in science-making.

Most students of human behavior know the distinction between cardinal numbers, which express amount, and ordinal numbers, which express degree, quality, or position in a series. One, two, and three are cardinal numbers, whereas first, second, and third are ordinals. In measurement, cardinal numbers are more precise, or at a higher level, than ordinal numbers.

A more detailed breakdown of numbers into *scales of measurement* was provided by S. S. Stevens (1951). Stevens characterized the degree of refinement or precision by which physical and psychological variables are measured in terms of four scales:

1. Nominal,
2. Ordinal,
3. Interval,
4. Ratio.

The first and lowest level of measurement is the *nominal scale*. On a nominal scale, numbers are used to designate or classify, rather than to indicate order or magnitude. For example, the numbers on athletic uniforms reveal nothing about the skills of the players, but they provide a way of identifying them and tracking their performances. Nominal scales are applied to demographic variables, such as sex (female = 0, male = 1), ethnicity (black = 1, white = 2, other = 3), and marital status (single = 1, married = 2, divorced = 3, widowed = 4). These numbers represent convenient ways of identifying individuals or groups for comparison purposes, but the numbers cannot be compared in terms of direction or magnitude.

The second level of measurement is an *ordinal scale*. In this scale, numbers represent the ranks or orders of merit of objects, persons, or situations on a variable of interest. An example of measurement on an ordinal scale is the order of finishers in a contest (first, second, third, and so on). Scales that rate behavior and personality characteristics also represent measurement on an ordinal scale. Many items on checklists are ordinal variables (e.g., more vs. less, stronger vs. weaker, like vs. dislike), but the response options on most checklist items are nominal categories.

Although many psychological and sociological variables are measured on ordinal scales, this level of measurement is rather limited. Numbers can be compared, but they yield only judgments of greater than (>), less than (<), or equal to (=). For example, if Paul finishes second, Louise finishes fourth, and Frank finishes sixth in a race, the ratings indicate that Paul was faster than Louise and Frank, and Louise was faster than Frank. Although it is true that $4 - 2 = 6 - 4$, it cannot be concluded that the difference in speed between Paul and Louise is the same as the difference in speed between Louise and Frank. This is because, on an ordinal scale, equal numerical differences do not necessarily translate into equal differences in whatever characteristic is being measured.

The *interval scale* is the third level of measurement discussed by Stevens. This scale allows some comparisons between different attributes of measured items, unlike the nominal and ordinal scales. The interval scale validates the statement, "The difference between a score of 4 and a score of 2 is equal to the difference between a score of 6 and a score of 4." Illustrative of measurement on an interval scale is temperature in degrees Celsius. If the temperature is 10° Celsius on Monday, 15° Celsius on Tuesday, and 20° Celsius on Wednesday, then we can say that the difference in temperature on Monday and Tuesday is equal to the difference in temperature on Tuesday and Wednesday. Because measurements of the attribute *temperature* in degrees Fahrenheit or Celsius are on an interval scale, the difference between 10 and 15 equals the difference between 15 and 20. However, interval scale numbers cannot be multiplied or divided, so we cannot conclude that it was twice as hot on Wednesday as it was on Monday—20 cannot be set equal to twice 10. A fourth scale of measurement is required to draw this conclusion.

The highest, or most refined, level of measurement is a *ratio scale.* A ratio scale possesses all the qualities of an interval scale, plus a true zero—a point indicating zero amount of whatever is being measured. Measurement on a ratio scale permits meaningful interpretation of equal ratios. If the temperatures in the previous example had been measured in degrees Kelvin, a ratio scale, instead of in degrees Celsius, an interval scale, it could be concluded that it was twice as hot on Wednesday as it was on Monday. Weight, height, response time, and many other physical variables are also measured on a ratio scale. If George weighs 180 pounds and Arlene weighs 90 pounds, it is correct to say that George weighs twice as much as Arlene, or that he is twice as heavy as she.

Scores on tests and other psychometric assessment instruments are usually ordinal or interval measurements. For this reason, a deviation IQ score of 150 cannot be interpreted as 1½ times a deviation IQ score of 100, or 3 times a deviation IQ score of 50. However, because deviation IQs are interval scale numbers, we can say that the difference between an IQ score of 150 and an IQ score of 100 is equal to the difference between an IQ score of 100 and an IQ score of 50.

Though the measurement of cognitive and affective variables is usually a combination of ordinal and interval scales, interval-scale statistics are often used in psychological assessment. Data may be summarized using interval-scale statistics, such as the arithmetic mean, the standard deviation, or standard scores, rather than ordinal-scale statistics, such as the median, the semi-interquartile range, or percentile ranks. This practice is generally accepted, recognizing that all measurements of psychological and sociological variables are fairly crude indicators and predictors. There are circumstances (e.g., a frequency distribution of scores that is markedly asymmetrical), when it is more appropriate to use statistics and statistical methods than assume measurement on an ordinal, rather than an interval or ratio, scale.

Psychometric Instruments

Psychometrics is concerned with research on psychological measurement, including the design and application of tests, checklists, rating scales, inventories, and other instruments for measuring abilities, personality, and behavior. The statistical and theoretical sophistication underlying the construction of these psychometric instruments has improved greatly during this century. The growth of psychological assessment as an applied science has led to the development of higher quality and more standardized instruments, as well as to a keener recognition of their limitations. Psychometric instruments, like checklists and rating scales, have increased the information obtainable through interviews and observations, and have provided a means for objectively recording that information.

Checklists

The simplest type of psychometric instrument to design and administer is a *checklist*, consisting of descriptive terms, phrases, or statements pertaining to certain objects, activities, or ideas. A checklist is a cost-effective and reliable method of describing or evaluating a person, object, or event. Answering the items on a checklist is simply a matter of checking, underlining, or otherwise indicating acceptance of those items pertaining to the subject of the checklist—the respondent him- or herself, someone with whom the respondent is acquainted, groups of people (teams, etc.), or other entities or events. The respondent makes a yes or no decision and indicates whether the term or statement is descriptive of the subject being judged or evaluated. Checklists are more efficient than rating scales, because the latter require decisions about the quality, frequency, or intensity of behaviors and characteristics. There is, however, a speed/accuracy tradeoff between rating scales and checklists: Rating scales can provide more detailed information than checklists, but they require more time to complete. More about checklists, including examples of commercially available and unpublished instruments in this category, will be presented throughout this text.

Rating Scales

Rating scales are a primary tool in contemporary assessment methodology (McReynolds, 1984), second only to teacher-made achievement tests in frequency of use for rating people, objects, and events. *Merit rating*, for example, is the most common method for evaluating employee performance (Landy & Farr, 1983; Muchinsky, 1990), and ratings of children's behavior are used extensively in intervention programs and developmental research (Witt, Heffer, & Pfeiffer, 1990; Piacentini, 1993). Rating scales are used in both applied and basic research contexts for a variety of purposes—to evaluate occupations, such as administrators, supervisors, students, teachers, and teams; commodities or products; institutions, such as colleges and universities; and concepts, such as ability, anxiety, and personality. Ratings are used for evaluating programs and publications, for designating educational achievement and health status, and for qualifying beauty and performances of all kinds. All countries use ratings for designating credit risk. Ratings are used both for selection purposes and for outcome (performance) criteria. In the workplace, ratings contribute to decisions concerning hiring, salary, promotion, transfer, termination, counseling, and other personnel actions resulting from performance appraisal (see Table 1.1). Ratings can reduce the subjectivity in observational and interview judgments by describing whatever is to be rated in more objective, standardized terms.

TABLE 1.1. Examples of Things That Are Rated

administrators	lawyers
athletic performance, teams	legislators
beauty	localities (cities, towns, suburbs)
bonds (industrial, local, municipal, revenue, state, treasury)	markets
	merchants
building materials	motion pictures
business climate	officers (military, police)
city managers	personality
colleges and universities	physicians
correctional personnel	principals
cost-of-living	programs (radio, television)
counselors	quality of life
credit risk	retirement climate
employees	sales (managers, personnel)
executives	soldiers
foodstuffs	stocks
funds (money market, mutual)	students
health (mental, physical)	supervisors
health workers	teachers (college and university, school)
insurance (companies, mortgage)	
judges	

Most consumer products are graded rather than rated. Many marketed foodstuffs are graded by the U.S. Department of Agriculture. These grades are usually in terms of quality ranks, but products may also be assigned category grades relative to characteristics other than a measure of quality. Examples of products that are graded by a quality variable are listed in Table 1.2.

Human beings have judged and evaluated other humans, objects, and events since time began. The thousands of languages spoken by people are replete with positive terms, such as good, better, best, and negative terms, such as bad, worse, and worst. A sequence of such terms constitutes a crude rating scale.

Francis Galton is frequently credited with introducing the rating scale into psychology. Galton, who also pioneered the use of questionnaires, word association techniques, and test batteries, proposed the use of ratings to assess good temper, optimism, and other personality traits by observing people in contrived social situations. However, almost 200 years before Galton, Christian Thomasius developed the first system of

---

TABLE 1.2. Examples of Graded Products and Grades

Beef: prime, choice, select, standard, commercial, utility, cutter, canner; depends on maturity and degree of marbling

Cognac: *, **, *** (in ascending quality); or C (Cognac), E (Extra or Especial), F (Fine), O (Old), P (Pale), S (Superior), V (Very), X (Extra), VO, VSOP, or Réserve (cognac aged in wood at least $4\frac{1}{2}$ years)

Fresh fruits and vegetables: trading grades—U.S. Fancy, U.S. No. 1, U.S. No. 2, U.S. No. 3); consumer standards—U.S. Grade AA (premium grade), U.S. Grade A (basic grade), U.S. Grade B (lower grade)

Hardwood: Firsts, Seconds, Selects, No. 1 Common, No. 2 Common, Sound Wormy, No. 3A Common, No. 3B Common, Below Grade

Padlocks: grades 1, 2, 3, 4, 5, 6

Steel doors: grades I (Standard-duty), II (Heavy-duty), III (Extra heavy-duty)

Textile colorfastness: to light—grades 1, 2, 3, 4, 5, 6, 7, 8, 9; alteration in lightness, hue, and saturation of color—grades 1, 2, 3, 4, 5; degree of staining—grades 1, 2, 3, 4, 5

Wood veneer: grades N, A, B, C, D

Source: From *Consumers' Guide to Product Grades and Terms* by T. L. Gall and S. B. Gall, 1993. Detroit: Gale Research Inc.

rating scales in the history of psychology. Thomasius's system involved 60-point scales, set off in 5-point intervals, for assessing what he considered to be the four basic characterological dimensions—(1) sensuousness, (2) acquisitiveness, (3) social ambition, and (4) rational love (McReynolds, 1984). By 1845, phrenologists—who believed that different psychological capacities are located in different brain areas, and that individual differences in these capacities can be measured by small differences in the topography of the skull—had developed forms that included systematic 9-point and 7-point rating scales, with detailed descriptions of each value (Bakan, 1966).

The early years of the twentieth century witnessed a scattered use of rating scales and checklists, but standard scales were not used extensively until the century was well advanced. During the past fifty years, paper-and-pencil scales for rating people have become popular psychological assessment devices in mental health, business/industrial, and educational contexts. Like checklists, they are easy to construct, administer, and score, and quite versatile in their applications. Also like checklists, raters may rate themselves (*self-ratings*) or other people (*ratees*) with whose behavior, abilities, and/or personality characteristics they are familiar. Unlike checklists, on which the responses are discrete categories (yes, no, ?, etc.), ratings are made on a continuum consisting of a series of numerals or descriptive designations (Excellent, Good, Fair, Poor, etc.). The rater marks the word or phrase that best describes the ratee's standing on the behavior or characteristic described in the item.

Both applied and theoretical research on ratings has increased since the 1960s, leading not only to more sophisticated instruments, but also to better standardization of these instruments and a clearer awareness of their advantages and limitations. One reason for the increased interest in the development and use of rating scales and checklists is the recognition that the effectiveness of educational and public health programs, as well as other social interventions, must be maintained through frequent reevaluation. The need to ensure that these public and private programs produce appropriate changes in behavior, attitudes, and other variables of concern has led to continued research and development of better evaluation instruments. When a particular program requires repeated, periodic evaluations, variations of the same instrument are required. This need is met through carefully designed rating scales and checklists.

Ranking and Pair Comparisons

Related to ratings are ranking items, on which the respondent places a group of people or things in rank-order according to their judged standing on the item. Unlike a rating scale, on which many people may receive the same rating, unless ties are permitted, ranking items "force" the respondent to assign a different numerical rank to each person. Supervisors rank their subordinates from highest to lowest or from best to worst on a list of behaviors or characteristics as well as on overall job performance; coaches rank their players on athletic ability, teachers rank students on cooperativeness, promptness, and neatness, and voters rank candidates for offices (see Box 1.1). Ranking is a fairly simple procedure, but it is cumbersome and quite time-consuming when more than a few persons or things must be ranked.

Related to ranking is the pair comparisons technique. It is also a tedious process, in that every person must be compared with every other person on a list of abilities, behaviors, or personality traits. This means that if n people are to be compared, then $n (n - 1)/2$ comparisons must be made. For example, if there are 10 people, then $10(9)/2 = 45$ comparisons must be made.

Ranking and pair comparisons involve only relative judgments—comparing one person with another. A variation of ranking known as the *point allocation technique* combines relative and absolute judgments (Duffy & Webber, 1974). In this method, a certain number of points, say 100, is given to the rater for each person to be rated. Then the rater assigns as many of the total number of points, say 1000 for 10 ratees, as he or she wishes to each ratee. The resulting rank orders of the points assigned represent relative judgments, and the differences between the points assigned to each ratee represent absolute judgments.

Inventories

An inventory is a kind of checklist or rating scale consisting of a fairly long list of questions or statements pertaining to personality, interests, or other characteristics and behaviors. The items on most inventories can be answered in the affirmative (True, Yes, etc.) or negative (False, No, etc.) or left unanswered (?, Don't know, etc.). On some inventories, however, the items are in multiple-choice or rating scale format. An inventory is scored by adding the numerical weights assigned to responses made by the respondent. For inventories that assess several variables or factors, a series of part scores must be determined.

Box 1.1
Voting Methods

Voting is a serious enterprise in democratic organizations and societies, but the procedures for determining the winners and losers are not always efficient, clear, or even fair. The two most common voting procedures employed in elections are *plurality voting*, in which the winner is the candidate who receives the largest number of votes, and *plurality voting with runoff*. In the latter case, if no candidate receives a designated percentage of the vote on the first ballot, a runoff election is held between the two candidates who received the most votes. The final winner is the candidate who gets the larger number of votes in the runoff. Although a runoff election presumably helps ensure that the candidate who is preferred by a majority of the voters actually gets elected, some form of ranking of candidates has been considered superior to plurality voting (with or without runoff).

One of the oldest ranking systems used in voting is the *Borda count.* This procedure begins by ranking all m candidates on a scale of 1 to m, where 1 is the first choice, 2 the second choice, and so forth. Then the points (p) obtained by each candidate are computed as $p = mn - \Sigma i n_i$, where n_i is the number of voters who assigned a rank of i to the candidate, $n = \Sigma n_i$, and the range of the summation is from 1 to m. For example, if 10 voters ranked 3 candidates according to first, second, or third place, a candidate who receives 3 first-place votes, 5 second-place votes, and 2 third-place votes obtains $p = 3(10) - [3(1) + 2(5) + 3(2)] = 11$ points. The candidate with the largest number of points wins the election.

More popular than the Borda count is the *Hare system* of single transferable vote. As with the Borda count, the process begins with rankings of the available candidates. For example, assume that one out of four candidates is to be elected and that the candidates (W, X, Y, Z) are ranked as follows by 21 voters:

	7 voters	6 voters	5 voters	3 voters
Rank 1	W	X	Y	Z
Rank 2	X	W	X	Y
Rank 3	Y	Y	W	X
Rank 4	Z	Z	Z	W

We begin by determining the integer component of q (quota) = $n/(m + 1) + 1$, where n is the total number of voters and m the number of candidates to be elected. If only one candidate is to be elected, then $q = 21/(1 + 1) + 1 = 11.5$, which truncates to 11. Thus, $q = 11$ is the minimum number of votes that a candidate must receive in order to be elected. Because no candidate received 11 or more rank 1 votes, the candidate (Z) with the lowest number of rank 1 votes is eliminated on the first round. Candidate Z's three rank 1 votes are transferred to candidate Y, who now has $5 + 3 = 8$ votes. Because

(Continued)

Box 1.1 *(Continued)*

none of the three candidates remaining (X, Y, Z) has 11 or more votes, the candidate with the smallest number of votes (X) is eliminated. X's 6 votes go to W, who now has 7 + 6 = 13 votes and is therefore elected. A similar procedure is followed when more than one candidate is to be elected (see Aiken, in press).

Even though it has been employed extensively since the mid-1900s, the Hare system has a number of problems. Two of these are its vulnerability to "truncation of preferences" and "nonmonotonicity." When voters truncate their preferences, that is, they do not rank all candidates in order of preference, an advantage may accrue to the candidate(s) whom those voters wish to see elected. Perhaps even more serious is the problem of nonmonotonicity, as seen in the paradoxical situation in which raising a candidate in one's preference order can actually hurt the candidate. The Borda count is also not without difficulties; for example, voters can gain by ranking the most serious rival to their favorite candidate last in order to lower his point total.

Perhaps more democratic than either the Borda or Hare systems is the Condorcet procedure, in which the winning candidates are those who can defeat all other candidates in separate pairwise contests. In the above problem 6 + 5 + 3 = 14 voters preferred candidate X to candidate W, but only 7 voters preferred candidate W to candidate X. Whereas application of the Hare procedure resulted in the election of candidate W, under the Condorcet procedure candidate X would be elected.

A number of other voting procedures, including cumulative voting, adjusted district voting, and approval voting, have been devised. In *cumulative voting*, each voter is given a fixed number of votes to distribute among one or more candidates. For example, if there are six candidates and the voter has six votes, he or she may give all of them to a single candidate, give two votes each to three candidates, or make any other assignment of the six votes to the six candidates. In *adjusted district voting*, the number of seats (i.e., votes) given to a minority group is adjusted to the proportion of minority members in the electorate. Finally, in *approval voting*, voters can vote for or approve of as many candidates as they wish. The number of votes received by a candidate is determined by the number of people who approve of him or her, and the candidate who receives the most "approvals" is elected (see Brams & Fishburn, 1991).[1]

The first personality inventory, the Woodworth Personal Data Sheet, was introduced in 1918 to screen U.S. Army recruits for emotional problems during World War I. This single-score instrument consisted of 116 yes-no questions concerning abnormal fears, obsessions, compulsions, tics, nightmares, and other feelings and behaviors. Examples of items on this inventory are:

Do you feel sad and low-spirited most of the time?

Are you often frightened in the middle of the night?

Do you think you have hurt yourself by going too much with women?

Have you ever lost your memory for a time? (DuBois, 1970, pp. 160–163)

Today, dozens of personality and interest inventories are commercially available. The most popular of all personality inventories is the Minnesota Multiphasic Personality Inventory (MMPI), which is administered for psychodiagnostic purposes and can be scored on many different clinical and special scales. The most popular vocational interest inventory, the Strong Interest Inventory, is scored on dozens of scales and used extensively in career counseling.

Tests

Generally the term *test* is associated with a systematic procedure for evaluating the knowledge, skills, or other abilities of a person in some area of endeavor. Such measures of *achievement* may be of the objective, essay, oral, or performance type. Until the twentieth century, most achievement tests consisted of a series of oral or essay questions. During the past half century, however, multiple-choice, true-false, and other objective tests have become the preferred method of assessing the extent to which students have attained the objectives of instruction in formal course work. These cognitive objectives are not the only kinds: the attainment of certain affective (motivation, attitudes, values, interests, etc.) and psychomotor skills are also objectives of educational programs. Many of these "tests" are informal devices or procedures devised by classroom teachers or other persons for a specific or one-time purpose.

During this century, *test* has also come to refer to published, standardized measures of intelligence, special aptitudes, interests, and personality. Such tests are administered for psychodiagnostic and counseling purposes as well as educational admissions and job selection rather than to ascertain the attainment of a set of instructional objectives. Familiar to most college students are standardized tests such as the Scholastic Assessment Test (SAT), the Graduate Record Examinations (GRE), the Graduate Management Aptitude Test (GMAT), the Law School Admissions Test (LSAT), and the Medical College Admissions Test (MCAT). These tests are *standardized* in the sense that they are administered with standard directions and have norms for evaluating scores on the test. In addition to being standardized, a good, commercially-available test is reliable and valid. These psychometric concepts are discussed in Chapters 3 and 4.

Rating scales and checklists, especially those that have been standardized and are commercially available, are sometimes called *tests*. Such instruments are not tests in the same sense as tests of achievement and aptitude. They are not designed to assess the ability of a person to perform some task or to profit from training or educational experiences. Nevertheless, whether completed by the ratee himself (herself) or by another rater, rating scales and checklists are often used to evaluate people for purposes of selection, training, psychotherapy, and other interventions. Applicants who receive poor ratings from others or whose responses to a rating scale or checklist indicate that they are unsuitable are not likely to be selected for the job or program. Patients who rate highly on one scale are more likely to be treated differently from patients who rate low. As these illustrations indicate, rating scales and checklists may serve purposes similar to those of traditional *tests* of ability.

OVERVIEW OF THE BOOK

The philosopher Immanuel Kant believed that psychology could never become a science, because science is concerned with objectively observable phenomena and psychology deals with subjective matters. It is often maintained that the research of Gustav Fechner, Francis Galton, and other pioneers in psychometrics refuted Kant's assertion—and so it may be. However, it would be foolish to claim that the status of psychology as a science is secure. Psychology involves human judgment and evaluation; the ultimate measuring instrument is the brain itself. Psychologists try to make their judgments more objective by operationally defining their variables, by training observers or evaluators to be more aware of their personal biases and their limited abilities to make accurate judgments, and by developing measuring instruments that are easy to use and reliable and valid indices of whatever they want to assess. But it is not an easy task.

This book focuses on rating scales and their derivatives—checklists, rankings, attitude scales, inventories, and other psychometric devices and procedures designed to make the assessment of people, objects, and events more objective and meaningful. Chapters 2, 3, and

4 are theoretical or methodological chapters. Chapters 2, 3, and 4 deal with methodological matters. Quite a bit of statistics and some complex concepts are considered in those chapters, but they are important to a thorough understanding of the chapters that follow. Chapters 5, 6, and 7 are applied chapters, dealing with the use of rating scales and checklists in industrial/organizational, research, and clinical situations, as well as other applied contexts. Many different psychometric instruments are described in these chapters, along with the details of how they are used in specific contexts. Chapter 8 is perhaps more comprehensive than any other chapter; it deals with theory, methodology, and applications in the measurement of attitudes and values.

Appendix A contains a glossary and Appendix B describes the computer programs accompanying the book. At the end of each chapter is a set of Questions and Exercises, at least two of which are concerned with using the Glossary and the computer programs. Descriptions of these programs and directions for using them are also given in Appendix B and on the diskette. Even if you are a computer expert, you should read the instructions and descriptions for the programs before attempting to run them.

SUMMARY

Scientific research may involve observations, interviews, correlations, experiments, and other methods of determining the relationships among variables. The only method that can identify cause-and-effect relationships between independent and dependent variables, however, is experimentation. In an experiment, extraneous or confounded variables are controlled by matching or randomization procedures. Because they cannot always control for extraneous variables, research psychologists and other behavioral scientists depend on careful observations, surveys, developmental studies, and correlational studies to identify significant relationships among variables.

Scientific research involves measurement, which varies in precision with the way in which the measurements are generated. It is convenient to classify measurement in four levels or scales—nominal, ordinal, interval, and ratio. In terms of precision of measurement, these four levels range from the simple descriptive or classificatory numbers of a nominal scale, through the ranked numbers of an ordinal scale and the equal-interval numbers of an ordinal scale to the highest level of measurement—a ratio scale. On either an interval scale or a ratio scale, equal numerical differences imply equal differences in the variable being measured, but only on a ratio scale do equal numerical ratios imply equal ratios in the measured variable. Most measurements in the behavioral sciences are no higher than an ordinal scale, or at best an interval scale level.

Psychometric instruments designed to measure behavioral and cognitive variables include (1) checklists, (2) rating scales, (3) ranking questionnaires, (4) inventories, and (5) tests. Of these, rating scales and tests are the most common. The rating scale method was introduced into psychology by Francis Galton and is now widely used in industrial/organizational, educational, clinical, and other contexts.

An inventory consists of a set of questions or statements designed to elicit responses indicative of certain personality characteristics, interests, or styles; responses to the items on a personality inventory or vocational interest inventory are in terms of agreement or disagreement with the item. These inventories are often labeled, somewhat loosely, as "scales." They consist of a series of checklists and rating scales.

A test is a form of examination for evaluating performance, capabilities, characteristics, or achievements. Most tests are of the objective (multiple-choice, true-false, etc.) or essay type, but the term *test*, as well as *technique*, has been used to label projective devices. Rating scales are not tests in the same sense as these instruments, but they serve many of the same purposes.

Advances in instrumentation, theory, and methodology have resulted in a science of psychology that deals with quantifiable variables. Psychology promises to produce even greater understanding of how people acquire both adaptive and maladaptive, behavioral and cognitive responses, and how those responses can be modified. Psychological assessment by means of rating scales and other psychometric techniques has and will continue to play an important role in attaining that goal.

QUESTIONS AND ACTIVITIES

1. Define each of the following terms used in this chapter. Consult Appendix A and/or a dictionary if you need help.

   area sampling   correlation coefficient
   assessment   dependent variable
   confounded variable   extraneous variable
   correlation   incident sampling

independent variable	ranking
interval scale	rating scale
measurement	ratio scale
merit ratings	representative sample
nominal scale	scale
objective test	stratified random sample
ordinal scale	target population
random sample	test

2. Run programs 1, 2, and 3 in category F ("Selecting and Assigning Samples") of the diskette of *Computer Programs for Rating Scales, Checklists, and Other Psychometric Instruments* accompanying this book. Use various sample sizes and various numbers of clusters and strata.

3. Make a series of 15-minute unobtrusive observations of a subordinate or coworker over a period of several days. Record your observations each day in diary format, and analyze them for similarities and differences at the end of the observation period. What did you learn about the person that you did not know before? Was the observed behavior consistent across time and situations? Why or why not?

4. Design a correlational study to determine whether women and men have different supervisory styles.

5. Design an experiment to determine the effects of positive reinforcement on productivity on various types of jobs.

6. Select several of the variables listed in Tables 1.1 and 1.2, and consult appropriate sources to determine on what categories and scales the variables are rated.

2

Constructing and Scoring Rating Scales and Checklists

onstruction of any effective psychometric instrument begins with a purpose, leading to a plan. As with tests of cognitive abilities, rating scales and checklists can serve many different purposes. Two of the most common purposes are evaluation of the adaptive or emotional behaviors of children and appraisal of the performances of working adults.

The purposes for which a rating scale or checklist is designed vary with the persons, organizations, objects, or events to be evaluated and how the responses will be used. For example, if a rough indication of behavior or performance is required, one need not spend much time refining an instrument to supply detailed information. If fine differentiations among individuals, organizations, or objects need to be made, greater care must be exerted in planning and constructing the instrument.

Rating scales can be used for evaluating almost anything. Many scales are designed to measure more than one entity or event (see Table 1.1). Instead of measuring only depression, anxiety, or hostility, a rating scale may consist of several subscales for measuring all three variables. Whatever the characteristic or trait to be evaluated, the behaviors defining those traits should be specified as objectively as possible to ensure that the instrument will be a reliable and valid measure of what it is designed to measure.

SOURCES OF INFORMATION

Once the purposes of a psychometric instrument have been clearly stated, one should not rush into the construction process. Hundreds of rating scales and checklists are commercially available. The twelve editions of *The Mental Measurements Yearbook* (Buros, 1978 and earlier editions; Conoley & Kramer, 1989; Conoley & Impara, 1995; Kramer & Conoley, 1992; Mitchell, 1985), a standard source of descriptive and evaluative information concerning psychological tests and other assessment devices, and *Tests in Print IV* (Murphy, Conoley, & Impara, 1994) contain many entries concerned with rating scales and checklists. Information and reviews may also be found in *Tests* (Sweetland & Keyser, 1991) and in *Test Critiques* (Keyser & Sweetland, 1984–1994). These reviews contain:

- A detailed description of the content of the instrument: title, author, publisher, data, and place of publication, forms available, type of instrument, cost, parts or sections, kinds of items and how selected, theory or conceptual basis of the instrument and the mental operations or characteristics it was designed to measure.
- Information on administering and scoring the instrument: instructions, time limits, whole or part scoring, clarity of directions for administration and scoring.
- Description of norms: size and composition of the standardization group and how it was selected, kinds of norms reported, overall adequacy of standardization.
- Reliability data: kinds of reliability information reported in the manual, nature and sizes of samples on which the reliability information was obtained and whether adequate.
- Validity data: kinds of validity information available and whether it is satisfactory in terms of the stated purposes of the instrument.

Among the many other sources of annotated lists and reviews of published tests are *Tests and Measurements in Child Development* (Johnson

& Bommarito, 1971; Johnson, 1976), *Tests in Education: A Book of Critical Reviews* (Levy & Goldstein, 1984), *Testing Children* (Weaver, 1984), *Testing Adolescents* (Harrington, 1986), *Testing Adults* (Swiercinsky, 1985), *A Consumer's Guide to Tests in Print* (Hammill, Brown, & Bryant, 1992), and the *ETS Test Collection Catalog*.

Information on available computer software and test-scoring services may be found in *Psychware Sourcebook* (Krug, 1993) and *Computer Use in Psychology: A Directory of Software* (Stoloff & Couch, 1992). Computer databases containing information on published tests include the *Mental Measurements Online Database* (Buros Institute of Mental Measurements, Lincoln, NE) and the *ETS Test Collection Database* (The Test Collection, Educational Testing Service, Princeton, NJ).

In addition to the published instruments cited in these volumes are the unpublished inventories, checklists, rating forms, attitude scales, and other affective instruments listed in *Dissertation Abstracts*, the several volumes of the *Directory of Unpublished Experimental Mental Measures* (Goldman & Busch, 1978, 1982; Goldman & Mitchell, 1990; Goldman & Osborne, 1985; Goldman & Saunders, 1974), the *Measures for Psychological Assessment* (Chun, Cobb & French, 1976), *Measuring Human Behavior* (Lake, Miles, & Earle, 1973), and *Tests in Microfiche* (Educational Testing Service).

Information on published and unpublished measures for clinical situations is given in *A Source Book for Mental Health Measures* (Comrey, Bacher, & Glaser, 1973) and the *Handbook of Psychiatric Rating Scales* (Lyerly, 1978). For information on unpublished measures of attitudes, the series of volumes from the University of Michigan's Institute for Social Research (Robinson, Athanasiou, & Head, 1974; Robinson, Rush, & Head, 1973; Robinson, Shaver, & Wrightsman, 1991) should be consulted. The HAPI (Health and Psychosocial Instruments) and PsycINFO databases are other useful sources of information on unpublished psychometric instruments.

Reviews of selected tests are also published in professional journals such as *Measurement and Evaluation in Counseling and Development, Personnel Psychology,* and *Psychoeducational Assessment.* Articles on the development and evaluation of psychological tests and measures are included in professional journals such as the *Journal of Clinical Psychology, Psychological Assessment: A Journal of Consulting and Clinical Psychology,* the *Journal of Counseling Psychology,* and the *Journal of Vocational Behavior.* Books have been written on single psychometric instruments, such as the Minnesota Multiphasic Personality Inventory (MMPI) and the Rorschach Inkblot Test.

Perhaps the most important source of information on rating scales and checklists consists of specimen sets of the instruments themselves and the accompanying manuals. A fairly comprehensive listing of the names, addresses, and telephone numbers of commercial publishers and suppliers of measures of this type is given in Appendix C. The development and marketing of psychometric instruments by these organizations is a sizable enterprise. Although more standardized achievement tests are sold than any other type of psychometric device, sales of rating scales, checklists, and inventories are still appreciable. Thousands of practicing psychologists and other professionals in private offices, public mental health clinics, educational institutions, business and industry, government, and other organizations use instruments of these kinds in their work.

Publishers and distributors of psychometric materials should require their customers to demonstrate some competency in psychological assessment. All too often, such materials are made available to individuals without adequate knowledge or training. The Ethical Principles of Psychologists and Code of Conduct stresses that evaluation and diagnosis should be provided only by trained, competent users of appropriate psychometric instruments and only in a professional context (American Psychological Association, 1992).

When deciding what assessment materials to order, potential users should not be misled by the *jingle fallacy*, that instruments having similar names necessarily measure the same characteristic, or the *jangle fallacy*, that instruments having different names necessarily measure different characteristics. A specimen set, which typically includes a copy of the instrument, an answer sheet, and perhaps a scoring key, can be ordered by professional psychologists and counselors to help them determine whether the instrument is applicable to the individuals and for the purpose which the potential purchaser has in mind.

The manual accompanying a rating scale or checklist, containing a description of how the instrument was constructed, directions for administering and scoring it, and perhaps norms, is usually not included in a specimen set and must be ordered separately. For some psychometric instruments, administration and scoring are covered in one manual, and the statistical details of norms, reliability, and validity are included in a separate technical manual. However, even a technical manual does not always provide up-to-date information on the validity of the instrument. Much of that information is contained in reports of research investigations published in professional journals.

PLANNING AND CONSTRUCTION

Once the purpose of the proposed rating scale or checklist has been spelled out and a suitable published or unpublished instrument cannot be found, the task of designing and constructing one begins. A number of questions concerning construction, administration, scoring, and interpretation, in addition to the analysis of results, should be considered before proceeding with the process of putting the instrument together. Not all of these questions can be answered completely at this stage. But since the nature of the instrument affects the answers, the instrument designer should at least keep the following questions in mind:

1. Considering the time and resources available, what type of instrument is best for the stated purpose—a checklist, rating scale, inventory, test, or some other kind of psychometric device or procedure?

2. What theories, empirical studies, personal experiences, and other sources of information will serve as guides to the development of the instrument?

3. If the instrument is to be of the paper-and-pencil type, what kinds of items will it contain? That is, how will they be worded, what format will be used, and how will they be arranged on the forms? How long will the list or scale be, who will the respondents be, and how long will it take them to respond to the items?

4. Where, when, to whom, and by whom will the instrument be administered? Will special directions or materials be needed to administer the instrument? If there is more than one section, are special directions required for each section? Will the instrument be standardized, that is, will data be collected from a representative sample to serve as a frame of reference for interpreting scores? Will a pilot study be conducted to identify problems in administration and scoring?

5. In preparing the directions or instructions for making ratings, what reference group should be specified, for example, all employees in an organization or all employees with whom the rater is acquainted, all teachers in this school or all teachers known by the rater? This will depend on why the ratings are being made, that is, what they are to be used for. It is important to make the reference group explicit, because raters often have some implicit standards of good and poor job performance that

affect their ratings in any case. If the directions for completing a rating scale do not specify a particular reference group, those internal standards—which vary from rater to rater—may have a disproportionate effect on the ratings.

6. How, when, and by whom will the instrument be scored? Will the scores to transformed in some way? Will the possibility of response sets be taken into account in scoring? To whom will the scores be reported?

7. How will it be determined that the instrument is actually measuring what it was designed to measure? Will item analysis, reliability studies, and validity studies be conducted?

Objective Observations and Interviews

As a preliminary step in instrument design, it is almost always worthwhile to make careful observations of the behaviors of interest and to interview potential subjects and people who know them well. Enough data may be obtained by means of observations or interviews to encourage a decision to forego the process of instrument development altogether. Information derived from observations and interviews can, in combination with certain theoretical preconceptions or experiences and other data, provide ideas about what type of instrument is best and how the items should be structured. Dictionaries, thesauri, and other reference works, as well as articles in magazines and newspapers, television programs, and other popular and professional sources of facts and suggestions can also contribute to the design of psychometric instruments.

Construction Strategies

Burisch (1984a) describes three major strategies for constructing rating scales and personality inventories—deductive, inductive, and external. The *deductive*, or content-based strategy (also referred to as the rational, intuitive, or theoretical approach), is based on à priori or theoretical conceptions of the behavioral or personality domain that the instrument is being designed to measure. The conceptions or judgments may be those of a single instrument-developer working alone or those of a group of experts. Wherever they may come from, these conceptions serve as a starting point. Then the instrument designer collects or constructs items that hopefully will measure the psychological construct(s) under consideration. Consider, for example, the rating

Directions: Circle the number corresponding to the extent to which each of the following adjectives is descriptive of the instructor of this course.

1 = Not descriptive at all
2 = Not descriptive
3 = Neither or uncertain
4 = Descriptive
5 = Very descriptive

	1	2	3	4	5
1. Considerate	1	2	3	4	5
2. Courteous	1	2	3	4	5
3. Creative	1	2	3	4	5
4. Friendly	1	2	3	4	5
5. Interesting	1	2	3	4	5
6. Knowledgeable	1	2	3	4	5
7. Motivating	1	2	3	4	5
8. Organized	1	2	3	4	5
9. Patient	1	2	3	4	5
10. Prepared	1	2	3	4	5
11. Punctual	1	2	3	4	5

Figure 2.1.   Eleven-item instructor rating scale.

scale in Figure 2.1; it was constructed by the deductive or content-based strategy. It was reasoned that a good teacher should know his or her subject-matter, be considerate or courteous, and motivating or stimulating—three characteristics that are encompassed by the adjectives in Figure 2.1. More formal theories of personality and behavior may also guide the process of instrument development. For example, Henry Murray's need-press theory of human motivation has served as a stimulus and outline for the construction of several personality tests. Included among these are the Thematic Apperception Test, the Edwards Personal Preference Schedule, and the Adjective Check List. Another illustration of theory-based construction is provided by Carl Jung's type theory of personality, which served as a guide in the development of the Myers-Briggs Type Indicator and the Singer-Loomis Inventory of Personality.

A second strategy, the *inductive* one, involves the use of factor analysis or other correlation-based procedures. Although designers of rating scales and personality inventories typically have some initial ideas about what they desire to measure, the major feature of the inductive approach is to let the data speak for themselves. In other words, a large collection of items is administered to an appropriate sample of examinees. Then a statistical and/or rational analysis of the responses reveals the number and nature of the variables being measured by the item aggregate and which items contribute to the assessment of which variables. This approach to constructing rating scales, checklists, and inventories has also been labeled internal, internal consistency, or itemetric. As an illustration of the inductive approach, a factor analysis of the ratings given by 90 college students to a professor in one of their classes confirmed that the scale in Figure 2.1 measures three factors— (A) consideration or interpersonal sensitivity, (B) preparation or knowledge, and (C) motivating or stimulating. Note that in the rotated factor matrix of Table 2.1, items 1, 2, 4, and 9 have high loadings (i.e., over .50) on Factor A, items 6, 8, 10, and 11 have high loadings on Factor B, and items 3, 5, and 7 have high loadings on Factor C.

Items from another scale developed by the inductive approach, in this case by computing the item-total correlations as a measure of internal consistency, are listed in Figure 2.2. The higher the corresponding correlations are, the greater the likelihood that the items are measuring the same variable or factor, and hence the more internally consistent the scale is. The low item-total correlation for Item 10 in Figure 2.2 indicates that this item is measuring something different from the other items, that is, a trait other than "distractibility."

Although the mathematical sophistication of the statistical procedures for developing rating scales by the inductive approach is impressive, factor analysis and related statistical methods do not provide an unerring path to the truth. Such methods are complex but not magical, and the results are often difficult to interpret.

TABLE 2.1. Rotated Factor Matrix for Items on Instructor Ratings Scale

Item	Factor A	Factor B	Factor C
1	.783	.090	.288
2	.853	.089	.131
3	.303	.015	.786
4	.790	−.041	.280
5	.148	.243	.792
6	.353	.669	−.113
7	.298	.009	.838
8	−.082	.649	.392
9	.691	.102	.120
10	.011	.867	.100
11	.052	.822	.048

Item Number	Item	Item-Total Correlation
7	Child is easily drawn away from his/her work by noises.	.72
10	If child is in a bad mood, he/she can easily be "joked" out of it.	.24
13	If another child has a toy he/she wants, this child will easily accept a substitute.	.75
20	If another child tries to interrupt when this child is engaged in an activity, he/she will ignore them.	.46
28	Child cannot be distracted when he/she is working (seems able to concentrate in the midst of bedlam).	.66
33	If other children are talking or making noise while teacher is explaining a lesson, the child remains attentive to the teacher.	.82
39	This child is easily sidetracked.	.73
47	Teacher may have to speak to the child several times before the child hears or responds if he/she is engaged in a task.	.41

Figure 2.2. Distractibility Scale—Teacher Form. From Martin, 1988. Reprinted with permission.

A third strategy, known as the *external, empirical,* or *criterion group* approach, has been characterized as the most accurate and most generally valid. Various statistical procedures, including correlation and regression analysis, chi square, and factor analysis, have been used in selecting items in the empirical method of constructing scales and inventories. In the empirical strategy, as exemplified in the construction of the Minnesota Multiphasic Personality Inventory (MMPI) and the Strong Vocational Interest Blank, items are selected or retained according to their ability to differentiate between two or more criterion groups of people. In designing the schizophrenia scale on the MMPI, for example, an item was selected for the scale if a significantly larger percentage of a sample of known schizophrenics than normal people gave a particular answer to the item. The other clinical scales on the MMPI were constructed in a similar manner. In constructing the Strong Vocational Interest Blank, an item became part of a particular occupational scale (e.g., the banker scale) if a significantly larger number of the criterion group (bankers) than men in general gave a particular answer.

Similarly, if it were found that delinquent children tended to watch television significantly more hours per week than nondelinquent children, the following item might be included on a scale designed to measure delinquency-proneness:

How many hours a week do you watch TV? 0–4 5–9 10–14 15–19 20–24 25+

Although rating scales and inventories based on the criterion-group approach do not require much psychological sophistication to construct, the validity of such scales depends greatly on the accuracy with which the groups are selected. The internal consistencies of such instruments are usually not very high, and they are designed to differentiate between two groups rather than among several groups (Martin, 1988).

It is not always clear whether any one of the three approaches to the development of rating scales is better than another, but it seems reasonable that a combination is best. Burisch (1984a) maintained that scales developed by the deductive approach are more economical to construct and communicate information more directly to the personality assessor. The majority of rating scales in use today were constructed primarily by the deductive approach. It is the starting point for most other scales. Burisch admits, however, that deductively developed scales can also be more easily faked and may not be as appropriate as empirically derived scales when it is advantageous for the examinee to dissimulate. Another disadvantage of the deductive approach is that items which experts view as measuring the same trait may actually be unrelated, resulting in low internal consistency when a scale is constructed with them. Finally, traits measured by instruments constructed by the deductive approach are generally viewed as normally distributed, making a normal-abnormal cutoff point rather arbitrary (Martin, 1988). A combination of the three strategies has been employed in the construction of many rating scales.

In another article on constructing rating scales and inventories, Burisch (1984b) emphasized that "You don't always get what you pay for." According to classical reliability theory, scales containing more items of the same general type are more reliable, and hence more valid, than scales having fewer items. But in assessing depressiveness by a variety of instruments, Burisch found that, on average, short scales were just as valid as long scales, simple scales were just as valid as sophisticated scales, and self-rating scales were just as valid as questionnaire scales. So in constructing a rating scale, Burisch's advice to "Make it simple." seems well-taken (also see Wolfe, 1993).

Types of Rating Scales

One way of classifying rating scales is according to whether they are unipolar or bipolar. On a *unipolar scale,* a single term or phrase referring to a behavior or trait is used; the rater indicates the extent to which the ratee possesses that behavior or trait. For example, degree of dominance may be rated on a scale of 1 to 7, where 1 is the lowest amount and 7 the greatest amount of dominance. This unipolar scale can be converted to a *bipolar scale* by using two adjectives—submissive and dominant—to designate the two extreme categories; the middle category represents equal amounts of dominance and submission. Because raters are ostensibly making judgments on longer continua in the case of bipolar scales than on unipolar scales, 5–9 intervals is recommended for the former and 4–5 intervals for the latter. If, on a bipolar scale, there is a tendency for responses to pile up in the middle ("undecided" or "neutral") category, that category should probably be omitted to make respondents commit themselves in one way or the other. Furthermore, in constructing a bipolar scale, the position of the "negative" and "positive" poles, if they can be designated as such, should be randomized or at least staggered in some way across items to cope with superficial responding or a position response set.

Rating scales may be classified in ways other than unipolar or bipolar. For example, there are numerical rating scales, semantic-differential scales, graphic rating scales, standard rating scales, behaviorally anchored scales, and forced-choice scales.

Numerical Rating Scale

On a *numerical rating scale,* the ratee is assigned one of several numbers corresponding to particular descriptions of the characteristic to be rated, such as "sociability" or "intelligence." All that is required is that the ratings be made on a series of ordered categories, with different numerical values being assigned to different categories. For example, in rating a person on "sociability," five categories, ranging from very unsociable (1) to very sociable (5), may be used. Figure 2.3 is a numerical scale designed to evaluate college courses and instructors. Notice that items 1–5 and 10 are concerned with the course and items 6–9 with the instructor. Therefore, at least two part scores as well as a total score may be determined.

Rather than using numbers to designate the scale categories, a set of adjectives (such as excellent, very good, good, average, poor, and very poor) or adverbs (such as always, very often, fairly often, sometimes,

Directions: Circle or check the appropriate number to the right of each statement to indicate how descriptive the statement is of this course or instructor. Circle any number from 1 (Not at All Descriptive) to 5 (Very Descriptive). Circle NA if the statement is not applicable to this course.

1.	The course is well organized.	1	2	3	4	5	NA
2.	The course objectives have been defined and met.	1	2	3	4	5	NA
3.	The textbook and other reading assignments are appropriate in content.	1	2	3	4	5	NA
4.	The papers, reports, and/or other written or oral assignments are reasonable and fair.	1	2	3	4	5	NA
5.	The tests and other evaluations are reasonable and fair.	1	2	3	4	5	NA
6.	The instructor has a thorough knowledge of the subject matter.	1	2	3	4	5	NA
7.	The instructor shows interest in and enthusiasm for the course.	1	2	3	4	5	NA
8.	The instructor has been available when needed outside of class.	1	2	3	4	5	NA
9.	Overall, the instructor is an excellent teacher.	1	2	3	4	5	NA
10.	Overall, this is an excellent course.	1	2	3	4	5	NA

Figure 2.3.   College course and teacher evaluation scale.

seldom, and never) corresponding to a series of numbers may be attached to each item phrase or statement. Responses in terms of these adjectives or adverbs may then be converted to the corresponding numbers and summed after administration. Bass and Barrett (1982) found that the six adverbial expressions of frequency listed above roughly bear order-of-merit ratios to one another of 5:4:3:2:1:0.

Semantic Differential Scale

A special kind of numerical rating scale is a *semantic differential.* This type of scale was employed initially in research concerned with the connotative (personal) meanings of concepts such as father, mother, sickness, sin, hatred, and love (Osgood, Suci, & Tannenbaum, 1957; Snider & Osgood, 1969). The procedure begins by having a person rate a series of concepts on several seven-point, bipolar adjectival scales.

For example, the concept of mother might be rated on the following seven-point scales:

Mother

Bad	____	____	____	____	____	____	____	Good
Weak	____	____	____	____	____	____	____	Strong
Slow	____	____	____	____	____	____	____	Fast

A semantic differential instrument typically consists of ten or more bipolar scales of this sort.

After all concepts of interest have been rated on the various scales, the rater's response to each concept is scaled on several semantic dimensions and compared with his or her responses to the remaining concepts. The principal connotative meaning (semantic) dimensions that have been determined by factor analyses of ratings given to a series of concepts on many different bipolar adjectival scales by different raters are evaluation, potency, and activity. A *semantic space* may be constructed by plotting the rater's scores on the rated concepts on these three dimensions. Concepts falling close to each other in the semantic space presumably have similar connotative meanings for the rater.

Graphic Rating Scale

One of the most popular types of rating scales is a *graphic rating scale.* At the two end points, and perhaps at intermediate points on the scale continuum as well, are graphic descriptions of the magnitude of the designated variable corresponding to those points. In addition to the behavior or attribute being assessed, these points, or *anchors*, should be worded as objectively as possible so they will have the same meaning for all respondents. An example of a graphic rating scale is:

What grades is the student expected to make in college courses?

|_____|_____|_____|_____|_____|

Below C	Below C	C in	Above C	Above C
in all	in most	most	in most	in all
courses	courses	courses	courses	courses

The rater makes a mark on each of a series of lines such as this one containing descriptive terms or phrases pertaining to a certain behavior or characteristic. The verbal description at the left end of the line usually represents the lowest amount or frequency of occurrence. The description at the right end represents the highest amount, intensity, or frequency of occurrence.

Standard Rating Scale

On a *standard rating scale,* the rater supplies, or is supplied with, a set of standards against which ratees are to be compared. An example of a standard rating scale is the *man-to-man* (or *person-to-person*) *scale* for rating people on a specified characteristic or behavior. Raters begin by thinking of, say, five people who fall at different points along a hypothetical continuum of the characteristic. Then they compare each person to be rated with these five individuals and indicate which one the ratee is most like with respect to the characteristic. The standards need not be persons: they can be any set of brief, behavioral descriptions falling on a "worst to best" or "lowest to highest" continuum.

In a *mixed standard scale,* raters are presented with concrete examples of good, average, and poor performance and then asked to judge whether the ratee's performance is "worse than," "as good as," or "better than" that described in the example. Because the examples are concrete or objective and the judgments required of the raters are fairly simple, mixed standard scales would seem to be demonstrably superior to other types of rating scales. Unfortunately, there are problems with scales constructed in this way, perhaps the most serious being the inconsistency with which raters respond to them (Murphy & Davidshofer, 1994).

Behaviorally Anchored Scales

Behaviorally anchored rating scales (BARS) represent attempts to make the terminology of ratings scales more descriptive of actual behavior and therefore more objective. Understandably, the meanings of concepts such as anxiety, self-confidence, and aggressiveness, as rated on traditional trait-oriented rating scales, are somewhat different for different raters. This is particularly so when the raters have received little or no training in what these terms mean in the specific context in which the judgments are made. An illustration of a behaviorally anchored scale for rating employees on knowledge and judgment is given in Figure 2.4.

Construction of a behaviorally anchored rating scale (BARS) begins by convening a group of people who possess expert knowledge of a particular job or another situation of interest. By means of discussion and painstaking deliberation, the group attempts to reach a consensus on a series of behaviorally descriptive statements on several dimensions,

Extremely good performance	7	By knowing the price of items, this checker would be expected to look for mismarked and unmarked items.
Good performance	6	You can expect this checker to be aware of items that constantly fluctuate in price. You can expect this checker to know the various sizes of cans—No. 303, No. 2, No. 2½.
Slightly good performance	5	When in doubt, this checker would ask the other clerk if the item is taxable.
		This checker can be expected to verify with another checker a discrepancy between the shelf and the marked price before ringing up that item.
Neither poor nor good performance	4	When operating the quick check, the lights are flashing, this checker can be expected to check out a customer with 15 items.
Slightly poor performance	3	You could expect this checker to ask the customer the price of an item that he does not know.
		In the daily course of personal relationships, this checker may be expected to linger in long conversations with a customer or another checker.
Poor performance	2	In order to take a break, this checker can be expected to block off the checkstand with people in line.
Extremely poor performance	1	

Figure 2.4. A behaviorally-anchored rating scale on knowledge and judgment. From "Development of First Level Behavioral Job Criteria" by L. Fogli, C. L. Hulin, and M. R. Blood. *Journal of Applied Psychology, 55,* p. 6. Copyright 1978 by the American Psychological Association. Reprinted with permission.

from which an objective, highly reliable rating scale can be constructed. These descriptions may refer to behaviors—on the job or in the classroom, for example—that are considered critical for effective performance in the specific situation. Such *critical incidents* in employment contexts have been identified by supervisors as distinguishing between good and poor workers. Examples are "secures machinery and tidies up place of work when finished" and "follows up customers' request promptly." Whether or not the behavioral descriptions are based on critical incidents, in constructing a rating scale by the BARS technique, the descriptions surviving repeated reevaluation by the group are then prepared as a series of items to be rated.

In a variation on the BARS technique known as a *behavioral expectation scale* (BES), critical behaviors are rated in terms of expectations rather that actual behaviors. Because the criteria on which workers are evaluated with the BARS and BES approaches refer to on-the-job performance, both approaches meet federal fair employment guidelines.

One might expect that the emphasis on objectively observable behavior and the concentrated group effort, which are features of behaviorally anchored scales, would make these scales psychometrically superior to other rating methods. In addition, the fact that the technique requires group involvement and consensus in constructing the scale, and hence a greater likelihood of group acceptance, would seem to be an advantage. After reviewing the research literature on the topic, Murphy and Constans (1987) concluded, however, that the results from the use of the BARS technique are mixed. Some studies have found fewer errors in ratings—the leniency error in particular—with BARS, whereas other studies have not found it to be any better than graphic rating scales (Champion, Green, & Sauser, 1988; Kinicki & Bannister, 1988). In short, behaviorally anchored ratings scales do not necessarily represent an improvement over graphic or other types of rating scales (Muchinsky, 1990).

Behavioral observation scales (BOS) are similar to behaviorally anchored scales in that ratings are made with respect to critical incidents on several performance dimensions. However, unlike the BARS approach, BOS ratings are in terms of the frequency (never, seldom, sometimes, generally, always) with which each of a set of critical behaviors is observed during a specified time period. Some research studies have found that the BOS method is preferred over the BARS method in employment contexts (Wiersma & Latham, 1986).

Forced-Choice Rating Scale

On the simplest type of *forced-choice rating scale*, the rater is provided with two descriptive words, phrases, or statements that are closely matched in desirability. The rater is told to indicate which description best applies to the ratee. When the rating scale contains three or more descriptions, the rater is asked to indicate which is most applicable and which is least applicable. In the case of a scale containing four descriptions, say an item consisting of two equally desirable and two equally undesirable descriptions, the rater is instructed to mark the one that is most applicable and the one that is least applicable to the ratee. Only one desirable and one undesirable statement discriminate between high and low ratees on the criterion (behavioral adjustment, etc.), but the rater presumably does not know which statements these are. A hypothetical example of a four-statement, forced-choice item that might be useful in evaluating supervisors or other leaders is:

> Assumes responsibility easily.
> Doesn't know how or when to delegate.
> Has many constructive suggestions to offer.
> Doesn't listen to others' suggestions.

Notice that the first and third statements are positive, and the second and fourth statements are negative. Which statement is most positive and which is least negative? Presumably, only the scale designer knows for sure.

When the forced-choice rating method was first introduced, it was viewed as a way of controlling for deliberate distortion and for personal biases, such as *response* sets. Response sets such as acquiescence (agreeing rather than disagreeing) and social desirability (responding in a more socially desirable direction) are tendencies to respond on the basis of the form rather than the content of items on assessment instruments. Unfortunately, raters often find the forced-choice format difficult and frustrating and it has proved cumbersome in practice. Consequently, some people who were initially enthusiastic about the forced-choice format went back to the man-to-man scale or another rating scale format. After reviewing its use, Bowmas and Bernardin (1991) concluded that the forced-choice method has several disadvantages and is not a popular technique among raters.[1]

Q-Sorts

Similar to rating scales, but also possessing certain features of checklists are Q-sorts. The *Q-sort technique,* pioneered by Stephenson (1953), requires the respondent to sort a set of statements descriptive of personal or social characteristics into a series of piles ranging from "most characteristic" to "least characteristic" of himself (herself) or an acquaintance. The respondent arranges the statements so a specified number will fall in each pile and yield a normal distribution of statements across piles.

Q-sort statements may be written specifically for a certain investigation, but standard decks of statements are available. A commercially distributed set is the California Q-Sort Revised (Adult Set), consisting of 100 cards containing statements descriptive of personality; a child set is also available.

Certain investigations of changes in self-concept resulting from psychotherapy or other interventions have required the research subjects to make before-and-after Q-sorts of a series of statements to describe their feelings and attitudes (e.g., Rogers & Dymond, 1954). If the real- and ideal-self sorts are more alike after than before intervention, it is concluded that the intervention experience was effective.

Self- and Other-Ratings

Rating scales and checklists are not limited to the appraisal or evaluation of others. You can rate things as well as other people, and you can also rate yourself. In self-ratings, which are not as common as other-ratings, both the rater and the ratee are the same person. Even when the rater is someone other than the ratee, the relationship of rater to ratee can have a pronounced effect on ratings. Ratings made by peers or colleagues, for example, may be different from those made by superiors or subordinates.

Ratings made by supervisors and other superiors are the most common evaluation procedure in employment contexts, but peer ratings have received favorable reviews in many situations. Peer ratings of job-related behaviors are fairly reliable and apparently less subject to error than ratings made by supervisors (Wexley & Klimoski, 1984). For these and perhaps other reasons, managers tend to have positive attitudes toward peer ratings (McEvoy & Buller, 1987). Peer ratings have been found to be very useful for evaluating industrial supervisors, military personnel, Peace Corps volunteers, and even college students (Kane & Lawler, 1978, 1980; Wiggins, 1973). In research conducted with U.S. Army personnel, it was found that supervisors' ratings were more closely related than peer ratings to actual job performance (Oppler, Campbell, Pulakos, & Borman, 1992). Perhaps the supervisors in this situation had a better opportunity to observe the performance of ratees than the typical supervisor in nonmilitary employment situations and were less influenced by interpersonal factors than the peer raters.

It is understandable why self-ratings tend to be higher than ratings made by other people. One way of making self-ratings more realistic is to ask people to rate themselves on a relative scale in which they compare themselves or their performances with other people rather than absolutely (Farh & Dobbins, 1989).

Mixed results have been obtained in studies of the relationships between peer ratings and ratings made by superiors or subordinates (Fox & Dinur, 1988; Harris & Schaubroeck, 1988). Some of the peer/superior and peer/subordinate correlations are significantly positive, but in general they are not very high. Likewise, the results of research on ratings made by subordinates have been rather inconsistent, varying with the specific situation, the personalities of the two parties, and the personal relationship between them. The accuracy of such ratings also varies with whether they are made anonymously: in general, anonymous ratings tend to be more candid than those in which raters are required to put their names on the rating forms (Bernardin, 1986).

One intriguing finding is that the correlation between self- and subordinate ratings is higher for women managers than for men managers (London & Wohlers, 1991). Perhaps women are more self-perceptive (or perhaps more honest!) than men, and hence their self-ratings agree more closely with those of their superiors than do those of men. Furthermore, women may be better acquainted with each other than men usually are.

Whether combining ratings from several sources—self, subordinates, peers, superiors—yields a more accurate picture of the ratee's behavior also depends on the situation: sometimes it does, sometimes it doesn't.

Computer Programs for Constructing Scales and Checklists

Three programs on the diskette accompanying this book can facilitate the process of constructing rating scales and checklists. These are programs 1, 2, and 4 in Category A ("Constructing and Scoring Rating Scales and Checklists").

Program A-1

This program assists in constructing a checklist or a rating scale having any desired number of rating categories and items. It is somewhat more flexible than program A-2, and is the best program if the user wishes to custom-design a rating questionnaire or checklist. The user enters the name of the scale, the directions, the number of rating categories, the label and definition of each category, the number of items to be rated, and each item. The completed scale can be printed at run time, or file "results" containing the output may be retrieved with and edited with an editor (edit, edlin) or a word processing program. The latter option permits further editing and embellishment (by including special fonts, graphics, etc.) of the scale before printing it.

Program A-2

This program consists of a set of 11 subprograms or procedures for constructing: (1) bipolar, forced-choice, graphic, numerical, semantic differential, and standard rating scales; (2) Likert attitude scales; (3) questionnaires for comparing and ranking persons; (4) checklists for rating the behaviors or characteristics of persons on several variables across several occasions. Option 11, which is discussed later in the chapter, is used in scoring rating scales and checklists.

Procedure 1 constructs a set of *bipolar rating scales* having a specified number of categories. Line segments, numerals, or a combination of line segments and numerals between the left and right ends of the bipolar continuum may be selected.

Procedure 2 constructs a set of *forced-choice rating scales,* each consisting of a stem statement and two or more descriptive options. Respondents may be asked to select one option or to select one option and reject any other one.

Procedure 3 constructs a set of *graphic rating scales,* each consisting of a vertical line marked by graphic descriptions at equidistant points along a line.

Procedure 4 constructs a set of *numerical rating scales* on which a series of designated numerical categories indicate points on a hypothetical continuum.

Procedure 5 constructs a series of *semantic differential scales* for rating a series of concepts on a set of bipolar adjectival scales. Between the polar adjectives of each scale are several numbered or unnumbered line segments separated by vertical markers. Any reasonable number of segments may be designated, but seven is typical.

Procedure 6 constructs a *standard rating scale* in which a group of applicants, candidates, or other persons are compared with a standard set of persons, characteristics, or behavioral descriptions.

Procedure 7 constructs a *Likert attitude scale* for assessing attitudes toward a designated object, person, or situation. The respondent marks the appropriate letter(s) (SD, D, U, A, or SA) appearing opposite each item to indicate the extent of his (her) agreement or disagreement with each item statement.

Procedure 8 constructs a *questionnaire for comparing persons* with each other. Each person is paired with every other person in the group. For each pair of persons, respondents indicate which one (a or b) possesses more of the specified characteristic or behavior.

Procedure 9 constructs a *questionnaire for ranking persons* on several specified behaviors or characteristics. The ranks range from 1 to n, where n is the number of persons to be ranked.

Procedure 10 constructs a *checklist* for evaluating: (1) one person on several behaviors or characteristics on multiple occasions or at different times; (2) several persons on one behavior or characteristic on multiple occasions or at different times; (3) several persons on several behaviors or characteristics on one particular occasion or at one time.

After a given procedure has been run, the user is asked whether the output file should be printed. If the answer if affirmative, the file is then printed on an associated printer. Otherwise, the output file can be printed later by typing and entering "copy (name of output file) (output port designation)" or by means of an appropriate editor or a wordprocessing program. The output of procedures 1–10 consists of a printed rating scale, an attitude scale, a questionnaire, or a checklist, with appropriate one-inch margins and otherwise appropriately formated.

Program A-4

This program (Aiken, 1992) generates and prints an intragroup ratings questionnaire from the names of the members of any kind of group (see Figure 2.5). The members' names are entered by the user, and the completed questionnaire is printed immediately. Alternatively, the questionnaire, which is in file "results," can be edited and printed through WordPerfect or another wordprocessing program. In administering the questionnaire, respondents are directed to fill out the printed questionnaires by rating each name on a scale of 1 to 7 according to how much they would like or dislike to engage in some activity with the person, how important the person is to the group, how close the respondent feels toward the person, likes to cooperate with him or her, considers the person important to the successful function of the group, or any other interpersonal perception or attitude. By omitting the "Me" category, this becomes a type of 360-degree rating

Directions: For each of the names listed below, indicate how much you like or dislike interacting with the person. Use the following key:

1 = Dislike strongly
2 = Dislike moderately
3 = Dislike mildly
4 = Undecided
5 = Like mildly
6 = Like moderately
7 = Like strongly
Me = The person is you

If you do not know a person well enough to rate him or her, circle number 4. Circle "Me" if the person is you.

	Dislike ⟶ Like							
Jennifer Brown	1	2	3	4	5	6	7	Me
Dennis Coltrane	1	2	3	4	5	6	7	Me
Kristy Kantorwitz	1	2	3	4	5	6	7	Me
Stacey Logan	1	2	3	4	5	6	7	Me
Matt Moore	1	2	3	4	5	6	7	Me
James Rogers	1	2	3	4	5	6	7	Me

Figure 2.5.   Student interaction inventory.

scale in which everyone rates everyone else on a designated characteristic or behavior. Multiple questionnaires may be constructed if everyone in a group is to be rated on several characteristics. The completed questionnaires may then be scored by program A-5, which is described later in the chapter.

Rating Errors

Cumbersome as it may be to select one of four descriptions that is most characteristic and one that is least characteristic of a person, forced-choice ratings have the advantage of controlling for certain errors in rating, such as *constant errors*, the *halo effect*, the *contrast error*, and the *proximity error*. Not all raters are equally prone to these errors, because, as with any other evaluation method that relies on observations, the background and personality of the rater affect his or her perception, judgment, and style of responding. However, one type of error to which all raters are susceptible is the *ambiguity error* caused by poor descriptions of the various locations on the scales and by scales consisting of items about which the rater has insufficient information (Kleinmuntz, 1982).

Constant Errors

Constant, or range restriction, errors occur when the assigned ratings are higher (*leniency* or *generosity error*), lower (*severity error*), or more often in the average category (*central tendency error*) than they should be. Perhaps the simplest way to determine the presence of a constant error on a particular scale is to compare each rater's rating on that scale with the mean ratings of all other raters on that scale. Transforming ratings to standard scores or other convenient units can assist in coping with such constant errors, but making raters aware of the various types of errors that can occur in rating is probably more effective. Having the respondent rank the target persons on a series of characteristics or attributes instead of rating them eliminates these kinds of errors but has other disadvantages.

Tendencies toward selection of either the middle or extreme categories on rating scales do not always constitute "errors" in ratings. For example, cultural differences in this practice were found in a cross-cultural study conducted by Chen, Lee, and Stevenson (1995). In this study, large samples of students in Japan, Taiwan, Canada, and the United States filled out a lengthy questionnaire consisting of 57 seven-point rating items concerned with ideas, values, attitudes, beliefs, and self-evaluations related to school and daily life. The results showed that the first two nationality groups were significantly more likely than the last two groups to use the middle category, whereas the U.S. students were significantly more likely than the other three groups to use the extreme categories in rating the items (see Figure 2.6). Furthermore, within each group, endorsement of individualism was positively related to the use of extreme categories and negatively related to the use of the middle category.

Halo Effect

The *halo effect* is the tendency of raters to respond to the general impression made by the ratee or to overgeneralize by assigning favorable ratings on all traits merely because the person is outstanding on one or two traits. A negative halo effect, in which one bad characteristic spoils the ratings on all other characteristics, can also occur. Similar to the halo effect is the *logical error* of assigning similar ratings on characteristics that the rater believes to be logically related.

Contrast Error

This term has been used at least two different senses. In one sense the *contrast error* refers to the tendency to assign a higher rating than

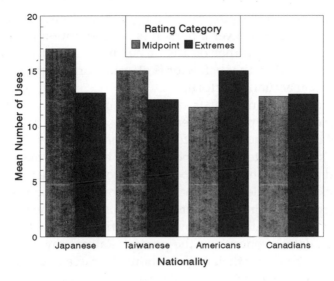

Figure 2.6. Mean number of uses of midpoint and extreme rating categories by four nationalities of students. Based on data from Chen, Lee, and Stevenson, 1995.

justified if an immediately preceding person received a very low rating, or to assign a lower rating than justified if the preceding person received a very high rating. In a second sense, contrast error refers to the tendency for a rater to compare or contrast the ratee with himself or herself (i.e., the rater) in assigning ratings on certain behaviors or traits.

Proximity Error

The actual location of a particular rating item on a printed page may affect the ratings assigned to it. In the *proximity error*, the rater tends to assign similar ratings to a person on items that are closer together on the printed page. Likewise, if a person is consistently rated high, low, or average on the majority of a set of items located close together, other items situated near those items may be rated in the same way—a kind of spread of response or response set.

Other Errors in Rating

Several other kinds of errors that may be made in ratings have been identified. Among these are the most-recent performance error, the inadequate information error, and errors due to certain cognitive or thought processes underlying raters' judgments. The *most-recent performance error* occurs whenever a person is judged not on his or her behavior as a whole but rather on his or her most recent performance. An error occurs when that behavior is atypical or unrepresentative of how the person actually performs.

Much of the rating that is done in employment, academic, and other contexts where periodic performance appraisals are conducted takes place despite inadequate information on the ratees. This is more likely to be so when raters are responsible for evaluating many different people and have not had an opportunity to observe each person at length. Lacking sufficient information, the rater may be overly influenced by irrelevant or incorrect communications about the ratee, stereotypes about human nature, and overly attentive to a few but relatively insignificant details concerning the person. Raters may recall only information that confirms their beliefs about the ratee and about human nature in general. Raters' judgments may also be influenced more by how they feel about the ratee than what they actually know about him or her.

Computer Programs for Analyzing Errors

Programs 1, 2, and 3 in Category B (Analyzing Errors in Ratings) on the computer diskette accompanying this book provide analytic information on the significance of various types of rating errors. Program B-1 compares items (across raters) or raters (across items) on eight different error coefficients: leniency, severity, leniency/severity, central tendency, homogeneity (halo), proximity, uniformity, and contrast. All of the coefficients except number 3 range from 0 to 1, with 0 being the least amount and 1 the greatest amount of the specific error; coefficient 3 (leniency/severity) ranges from -1 to $+1$, with -1 indicating the greatest degree of severity error and $+1$ the greater degree of leniency error.

To run program B-1, the user must enter the number of rating categories, the number of items or traits, the number of raters, the number of ratees, and whether the ratings are to be entered from the keyboard or from a separate file called *data*. The printout from this program lists the name of the error coefficient, its numerical value, and its mean and range. In addition to output for each rater, the average results for all raters combined may be computed and printed.

Program B-2 determines the discrete and right-tail probabilities of the eight error coefficients computed by program B-1. The user enters the number of the coefficient desired, the number of rating categories, and the number of observations (rating scales). The print-out consists of a table listing the value of the coefficient and the corresponding discrete and cumulative probabilities based on small samples of ratings.

Somewhat older, and therefore perhaps more time-honored, than the above methods for analyzing errors in rating is J. P. Guilford's (1954) analysis of variance procedure for determining the significance of certain constant errors in rating. As formalized in program B-3, a raters × ratees × traits analysis of variance is conducted to determine the presence of certain rating errors by examining the main effects for raters, ratees, and traits, as well as the raters × ratees, raters × traits, and ratees × traits interactions. Significant differences in main effects for raters points to differences between raters in the magnitude of the leniency or severity error, and hence low interrater reliability. Significant differences among ratees may reveal bona fide differences among ratees or may be indicative of a tendency on the part of the raters in general to be more lenient with some ratees than others. Significant differences among traits is less likely to be due to error than bona differences among traits, but more objective definitions on some traits than others can contribute to differences in ratings assigned to various traits. Perhaps even more interesting in examining the results of these three analysis of variance are the interactions between raters and traits, raters and ratees, and ratees and traits. A significant interaction between raters and traits indicates that differences in ratings given by different raters vary with the trait; Guilford interpreted this result as a tendency to overvalue or undervalue a certain trait in others, a type of *contrast error*. A significant interaction between raters and ratees indicates that some raters tend to overvalue or undervalue specific ratees, the so-called *halo effect*. Finally, a significant interaction between ratees and traits might point to a tendency to overvalue or undervalue a certain trait in some people more than in others.

The leniency, severity, leniency/severity, and central tendency errors, computed by program B-1, are types of range restriction errors. One other program that may provide analytic information on range restriction is program B-4. This program computes and evaluates the statistical significance of two coefficients (H and C) for determining the homogeneity or congruence of a set of n ratings. Tests for determining the statistical significance of the two coefficients in both small and large samples are conducted. More generally, these procedures may be used to evaluate the consistency of ratings made on n persons or in n

situations on one characteristic, or on one person or in one situation on *n* characteristics. Because the range of ratings to which the rater limits himself (herself) may be low, high, or medium, high intraindividual consistency in ratings across traits and/or situations is suggestive of a range restriction error.

Improving Ratings

It is not easy to make reliable and valid ratings of people under any circumstances and particularly so when the behaviors or personality characteristics are poorly defined or highly subjective. In addition, the meanings of the scale units may be unclear and hence interpreted differently by different raters. In general, errors in rating are smaller if each characteristic or behavior being rated is described as objectively as possible with reference to some actually observed activity. Rating statements should be short and clear, avoiding abstract, general terms such as honest, loyal, superior, and average.

Personal biases can obviously affect ratings: if you like someone you will probably give higher ratings to that person, and if you dislike him or her you will tend to give lower ratings than to someone whom you neither like nor dislike. Furthermore, raters are often not sufficiently familiar with the individual being rated to make accurate ratings, or they may be familiar with the person's behavior in certain situations but not in others. Training in how to make ratings more objective—by being aware of the various kinds of errors that can occur, by becoming more familiar with the individual and the characteristics being rated by the instrument, and by omitting items that the rater feels unqualified to judge, can improve the accuracy of ratings. In addition to training raters, selecting them is important. Some individuals are simply not interested, are clearly too biased, or are unwilling to invest the time required to become objective raters. Such people should not be used as raters if they cannot be motivated and trained to be conscientious and objective.

Another way of improving ratings is to balance out the biases of individual raters by combining the responses of several raters. And, as noted previously in this chapter, a combination of ratings by peers, subordinates, supervisors, and self may be better than either one alone. In addition, careful attention to the design of rating scale items can result in greater reliability and validity. Both the behaviors or traits being rated and the scale points should be designated in precise behavioral terms that will be interpreted in the same way by different raters. Also important in providing accurate, meaningful results are matters of format, such as arranging the items on the rating sheets so they can be easily completed and scored, making certain that bipolar scales are not all in the same direction, placing items far enough apart (one per page is preferable but probably impossible), and keeping the rating form reasonably short. Last, but not least, like any other measuring instrument, raters should be periodically "recalibrated" to make certain they are continuing to use the same criteria. This involves feedback to raters concerning their performance, the criteria on which the ratings should be made, and the need to be attentive to the task as well being aware of biases in ratings and how to avoid them.

SCORING CHECKLISTS AND RATING SCALES

Conventional scoring of checklists is dichotomous, in the sense that 1 point is assigned to each checked item and 0 points to unchecked items: $+1$ is given if checking that response is favorable and -1 if it is unfavorable toward whatever the underlying variable may be. In certain cases, as when the items have been scaled in some way according to importance, numerical weights other than 0 and 1 may be used. However, such differential item weighting usually has little effect on reliability and validity when the number of items comprising a checklist inventory is large.

Unless respondents are asked to check a specified number of items, different people will check different numbers of items. Such a response set can have a pronounced effect on the determination of scores, so some sort of grouping or statistical control is frequently used. In scoring the Adjective Check List, for example, the frequency distribution of scores on the "number checked" variable is divided into five groups and standard scores on the other variables are computed separately for each group. If the relationship of scores on a particular scale to the total number of items checked is approximately linear, differences between raw scores on the scale and scores predicted from the total number of items checked might be used as a measure of standing on the particular scale. When analyzing the relationship of scores on content variables to an external criterion or predictor variable, the number of items checked may be statistically controlled by partial or semi-partial correlational techniques.

Scoring Pair Comparisons and Ranks

With regard to the pair comparisons format, a rough score for an item is the number of other items over which it was preferred, considered superior to, etc. Again, if à priori weights have been assigned to items such that item B has a higher weight than item C, then preferring item A to item B may warrant a larger contribution to total score on item A than preferring item A to item C. If the preferences are transitive (i.e., if $a > b$ and $b > c$ implies that $a > c$, then the items may be rank-ordered according to preference and compared with the rank-orders of the same items made by other persons or with a set of standard ranks.

In scoring ranking items, items are ranked from 1 to n, where n is the total number of "things" ranked, 1 is the highest rank and n the lowest rank. To make higher scores on a ranking item indicative of a greater amount of the characteristic being measured, ranks (r) may be transformed to scores (s) by the formula $s = n - r + 1$. A set of ranks may be scored as a whole in comparison with some standard by using the formula

$$S = n[1 - 2\Sigma d_i/(n^2 - k)], \tag{2.1}$$

where n is the number of things ranked, k is 0 if n is even and 1 if n is odd, and the d_i are the absolute values of the differences of the differences between the obtained ranks and the keyed ranks. For example, if a "standard" set of ranks for five officers is 1, 2, 3, 4, 5, and if a rater ranks them as 2, 3, 1, 4, and 5, then $n = 5$, k = 1, $\Sigma d_i = |1 - 2| + |2 - 3| + |3 - 1| + |4 - 4| + |5 - 5| = 1 + 1 + 2 + 0 + 0 = 4$. So $S = 5[1 - 2(4)/(5^2 - 1)] = 5(\frac{2}{3}) = 3\frac{1}{3} \approx 3.^2$

Scoring Rating Scales

Various categories, segments, or anchors on rating scales are most easily scored by assigning successive numerical integers to them. In the case of a unipolar scale, it is probably best to assign a score of 0 to the lowest category and a score of $c - 1$, where c is the number of categories, to the highest category. Ratings closer to 0 indicate a lower rated amount of the characteristic, and ratings closer to $c - 1$ a higher amount of the characteristic. When several items or scales on a rating questionnaire measure the same variable, a composite score may be determined by adding the ratings on all the items.

In the case of bipolar scales, it is probably best to use an odd number of categories (c), assigning the consecutive integers from $(1 - c)/2$ for the lowest category to $(c - 1)/2$ for the highest category. These values may be converted to a *B*-coefficient scoring scale ranging from -1 to $+1$, providing information on both the magnitude and direction of a set of ratings. (see program A-6 and Aiken, 1985a). A *B* coefficient may be computed from the responses of one person to n items or from the responses of n persons to one item on a bipolar rating scale items. An appropriate formula is

$$B = 2\Sigma r_i / [n(c - 1)] \tag{2.2}$$

where c is the number of rating categories and r_i each of the obtained n ratings on a scale of $(1 - c)/2$ to $(c - 1)/2$. For example, if the five ratings on a seven-category bipolar scale are $-1, 0, 1, 1$, and 2, the corresponding B coefficient is $2(3)/[5(6)] = .20$.

Whether the rating scales are unipolar or bipolar scales, item scores need not be based on successive integers designating category responses but rather may be rational (à priori) weights or empirical weights determined by scaling procedures such as those discussed in Chapter 3. Hopefully the use of such response weighting procedures will result in scores that are more likely than arbitrary integers to represent measurement at something close to an interval level.

Computer Programs for Scoring

Programs 2, 3, 5, 6, and 8 in category A of the computer programs accompanying this book facilitate scoring of questionnaires containing checklist, ranking, and rating items. The user of program A-3 enters the number of questionnaires (examinees) to be scored, the number of response categories per item, the label for each category, the numerical value corresponding to category k for item j, and the examinee's response to each item on the questionnaire. A frequency distribution of each examinee's responses to all items and his or her total score on the questionnaire is printed.

The construction functions of program A-2 were described earlier in this chapter. With respect to the scoring function of this program, option 11 is selected from the menu. The designated name of the output file, the number of questionnaires, the number of items per questionnaire, the number of response categories per item, the label for each response category, whether or not the numerical values corresponding to the response categories are constant across items and what they are, and the response given by each respondent to each item are entered. Responses may be reentered if an error is made. The printout consists of the frequency distribution across response categories and the total score for each questionnaire, the overall frequency distribution across response categories for all respondents combined, and the overall mean and standard deviation of the scores.

Program A-5 scores the responses obtained from administering the questionnaire constructed by program A-4, which was described earlier. Using the numerical ratings (on a scale of 1 to c, the number of response categories), three sociometric or "cohesiveness" coefficients, ranging from 0 to 1, are computed: (1) a coefficient for each rater indicating how he or she feels toward the other members of the group, (2) a coefficient for each ratee indicating how the rest of the group feels toward him or her, and (3) a coefficient indicating how the entire group feels about itself. When the number of respondents (n) is small, the statistical significance of each coefficient is determined by computing the exact right-tail probability corresponding to the coefficient. When n is large, a normal approximation to the exact right-tailed probability is computed.

Program A-6 computes B coefficients for n ratings, using Formula 2.2. The program also provides a normal approximation test for the significance of B in large samples. For small samples of ratings, program A-7 calculates the right-tail probability, based on either a normal or a uniform distribution.

Program A-8 scores ranking items by Formula 2.1. The user specifies the number of categories (ranks), enters the correct (keyed) ranks by category, and the respondent's rankings by category. The scores, which range from 0 to c (the number of things ranked) may be printed in decimal form or rounded to the nearest whole number.

SUMMARY

Rating scales and checklists are designed to evaluate a wider range of attributes possessed by people, objects, and events than any other type of psychometric device. This is documented by the many sources of information on commercially available instruments of the kinds listed in this chapter. Such instruments are administered for purposes of selection, placement, and performance appraisal in educational and industrial/organizational contexts, for diagnostic and treatment progress evaluations in clinical/medical contexts, and for research purposes as independent, dependent, and control variables.

A number of questions need to be considered in planning or selecting a rating scale or checklist, depending on the nature of the situation and the purposes for which the instrument will be used and the resources available. The construction of rating scales involves one or more strategies—rational/theoretical, inductive, and empirical or criterion-group. Although the rational strategy is the most common, the inductive and criterion-group strategies are more sophisticated approaches from a statistical standpoint. Be that as it may, none of the strategies appears to be demonstrably superior to any other in terms of reliability and validity. In actual practice, a combination of the three strategies is often employed and appears to have the best results.

Various types of rating scale formats—numerical, semantic differential, graphic, standard, behaviorally anchored, forced-choice—have been devised. Depending on the nature of the attribute or characteristic being rated, any of these formats may be unipolar or bipolar; 4–5 rating categories are best for unipolar scales, and 5–7 categories for bipolar scales. The graphic and numerical formats are most popular, though behaviorally anchored and forced-choice formats would seem to be superior in terms of their objectivity and control over errors in rating. Evidence for the higher validity of behaviorally anchored and forced-choice scales is, however, unimpressive. Recent efforts to improve ratings have shifted away from experiments on scale format and toward an analysis of cognitive processes involved in making rating judgments.

A number of research studies in organizational settings have compared ratings by self, peers, subordinates, and superiors. Self-ratings tend to be higher than ratings made by other people. Several studies have found peer-ratings to be highly valid, and such ratings meet with the approval of both management and labor organizations. However, the validity of all rating systems depends on how well the raters know the persons whom they are rating and whether they can control their own biases and proneness to errors of various kinds. Among these are constant errors (severity, leniency), the halo effect, the contrast error, and the proximity error. Training raters to be aware of these errors and how to make their ratings more objective can improve the accuracy of ratings, but unfortunately not as much as desired.

Checklist responses are often scored on a numerical scale (−1, 0, +1), depending on whether the item is checked and, if checked, whether it receives a negative or positive weight on the variable to which it contributes. The most common method of scoring ratings is to assign successive plus or minus integers to responses in successive categories and to add the integers corresponding to the indicated ratings or categories on several items to produce a composite score. However, rational (à priori) or empirically-determined weights corresponding to the various scale categories are also applied in scoring certain scales.

Several computer programs for constructing and scoring rating scales and checklists are described in this chapter. These programs are included on the computer diskette accompanying this book.

QUESTIONS AND ACTIVITIES

1. Define each of the following terms in a sentence or two:

ambiguity error	jangle fallacy
anchors	jingle fallacy
behavioral expectation scale (BES)	leniency (generosity) error
	Likert attitude scale
behaviorally anchored rating scales (BARS)	logical error
	man-to-man scale
bipolar rating scale	mixed standard scale
central tendency error	numerical rating scale
constant error	pair comparisons
contrast error	proximity error
criterion group approach	questionnaire for comparing persons
critical incidents	
deductive approach	questionnaire for ranking persons
empirical approach	response sets
external approach	semantic space
forced-choice rating scale	semantic differential scale
graphic rating scale	severity error
halo effect	standard rating scale
inductive approach	unipolar scale

2. Using program A-2 on the computer diskette accompanying this book, construct a bipolar, forced-choice, graphic, numerical semantic differential, and standard rating scale. The scales

need not be long; three or four items will suffice, but include a title, directions, and other necessary information in your constructed scales.

3. Use program A-4 on the computer diskette accompanying this book to construct a questionnaire for assessing the cohesiveness of any moderate-sized group of which you are a member. Print your questionnaire, make multiple copies of it, and administer it to the members of the group.

4. Score the responses to the questionnaires in exercise 3 by using program A-5 on the computer diskette accompanying this book. How cohesive was the group? Did some group members like the group more than others? Were some group members liked by the group more than others? Would you expect the cohesiveness of the group to change over time? Why or why not?

5. What types of errors are most likely to cause problems on: (a) checklists, (2) numerical rating scales, (3) forced-choice rating scales?

6. Despite efforts to make behaviorally-anchored rating scales as objective and behaviorally-oriented as possible, such scales are really not much better than graphic rating scales in terms of their reliability and validity. How can this be so? What is the problem?

7. Construct a semantic differential scale to measure the connotative meanings of the constructs of COLLEGE, TEACHER, TEST, and GRADES. Use seven point scales and the bipolar adjectives of good-bad, weak-strong, fast-slow, high-low, and like-dislike. You may wish to use program A-2 on the computer diskette accompanying this book to construct your scale. Administer the scale to several people and compare their responses.

3

Item Analysis, Standardization, and Reliability

Before a questionnaire or an inventory composed of checklist or rating scale items can be viewed as a finished instrument, data on the functioning of the items and item composites must be obtained and analyzed. The purpose of collecting a representative sample of responses to items on a rating scale or checklist is to see whether those responses indicate that the items are measuring what they are supposed to measure and whether they are doing so efficiently. The goal in analyzing item composites is similar: Is the composite measuring what it is supposed to measure, and does it do so consistently? Of foremost importance is the question of validity: Does this psychometric instrument measure what it was designed to measure or some other construct? A second question pertains to the quality of the instrument—to its relative freedom from errors of measurement: Are the measurements made by the instrument reliable? Whatever the instrument may measure, does it do so consistently, regardless of temporal, situational, or other variations in personal and environmental circumstances? A psychometric instrument must measure *reliably* before it can be a valid measure of any variable or construct.

Reliable and valid items imply reliable and valid item composites. Consequently, the analysis of responses to checklists and rating scales—

as with test items in general—begins with item analysis and proceeds to an analysis of item composites. Once it has been established that the items and composites are reasonably reliable and valid, then the process of standardizing the instrument can be undertaken. Standardization results in norms which serve as a frame of reference for interpreting or making sense of the responses to the items and item composites.

ITEM ANALYSIS

Before a psychometric instrument is administered for the first time, it must be reviewed carefully and field-tested on a pilot sample of motivated respondents. Much work and a great deal of frustration can be avoided by clear, complete directions, careful editing of the instrument, and efforts to anticipate potential difficulties of administration and scoring by putting oneself in the place of examinees. Despite these precautions, unexpected problems still occur when the instrument is finally administered to a sizable sample. The respondents may not comprehend the wording of certain items; they may not understand or may misunderstand how they are supposed to mark their answers; they may not have enough time to complete the inventory or scale, and the like. Observing examinees carefully while they are responding to items and questioning them after they have finished filling out a checklist or rating scale can provide information for revising or fine-tuning the instrument. In addition to such subjective or semi-objective data, more objective, statistical information can be provided by analyzing the functioning of individual items and the instrument as a whole.

Item Response Proportions and Frequencies

A traditional item analysis of a test of achievement or aptitude begins with the computation of an item difficulty index and an item discrimination index. The item difficulty index (p) is a proportion reflecting the number of respondents who answered the item correctly. The magnitude of p varies inversely with the difficulty of the item: the lower the value of p, the more difficult the item is. The optimum p value also varies inversely with the number of options on a multiple-choice item, ranging from .85 for two-option items through .69 for five-option items.

Similar to the item difficulty index for an achievement test, the proportion of respondents who checked a particular item (p) is a useful statistic to compute when analyzing responses to a checklist. Although the optimum difficulty index for ability tests varies with the purpose of the test—screening, awarding scholarships, placement—we may not be able to say precisely what the optimum value of p is in the case of a checklist item. In general, items with p values close to .50 have larger variabilities and are potentially the most discriminating. That is, such items are most likely to differentiate accurately between people who possess a larger amount of the attribute being evaluated and those who possess a smaller amount of it.

The proportion of people in the population who possess the particular characteristic expressed in a checklist item is known as the *base rate* for that characteristic. Some characteristics, such as sociability or extroversion, have fairly high base rates, whereas other characteristics, such as psychoticism or suicidal behavior, have low base rates. Although it becomes increasingly difficult to detect and predict a particular characteristic or behavior as the base rate becomes increasingly deviant from .5, many attributes or events in which we may be interested have base rates substantially higher or lower than .5.

Many checklist items are endorsed by a fairly high or low proportion of respondents, and hence it can be assumed that the base rates of characteristics measured by those items are different from .5. The p values obtained in our sample of respondents are not precisely equal to the base rate of the corresponding characteristic of which the obtained responses are presumably a random sample. However, we can be approximately 95% certain that the population base rate falls within a range of $\pm t \sqrt{p(1 - p)/n}$, where n is the number of responses and t is two-tailed critical value of the t statistic at the .05 level with $n - 1$ degrees of freedom. For example, if the p value of a checklist item administered to 30 people is .70, we can be 95% certain that the population base rate is somewhere between $.7 \pm 2.045\sqrt{.7(.3)/30} = .53$ to .87.

Whether, in the final version of the checklist, we retain or eliminate items having very small or very large p values depends on what we are trying to measure and how accurate we want to be. As a rule of thumb, items with p values lower than .20 or higher than .80 should probably be revised or discarded.

Unless they have only two response categories, in the case of rating scale items there is no statistic exactly like the p value of items on an objective ability test or a checklist. We can compute the frequencies in each in the c categories of a rating scale and by inspection decide whether the resulting frequency distribution is too narrow, too skewed, too leptokurtic, too platykurtic, or otherwise irregularly shaped. We may have some à priori conception of what the frequency distribution should look like, and may feel justified in retaining or rejecting an item depending on whether our "eyeball analysis" shows that it meets or fails to meet our requirements. Programs B-1 and B-2 on the computer diskette accompanying this book should also prove useful in making this decision. Coefficients 1 (leniency), 2 (severity), 3 (leniency/severity), 4 (central tendency), 5 (homogeneity or halo) and 7 (uniformity) computed by program B-1 and analyzed for statistical significance by program B-2 can provide analytic information on the shape of the frequency distribution of responses to each item.

If we expect the frequency distribution of responses to be uniform across the c rating categories, then programs G-2, H-1, and H-2 can prove helpful in making this determination. If the sample size is fairly large, that is, $n \geq 5c$, a chi square goodness of fit test should be conducted using program G-2. In the case of small samples, a D coefficient may be computed using program H-1 and evaluated for statistical significance with program H-2.

Validity of Checklist Items

The proportion checking an item on a checklist is a useful statistic, but of even greater interest is the *validity index* of the item. This index is a measure of the relationship between responses to the item and scores on an internal or external criterion of whatever the item was designed to measure. The *internal criterion* consists of scores on a composite of items, of which the item of interest is a part. In the case of an achievement test item, the internal criterion consists of total test scores, which, for purposes of analysis, are usually divided into upper 27% and lower 27%. The lower group on this internal criterion consists of examinees whose composite scores fall in the lower 27% of the distribution of total test score, and the upper group consists of those who fall in the upper 27% of total test scores. Upper and lower halves (50%) may also be used when the sample is small.

The validity index, referred to as the *item discrimination index* in this context, is the difference between the proportion in the upper group (p_u) and the proportion in the lower group (p_l) who answer the item correctly ($D = p_u - p_l$). For example, if a total of 100 people take a test, there will be 27 people in the upper group and 27 in the lower group on total test score. If 15 of those in the upper group and 5 of those in the lower group get the item right, then D, the discrimination index, is $15/27 - 5/27 = .56 - .19 = .37$.

We can use this same procedure with checklist items that are part of a larger composite. Suppose that the checklist consists of 10 items and we wish to compute an item discrimination index for each item. We administer the checklist to, say, 200 people and assign scores of 0 to 10 to each person, depending upon how many of the 10 items he or she checks. From a frequency distribution of these scores, we determine the upper (highest 27%) and lower (lowest 27%) groups on total test scores—54 people in each group. Assume that 40 people in the upper group and 15 people in the lower group check item A. Then the D value for that item is $.74 - .28 = .46$. In general, D values of .30 or above are acceptable, although a value somewhat smaller than .30 may be satisfactory when the sample size is very large (Aiken, 1979). A low D value serves as a "flag" indicating that the item is not functioning properly and should be revised or discarded.

When devising a checklist to serve as a predictor variable for forecasting behavior or performance—in school, on the job, in an interpersonal relationship—we are usually more interested in an external criterion than in the internal criterion of total scores on the checklist itself. If the performance criterion is a dichotomous variable such as pass vs. fail, good vs. poor, present vs. absent, and the like, a nominal-level measure of association such as lambda, Cramer's V, or the phi coefficient may be satisfactory. Program C-3 on the accompanying diskette will compute all of these coefficients. If both the checklist and the criterion are considered to be artificial dichotomies with underlying normal distributions, then the tetrachoric coefficient is a more powerful statistic.

When the criterion is continuous and measured on an interval or ratio scale, such as the number of units produced, volume or dollar value of sales, supervisors' ratings of employee performance, or any other continuous criterion, the point-biserial coefficient is an appropriate validity index. The *point biserial coefficient* is computed as

$$r_{pb} = (\overline{Y}_c - \overline{Y}_n)\sqrt{p(1-p)}/s \tag{3.1}$$

In this formula p is the proportion of those who checked the item, $\overline{Y}_c$ is the mean criterion score of those who checked the item, $\overline{Y}_n$ is the mean criterion score of those who did not check the item, and s is the criterion standard deviation of both groups combined. If, for example, the mean criterion score of the 60 out of 100 employees who checked a particular item is 21.67, the mean criterion score of the 40 employees who did not check the item is 11.25, and the standard deviation of both groups combined is 9.15, then $r_{pb} = (21.67 - 11.25)\sqrt{.60(.40)}/9.15 = .56$.

The range of r_{pb} is -1 to $+1$, and its statistical significance can be determined by a t test with $n - 2$ degrees of freedom:

$$t = r_{pb}\sqrt{(n - 2)/(1 - r_{pb}^2)} \qquad (3.2)$$

For the above example, $t = .56\sqrt{(100 - 2)/(1 - .56^2)} = 6.69$. Because the two-tailed critical value of t at the .05 level with 98 degrees of freedom is 1.98, it can be concluded that the population value of r_{pb} is greater than zero. Program C-4 may be used to compute the point-biserial coefficient and test it for statistical significance.

Rather than being a continuous, interval-level variable, the behavioral or performance criterion may consist of ratings or rankings, which are ordinal-level scores. The point-biserial coefficient is the wrong statistic in such cases, but a modification known as the *rank-biserial coefficient* is appropriate (Glass, 1966). The computing procedure for this statistic begins by assigning the ranks 1 to n to the criterion scores, where 1 corresponds to the highest and n the lowest rating or ranking on the criterion. After eliminating tied ranks, the remaining m ranks are sorted into two groups: those made by respondents who endorsed the checklist item of interest, and those who did not. Then, after computing Y_c and Y_n, which have the same meaning as in formula 3.1, we find:

$$r_{pb} = 2(\overline{Y}_c - \overline{Y}_n)/m \qquad (3.3)$$

Program C-4 may be also used to compute the rank-biserial coefficient.

An alternative method for analyzing checklist items is to plot a graph relating the proportion of respondents who endorse the item at successively higher scores on an internal or external criterion. The resulting *item characteristic curve* is actually more informative than the methods described above because it reveals whether the item is functioning effectively at all levels of the criterion. Illustrative two-item characteristic curves against an external criterion is shown in Figure 3.1. Ideally, the characteristic curve for an item should rise or fall gradually—not too steeply or too flatly—across increasing criterion scores. The criterion score at which 50% of the respondents checked the item

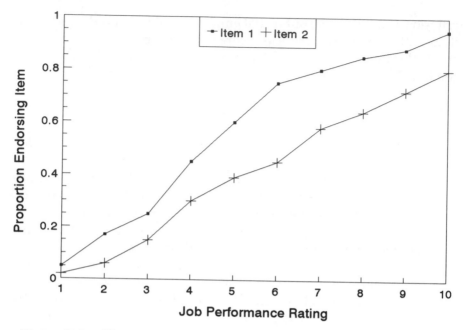

Figure 3.1. Characteristic curves for two checklist items.

is comparable to the item difficulty index described above, whereas the slope of the curve at $p = .50$ is comparable to the item validity index. Of the two-item characteristic curves depicted in Figure 3.1, the composite score (job performance rating) corresponding to an endorsement proportion of .5 is lower for item 1 than item 2, but item 1 also has a steeper slope at that point than item 2. Hence, the validity index of item 1 is greater than that for item 2.

Program C-2 on the computer diskette will plot item characteristic curves for a set of endorsement proportions and associated (mean) criterion scores. You must enter the total number of scores, the number of intervals for the criterion variable, and, for each interval, the midpoint of the interval, the number of scores on the interval, and the number of respondents endorsing the item whose criterion scores fall within the interval. This program can also be used to plot item response curves. More will be said about this later in the chapter.

Validity of Rating Scale Items

As with checklist items, determining the validity of items on rating scales is a matter of computing a measure of relationship between scores on each item and scores on an internal (item composite) or external criterion. If the criterion is dichotomous, we might use formula 3.3, with ranks being assigned to ratings. The only problem here is that there will be many tied ranks. Another possibility is to view the criterion as a two-category ordinal variable and then compute Kendall's tau or Spearman's rho coefficient, from an ordered contingency table (Aiken, 1975; Kendall, 1970; see program C-3). These statistics are even more appropriate indexes of item validity when the criterion consists of ratings or rankings. When the criterion is measured on an interval or ratio scale, one has something of a choice. If it can be assumed that the rating scale items constituting the predictor variable have an underlying normal distribution, then the Pearson product-moment coefficient is an appropriate statistic. Even if this assumption is not strictly tenable, the Pearson r is a robust statistic and will probably be satisfactory if the ratings are not markedly skewed (see program C-5). Perhaps a better solution is to convert the criterion scores to ranks by program D-4, and then use program C-3 to compute Kendall's or Spearman's coefficient relating ratings (ranks) on each item to ranked scores on the criterion measure.

TRANSFORMATIONS AND STANDARDIZATION

Initial scores assigned to responses on rating scales and checklists are expressed in arbitrary numerical units such as 0–1 or 1–2–3–4–5. A voluminous psychometric literature exists on procedures for expressing scores in more meaningful units, a process known as *scaling* or *calibration*. In this section, we merely touch on the various ways in which scores on individual items and item composites have been expressed. For more information on this topic, consult articles by Reckase (1990), Andrich (1978b, 1994), Weinberg (1991), and Wright and Masters (1982).

Transforming Proportions on Checklist Items

For purposes of statistical analysis, the proportions of respondents endorsing checklist items are sometimes transformed to normal deviates or arc sines. To transform a proportion to a normal deviate (z), a table of cumulative proportions under the normal curve (or program D-1) is consulted. The resulting z value may then be transformed to a convenient standard score (SS) scale having any desired mean (M) and standard deviation (s):

$$SS = M + sz \tag{3.4}$$

One such transformation, delta = 13 + 4z, yields an item score scale having a mean of 13 and a standard deviation of 4. Most items on this delta scale, which has been used primarily by the Educational Testing Service, fall within a range of 6 to 20. It can be argued that this kind of transformation changes item responses from an ordinal to an interval scale, but this assertion is questionable. However, it does provide a standard metric for comparison purposes.

Transformation of proportions to arc sines is accomplished by means of

$$X = 2 \arcsin \sqrt{p}, \tag{3.5}$$

a table of which is found in Weiner, Brown, and Michels (1991) (or program D-2). This transformation has the effect of stabilizing the proportion variances so they are not related to the means, permitting the resulting X scores to be used in parametric statistical analyses.

Calibrating Composite Scores with IRT

Total scores on a composite of checklist items may be converted to standard scores or normalized standard scores by procedures similar to those for single items. Assuming that items comprising the composite are responded to independently and that they measure the same dimension or construct, item response methodology can be used to calibrate item scores and composite scores and provide an estimate of each respondent's score on the resulting scale. The one-parameter BICAL program (Wright, Mead, & Bell, 1979), the two-parameter BILOG program (Mislevy & Bock, 1983), or the three-parameter LOGIST (Wingersky, Barton, & Lord, 1982) or ASCAL (Vale & Gialluca, 1985) programs can make these transformations. These programs also provide other useful information on the functioning of individual items and the item composite. The one-parameter logistic model assumes that the items vary only in their rate of endorsement, the BILOG program assumes that they also vary in their discriminating power, and the LOGIST program also assumes that there is a non-zero base rate (a guessing parameter) for positive responses to the items.

Converting Ranks

For analysis of ranked data, the ranks can be converted to proportions by the following formula and further transformed by the above procedures:

$$p = 1 - (r - .5)/n \tag{3.6}$$

In this formula, n is the number of things to be ranked, r the rank of a specific item, and p the corresponding proportion. For example, if 10 things are to be ranked, a rank of 2 is equivalent to a proportion of $1 - (2 - .5)/10 = .85$. This is equivalent to a normal deviate of $z = 1.04$, or, applying formula 3.9 and a 10-point scale, 7.06 (see program D-8).

Ratings and Scaling

Like ranks, ratings can also be transformed to proportions and treated as described previously. For purposes of comparing two sets of ratings of the same variable made on two scales having different numbers of categories, and perhaps different origins as well, ratings on one scale may be converted to the other scale by:

$$Y = Y_l + (X - X_l)(Y_h - Y_l)/(X_h - X_l) \tag{3.7}$$

In this formula X is the score on the X-scale, X_l and X_h are the low and high scale points on the X-scale, Y_l and Y_h are the low and high scale points on the Y-scale, and Y is the transformed score on the Y-scale. For example, to convert a rating of 4 on a scale ranging from 1 to 5 to a scale ranging from 1 to 7, we have $Y = 1 + (4 - 1)(7 - 1)/(5 - 1) = 1 + 18/4 = 5.5$. Program D-3 may be used to perform a series of such transformations.

Normal and Uniform Transformations

The above transformation is a linear one, in that the Y scores are linearly related to the X scores. This transformation also results in the high and low values on the transformed scale remaining fixed. By working with the frequency distribution of ratings to a specified item,

TABLE 3.1.   Transforming a Distribution of Ratings to Normalized Standard Scores

Rating	Frequency (n_r)	n_b	$n_b + \frac{1}{2}n_r$	p	z	Y
1	3	0	1.5	.03	−1.88	2.12
2	6	3	6	.12	−1.18	2.82
3	8	9	13	.26	−.64	3.36
4	12	17	23	.46	−.10	3.90
5	9	29	33.5	.67	.44	4.44
6	7	38	41.5	.83	.95	4.95
7	5	45	47.5	.95	1.64	5.64

we can also transform the ratings to normal curve or uniform (rectangular) equivalents. Table 3.1 illustrates the transformation of ratings on a 7-point rating scale to a standard normal z-score scale and a standard normal 7-point scale. To transform a specified rating, we add one-half the number of responses for the specified rating ($\frac{1}{2}n_r$) to the sum of the number of responses for all ratings below the specified rating (n_b). The result is divided by the total number of ratings (n_t) to yield:

$$p = (n_b + .5n_r)/n_t \tag{3.8}$$

Then the normal deviate (z) corresponding to the obtained p value is found from a table of areas under the normal curve or by using program D-1.

Standardized z-scores may be converted to a scale having any desired mean and standard deviation, such as the T score ($T = 50 + 10z$) or stanine scale ($S = 5 + 2z$). It may be convenient to convert the z-scores to a scale having approximately the same units as the original rating scale by using

$$Y = z(H - L)/6 + (H + L)/2, \tag{3.9}$$

where H is the highest and L the lowest rating category. The mean of the transformed scale is set equal to (H + L)/2 and the standard deviation to (H − L)/6.

To transform the ratings so that different ratings have equal response frequencies—that is, to a uniform or rectangular distribution—we compute

$$Y = 2c(r - L + 1)(n_b + n_r/2)/[n_t(2r - 2L + 1)] + L - 1 \tag{3.10}$$

where c is the number of rating categories, r is the rth rating, L is the lowest rating, n_b is the total number of ratings below those in the rth category, n_r is the number of ratings in the rth category, and n_t is the total number of ratings. When the lowest rating category (L) is equal to 1, formula 3.10 reduces to:

$$Y = 2cr(n_b + n_r/2)/[n_t(2r - 1)] \qquad (3.11)$$

Assume, for example, that we obtain the following distribution of ratings on a five-point scale:

Rating	Frequency
1	3
2	4
3	7
4	4
5	2

For these data, $c = 5$ and $n_t = 20$; for a rating (r) of 2, $n_b = 3$ and $n_i = 4$. Therefore, the transformed value of a rating of 2 is $2(5)(2)(3 + 2)/[20(4 - 1)] = 1.67$. A more comprehensive illustration of this procedure for seven rating categories is given in Table 3.2.

The computations in formula 3.10, which can made with program D-8, are applicable to both unipolar and bipolar scales. Any positive or negative numbers may be used to designate the rating categories as long as the successive categories are equidistant in numerical value.

TABLE 3.2.   Transforming a Distribution of Ratings to a Uniform (Rectangular) Distribution

Rating	Frequency (n_r)	n_b	$n_b + \frac{1}{2}n_r$	Y
1	3	0	1.5	.42
2	6	3	6	1.12
3	8	9	13	2.18
4	12	17	23	3.68
5	9	29	33.5	5.21
6	7	38	41.5	6.34
7	5	45	47.5	7.16

Scale Calibration

Item response theory can be used to calibrate rating scales so item parameters and total scores of the examinees on an item composite may be estimated. Depending on the particular item response model employed, this is a formidable task requiring a great deal of computer assistance. One appropriate program for scale calibration of rating items is MULTI-LOG, although there are others (see Thissen & Steinberg, 1986).

Older psychometric methods for scaling rating composites, such as those proposed by Guttman, Likert, and Thurstone, are discussed in Chapter 8 (also see Reckase, 1990). We can make both linear and nonlinear transformations of composite scores by the use of appropriate equations, but this is often unnecessary for purposes of statistical analysis. Parametric statistical procedures such as Pearson correlations, t tests, and F tests are quite robust and are not greatly affected by minor deviations from the assumptions underlying them.

Item and Part-Score Weighting

Another practice that may or may not be worth the effort is that of assigning various numerical weights to different items making up a composite. In general, if the composite consists of a fairly large number of items, the reliability of the composite scores are not significantly affected by differential item weighting (Aiken, 1966). It is important to realize, however, that the items comprising a composite are automatically weighted according to the variability of the responses to the items. Items exhibiting a wider range of responses, say from 1 to 7 instead of 1 to 5, automatically receive a greater weight when the ratings on several items are summed to yield a total score. Converting the ratings on all items to standard (z) scores before combining them eliminates the effect of different item variabilities, whatever its cause may be—constant errors or bona fide differences in rater perceptions. If desired, the resulting z-scores can be further transformed to T-scores to get rid of decimals or, by using formula 3.9, to the same c-point scale as the original ratings.

Although the effect of differential item weighting on total scores is relatively inconsequential when the number of items is large, it can be significant when the number of items is small or when a small number of part scores is summed to yield a total score. Separate scores may be assigned on several groups of items—for example, scores on items that presumably measure intelligence, motivation, leadership ability, cooperativeness, and so on. To predict a criterion of job performance, scores on each part are converted to standard scores and then the standard scores are multiplied by numerical weights proportional to the emphasis that one wishes to place on the part variables.[1] An optimum set of weights can be obtained by conducting a multiple regression analysis, the resulting partial regression coefficients (beta weights) being used subsequently in combining scores on those parts to yield a composite predictor of job performance.

Standardization and Norms

Item analysis is an important step in designing and evaluating rating scales and checklists, but it is by no means the last step. Before one can have some assurance that such instruments measure what they are supposed to, proof of their reliability and validity must be obtained. Furthermore, in order to make meaningful interpretations of individual and group responses, the instrument must be standardized.

Sampling

Standard directions for administration and scoring are necessary but not sufficient in standardizing a psychometric instrument. Standardization also requires administering the instrument to a large sample of people (the *standardization sample*) selected as representative of the *target population* for which the instrument is intended. The standardization sample, or *norm group,* should be fairly large, but sample size alone does not guarantee representativeness. To be truly representative of the population of interest, the sample must be selected carefully. The sampling unit may be people, responses, events, objects, or anything countable.

Sampling from Lists. One popular sampling procedure that is employed extensively in surveys and marketing studies is *sampling from lists.* In this procedure, a list of the names of individuals in the target population—say a list of telephone subscribers, heads of households, or other elements (people, objects, events, etc.) having specified characteristics—is obtained. Next we count the number of elements in the population (N) and divide it by the size of the sample (n) that we have decided for economic and statistical reasons to select. Rounding the resulting value of $m = N/n$, we randomly select a number between 1 and m, say s, as a starting point in the list. The element corresponding to s is the first member of the sample; the next element is $s + m$, the next $s + 2m$, and so on, successively adding m to the preceding number. For example, if $N = 1000$ and $n = 100$, then $m = 10$. Entering a table of random numbers, selecting a starting place at random, and reading down the table until we find a number between 1 and 10, let us say that we get 4. Then our sample will consist of the elements numbered 4, 14, 24, . . . , 94.

Though popular, sampling from lists has some serious drawbacks. A list of the population is not always available and too costly to compile, or if available it may not include the entire population of interest. Furthermore, the resulting sample may not be truly representative of the population. For these reasons, in standardizing tests and other psychometric instruments or in conducting psychological research other sampling procedures are usually preferred.

Random Sampling.   In *simple random sampling,* the probability of selecting a given member or element in the target population is the same as for any other one. Because randomness by itself does not ensure that a sample will be representative of the population, we usually begin by grouping the members of the target population on some variable(s) related to the measurements we are making. A popular way of stratifying people in survey studies is according to demographic variables, such as age, sex, socioeconomic status, geographical region. For example, we may stratify the population by socioeconomic status (SES) as upper, middle, and working class. The number of individuals who are selected at random from each of these three groups is made proportional to the total number of individuals who are in that group. Such a *stratified random sample* is more likely than a simple random sample to be unbiased and therefore representative of the population. For this reason, the responses of a carefully selected stratified random sample are quite similar to those that would be obtained in the entire target population.

Cluster Sampling.   More economical than stratified random sampling and more likely than simple random sampling to yield a sample that is representative of the population is cluster sampling. In selecting a *cluster sample,* a designated geographical area or composite population is first divided into a specified number of blocks or clusters. Next a certain percentage of the clusters is selected at random, and a certain number of subunits (schools, households, etc.) is chosen at random from each cluster. Finally, all individuals within each subunit, or at least a random sample of those having certain characteristics, are selected.

Four programs for selecting samples for survey, correlational, and experimental research are included on the diskette accompanying this text. These are programs F-1 (Random Sampling and Random Permutations), F-2 (Random Assigning of Observational Elements to Conditions), F-3 (Stratified Random Sampling-Selection and Assignment), and F-4 (Multistage Cluster Sampling). Program F-1 selects at random, with or without replacement, a sample of m numbers from a population of n numbers. When $m = n$, the numbers are selected without replacement and the result is a random permutation of the numbers. Program F-2 randomly assigns n observational elements to g groups. Program F-3 selects a sample of n observational units at random from (or assigns the observational units to) b strata, levels, or blocks, each consisting of g groups. The number of elements selected from or assigned to each stratum is proportional to the total number of elements contained in the stratum in the population of interest. Program F-4 selects, at each of 2 to 5 successive sampling stages, a designated number of subclusters from clusters randomly selected at the preceding stage. At the final stage, all observational elements, or a random sample selected by program F-1, may be examined.

Norms

After the sample has been selected and ratings obtained from each member of the sample, the ratings are summarized in the form of a frequency distribution and the scores or interval midpoints are then transformed in some way. These *derived scores*, or *norms*, serve as a basis for comparing and interpreting the scores. To illustrate the computation of several types of norms, consider a frequency distribution of the composite ratings given by 90 students to the 11-item Instructor Rating Scale in Figure 2.1. Table 3.3 lists the frequency distribution of these scores, along with the corresponding percentile ranks and T-scores—two common types of norms.

TABLE 3.3. Frequency Distribution and Norms for
Composite Scores on Instructor Rating Scale

Composite Score	Number of Students (Frequency)	Percentile Rank	T-Score
55	1	99	76
54	1	98	74
53	1	97	73
52	1	96	71
51	1	95	70
50	2	93	68
49	1	92	67
48	1	91	65
47	2	89	63
46	1	87	62
45	1	86	60
44	1	85	59
43	2	83	57
42	7	78	56
41	5	72	54
40	7	65	53
39	8	57	51
38	4	50	50
37	6	44	48
36	6	38	47
35	5	32	45
34	5	26	44
33	5	21	42
32	1	17	41
31	4	14	39
30	0	12	38
29	3	11	36
28	5	6	35
27	1	3	33
26	1	2	32
25	0	1	30
24	1	1	29

Percentile Ranks.   The *percentile rank* corresponding to a raw score or
the midpoint of a score interval is computed by the following steps:

1. Sum the frequencies on the intervals below the interval containing the designated score; call the result *cf*. For example, there are 67 scores below a score of 42, so in this case *cf* = 67.

2. To the value to *cf* add one-half the frequency (*f*) of the designated score (or score interval containing the designated score): $cf + \frac{1}{2}f = 67 + \frac{1}{2}(7) = 70.5$.

3. Multiply the result by 100, and divide the product by the total number of scores (*n*): $PR = 100[cf + \frac{1}{2}(f)]/n = 100(70.5)/90 = 78.33$.

In Table 3.3, the percentile ranks computed in this way have been rounded to the nearest whole number. The percentile rank corresponding to a given raw score or interval midpoint is the percentage of scores falling below that score or midpoint. Thus, 78% of this group of 90 students assigned composite ratings lower than 42 to the instructor.

Standard Score Norms. Percentile ranks are ordinal-scale numbers, so equal numerical differences in ranks do not correspond to equal differences on the variable measured by the instrument. *Standard scores* are more precise, in that they represent measurement on an interval scale. Determination of all standard score norms begins with z-scores, computed as

$$z = (X - \overline{X})/s \qquad (3.12)$$

Given that the mean ($\overline{X}$) and standard deviation (s) of the composite ratings in Table 3.3 are 38.09 and 6.59, respectively, if $X = 42$, then $z = (42 - 38.09)/6.59 = .59$. Because z-scores have a mean of 0 and a range of approximately -3 to $+3$, a z-score of .59 is slightly above average.

The negative signs and decimals of z-scores are somewhat inconvenient to work with, but we can get rid of them by converting the z-scores to a scale having any desired mean and standard deviation. Among the most popular of these standard score scales are *T*-scores, stanine scores, sten scores, and deviation IQ scores. The *T*-score scale has a mean of 50 and a standard deviation of 10, so to convert z-scores to *T*-scores we compute:

$$T = 10z + 50 \qquad (3.13)$$

If $z = .59$, $T = 10(.59) + 50 = 55.9$, which rounds to 56.

When interpreting percentile rank norms, remember that the scale ranges from 0 to 100, with an average of 50, and that the same difference between two percentile ranks does not have the same meaning on different parts of the scale. The further out you get on the percentile rank scale—on either the high or low end—the more significant a given numerical difference becomes. Thus, the difference between percentile ranks of 50 and 55 is not as significant—in terms of the attribute being measured—as the difference between ranks of 90 and 95 or ranks of 5 and 10.

When interpreting T-score norms, remember that the scale ranges from approximately 20 to 80, with an average of 50, and that equal numerical differences correspond to equal attribute differences—wherever you are on the scale. Thus, the difference between T-scores of 40 and 50 or 50 and 60 is equal to the difference between T-scores of 20 and 30 or 70 and 80.

Normalized Standard Scores.   The standard score norms discussed above are simple linear transformations of raw scores. They have different means and standard deviations from the raw scores, but the shapes of the frequency distributions of the raw and transformed scores are identical. In contrast, normalized standard scores have a normal distribution—whatever the shape of the raw score distribution may be. To convert a raw score to a normalized standard T-score, we begin by finding the percentile rank of the raw score and then use a table of areas under the normal curve to convert it to a z-score. Finally, we multiply the z-score by 10 and add 50 to the product. A raw score of, say, 42 in Table 3.3, has a percentile rank of 78.33. Consulting a table of areas under the normal curve in an elementary statistics books (or using program D-1), we find that $z = .78$ and, consequently, $T = 10(.78) + 50 \approx$ 58. Because the frequency distribution in Table 3.3 is not exactly normal, this normalized value of T is similar but not identical to that obtained for the non-normalized value of T.

Computer Programs.   Programs D-5, D-6, and D-7 can be used to determine the norms discussed above. Program D-5 converts raw scores to percentile ranks, deciles, and quartiles. Program D-6 converts raw scores to non-normalized z- and T-scores, and program D-7 converts raw scores to normalized z- and T-scores.

Parallel Forms and Equating

Research and practice involving psychological assessment often requires multiple forms of the same instrument. For example, ratings on various behavioral characteristics are made before and after a particular treatment or intervention program designed to change those behaviors. If two parallel forms of a rating scale are administered, the second (after) ratings are less likely to be biased by the first (before) ratings. Similarly, therapeutic intervention programs may require frequent evaluations of behavioral changes; in such cases, multiple forms of a behavioral checklist are needed.

Constructing parallel or equated forms of tests and scales is a rather expensive and time-consuming process. Two instruments having the same number and the same kinds of items, which yield the same means and standard deviations when standardized on the same sample of people, must first be constructed. Then the equating process begins. Traditionally, equating was done by the *equipercentile method*. This consisted of changing the scores on both forms of a test to percentile ranks. Then a table of equivalent scores on the two forms was prepared by equating the pth percentile on the first form to the pth percentile on the second form.

Tests and other psychometric instruments many also be equated, or rather made comparable, by anchoring them to a common test or pool of items. In recent years, the equating process has become even more sophisticated, involving item response methodology. The procedure is economical in that it involves *item sampling,* which consists of administering randomly selected subsets of items to different randomly selected groups of people. Then items and total scores on the several tests to be equated are calibrated by computer-based, iterative procedures and placed on a common scale.

Regardless of the equating method employed, strictly speaking psychometric instruments cannot be equated. About the best that can be done is to make the instruments comparable. For this reason, changes in scores on parallel forms of instruments administered before and after an intervention procedure is implemented should be interpreted cautiously.

RELIABILITY

Generally speaking, rating scales and checklists cannot be useful unless they measure whatever they measure consistently. Responses to the items on these instruments are reliable only if they are not significantly affected by temporary internal states (low motivation, temporary indisposition, etc.) or external conditions (a distracting or uncomfortable environment, etc.). More formally, we say that a psychometric measure or instrument is reliable if scores on it are relatively free from errors of measurement. Only when errors of measurement are low will the instrument consistently differentiate between the persons, objects, or events we are trying to measure—and therefore be reliable.

Classical reliability theory is based on the assumption that the observed variance of scores on a measuring instrument (s_o^2) is equal to the sum of true variance (s_t^2) plus error variance (s_e^2):

$$s_o^2 = s_t^2 + s_e^2 \qquad (3.14)$$

By definition, reliability (r_{11}) is the proportion of observed variance that is due to errors of measurement:

$$r_{11} = s_t^2/s_o^2 \qquad (3.15)$$

Cross-multiplying yields $s_t^2 = r_{11}\, s_o^2$, which, when substituted in formula 3.14 yields the error variance:

$$s_e^2 = s_o^2(1 - r_{11}) \qquad (3.16)$$

The square root of the error variance known as the *standard error of measurement*:

$$s_e = \sqrt{1 - r_{11}} \qquad (3.17)$$

Standard Error of Measurement

Because the reliability coefficient ranges from .00 to 1.00, the standard error of measurement ranges from a minimum of 0—which it equals only when reliability is perfect $(r_{11} = 1.00)$—to a maximum of s_o. In classical reliability theory, the standard error of measurement is used to establish a range of values within which one can say with $p\%$ confidence that the true scores of a group of individuals making the same observed score fall. Thus, the true scores of 68% of a group of people whose observed score is equal to a specified value fall within one standard error of measurement of the observed score. Likewise, the true scores of 90% fall within 1.645 standard errors of measurement of their observed score, 95% fall within 1.96 standard errors of measurement of their observed score, and 99% fall within 2.575 standard errors of measurement of their observed score.

To minimize the tendency to consider a score on a psychometric instrument as a fixed, unvarying measure of a characteristic but only as an approximation, that score may be expressed in terms of a score band, or *percentile band*. A percentile band consists of a range of scores which takes into account the standard error of measurement or its percentile-rank equivalent. When making a graphical plot of a person's responses or scores on several measures, it is accepted practice to draw a band of one or two standard errors of measurement on either side of the score points. Then small differences between the person's scores on two different variables or small differences between the scores of two people on the same variable are less likely to be interpreted as significant. As a general rule, the difference between the scores of two people on the same variable (instrument) should be interpreted as significant only if it is equal to at least twice the standard error of measurement of the variable. But the difference between the scores of the same person on two different variables should be greater than twice the standard error of measurement of *either* variable before it is interpreted as significant.

Coefficient of Stability

A coefficient of stability, otherwise known as *test-retest reliability coefficient,* indicates how consistent ratings or other measures are over time. A test-retest coefficient is obtained by correlating the scores obtained on the same instrument on two separate occasions. Because the conditions of administration are likely to be different over long time intervals than over short ones, the size of a test-retest coefficient tends to be larger when retesting takes place after a few days or weeks than after several months.

Coefficient of Equivalence

The magnitude of a test retest coefficient is affected by the fact that measures on certain persons, objects, or events are more consistent than others, and hence the rank order of the entities being measured changes over time. For example, some people remember more than other people about the content and/or responses to the items when completing a rating scale or checklist a second time. One way of controlling for the inconsistency with which a psychometric instrument differentiates among people or things is to construct a second form of the instrument and administer it on the second occasion. Then we can compute a parallel forms coefficient by finding the correlation between the scores or ratings on the two forms. Even better, we might divide our sample in half and administer instrument A on occasion 1 and instrument B on occasion 2 to the first half of the sample. The second half of the sample, on the other hand, would take instrument B on occasion 1 and instrument A on occasion 2. The resulting correlation between the scores on forms A and B is a measure of the stability and equivalence of the instrument.

Internal Consistency Coefficients

Because there are problems with both the test-retest and the parallel forms procedures for determining the reliability, quite early in the history of psychological assessment researchers began searching for a technique that would not involve the expense of constructing a parallel form or readministering the same or a different form of a test. One approach, the *split-half* or *odd-even method,* was to administer the test only once but to score it by halves. In other words, every examinee received two scores—one score on the odd-numbered items and another score on the even-numbered items. Then, by using the following formula, known as the *Spearman-Brown prophecy formula,* one could estimate the reliability of a test having twice as many items as the original:

$$r_{11} = 2r_{oe}/(1 + r_{oe}), \tag{3.18}$$

where r_{oe} is the correlation between scores on the even numbered items with those on the odd-numbered items and r_{11} is the estimated reliability of the full-length test. A generalized version of this formula can be used to estimate the increase in reliability that would be expected to result from adding more items to the instrument.[2]

The split-half method assumes that the two halves constitute parallel forms and hence the items are parallel. Although this assumption may be correct in some cases, not all of the hundreds of ways of dividing a test into halves produce parallel forms. A possible solution is to estimate the reliability of all half splits of a test and then compute the mean reliability, but this is cumbersome. For this reason, a more general procedure was developed for estimating the mean of the reliability coefficients obtained from all possible ways of dividing the test into split halves. The result was the following Kuder-Richardson formulas:

$$r_{11} = [k/(k-1)][1 - \Sigma(p_i(1-p_i)/s^2] \qquad (3.19a)$$
$$r_{11} = [k/(k-1)][1 - \overline{X}(k-\overline{X})/(ks^2)] \qquad (3.19b)$$

In these formulas, k is the total number of items, $\overline{X}$ is the mean of total scores, s^2 is the variance of total scores, and p_i is the proportion of examinees who gave the keyed response to item i. Formula 3.19(b), which assumes that all items are of equal difficulty, yields a more conservative estimate of reliability and is easier to use than formula 3.19(a).

The Kuder-Richardson formulas are applicable only with instruments on which the items are scored as 0 or 1. A more general formula for estimating the reliability of a rating scale or any other psychometric instrument on which responses to items are assigned two or more scoring weights is Cronbach's alpha coefficient

$$\alpha = [k/(k-1)][1 - \Sigma s_i^2/s_t^2] \qquad (3.20)$$

In this formula s_i^2 is the variance of scores on item i and s_t^2 is the variance of total test scores. The values of s_i^2 are summed over all items.

The Spearman-Brown, Kuder-Richardson, and Cronbach procedures yield estimates of the internal consistency of an instrument—in other words, the extent to which the items on the instrument measure the same thing. Because all three procedures overestimate the reliability of instruments in which speed is a factor, they are generally not recommended for estimating the reliability of speeded tests or whenever performance on a psychometric instrument is greatly affected by time pressure.

Interrater Reliability

In scoring rating scales and other instruments involving subjective scorer judgment, it is important to know the extent to which different respondents agree with each other in their evaluations or judgments of whatever or whomever they are evaluating. The most common procedure for determining an *interrater* or *interscorer reliability coefficient* is to have two evaluators or judges rate the behaviors or performances of a sizable number of persons; then the correlation between the ratings assigned by the two evaluators is computed. Another approach is to have several evaluators or judges rate the performance or behavior of one person, or better still, to have many evaluators rate the performances or behaviors of a number of people. The latter approach yields an *intraclass coefficient* or *coefficient of concordance*, which is a generalized interscorer or interrater reliability coefficient. Procedures for computing these coefficients are described by Winer, Brown, and Michels (1991) and in many other statistics or psychometrics textbooks. Special methods for computing test-retest and internal-consistency reliability coefficients from ratings and for conducting statistical tests of significance on the coefficients have also been provided by the author (Aiken, 1985b).

Interpreting Reliability Coefficients

The reliability coefficients of checklists, ratings scales, and inventories are usually lower than those of tests of achievement, intelligence, and special abilities. But what is meant by a low or high reliability, what factors influence reliability, and how can it be improved?

How high should a reliability coefficient obtained from scores on rating scales and checklists be in order for the instrument to be considered potentially useful? The answer depends on what one plans to do with the responses or scores. If the scores are used to determine whether two groups of people differ significantly on a variable of interest, a reliability coefficient as low as .65 may make a contribution to the decision. On the other hand, if the scores are being used to compare the performances of different individuals, then a reliability coefficient of at least .85 is needed. By these criteria, many rating scales and checklist might make a contribution to decisions concerning groups but not decisions concerning individuals.

Variability and Reliability

Like other measures of relationship, reliability is affected by the variance of the variables being measured: larger score variance promotes higher reliability. For this reason, efforts to improve the reliability of a psychometric instrument often focus on methods for increasing its variance. One way to increase score variance is to add more items of the same general type to the instrument. Score variance is also affected by the characteristics of the group of the people who are being evaluated. Reliability tends to be higher with more heterogeneous groups—in which there is a wide range of individual differences on whatever characteristic is being evaluated. The range of individual differences varies with the age, grade, sex, and other demographic and personal variables.

Errors of measurement are greater when uncontrolled situational factors are allowed to affect the precision of measurement. Efforts should be made to keep such situational or environmental conditions under which the instrument is administered as constant as possible. In addition, making item content and directions unambiguous and complete, making certain that parallel forms of the instrument are really comparable, and ensuring that examiners and evaluators are well-trained in the rating process all contribute to reliability.

Generalizability Theory

The error variance component of formula 3.14 may encompass errors due to many sources—differences in the items on an instrument, differences in instructions for completing the instrument, differences in times at which the instrument is administered, and other contextual or situational variations in the conditions under which a psychometric instrument is used. Traditionally, the test-retest method of reliability determination has been viewed as taking into account error variance due to differences in times at which an instrument is administered, whereas the parallel forms procedure takes into account differences among the items comprising the instrument. Finally, internal consistency approaches take into account differences among items purporting to measure the same construct and administered within the same time frame.

During the 1960s and 1970s, it became increasingly obvious that the classical approach to reliability, although useful, was too simplistic. Alternative approaches, based on the general notion that the utility of scores on psychometric instruments depends on the extent to which they are applicable or generalizable across different situations or contexts or under different conditions, were developed. Statistical methods were then devised to estimate the dependability or generalizability of test scores across different "domains." One such approach, known as *generalizability theory*, views a score or rating as a single sample from a universe of possible scores and the reliability of that score as the accuracy with which it estimates a more generalized universe value of the score (the "true score"). The computations involved in generalizability theory are based on analysis of variance statistical procedures. These procedures are applied in determining the generalizability, or *dependability*, of test scores as a function of changes in the person(s) taking the test, different samples of items comprising the test, the situations or conditions under which the test is taken, and the methods or people involved in scoring it. A *generalizability coefficient*, which is similar to a traditional reliability coefficient, is then computed as the ratio of the expected variance of scores in the universe to the variance of scores in the sample. Finally, a "universe value" of the score, similar to the "true score" of classical reliability theory, can be estimated (Cronbach et al., 1972). The effects of various samples of items, conditions of administration, or other *facets* on the accuracy with which the universe values of scores can be determined are of particular interest.

Generalizability theory, item-response theory, covariance structures analysis, and other modern statistical methods are certainly more technically sophisticated than classical test theory. Developments and applications in psychological measurement, however, still make extensive use of traditional concepts of reliability and validity and the procedures derived from them (see Feldt & Brennan, 1989).

Computer Programs

A number of programs for estimating the reliabilities of rating scales and checklists are included on the diskette accompanying this book. Programs for computing coefficient alpha (program E-1), the Kuder-Richardson reliability coefficients (program E-2), and coefficient kappa (program E-3) are included in category E of the program diskette. Kappa is a type of test-retest coefficient, used primarily with criterion-referenced tests but also appropriate for estimating the test-retest reliabilities of rating scales and checklists. In addition to computing kappa, this program conducts a statistical significance test on the obtained value and provides an associated probability value.

Computer programs for computing several other measures of reliability, including the intraclass correlation coefficient (program E-4), the concordance coefficient (program E-5), and the author's R and H coefficients (program E-6), may also be found in category E. An intraclass correlation coefficient is a measure of the consistency of the ratings assigned by several raters to the same ratees; this program also computes the intraclass correlation of a sum or average. A similar measure is the concordance coefficient, an index of the degree of agreement among the ranks assigned by several raters to the same ratees. In addition to the coefficient of concordance and the corresponding value of chi square, this program (E-4) computes the average rank correlation and the expected correlation among the set of rankings with a comparable set.

The package of programs under "Absolute Difference (V, R, and H) Coefficients" (program E-6) includes the author's R (repeatability) and H (homogeneity) coefficients for determining test-retest and internal consistency reliabilities of ratings. R is equal to one minus the ratio of the obtained sum of the absolute values of the differences between two sets of ratings to the maximum possible sum of those values. H is equal to one minus the ratio of the sum of the absolute values of the differences among all ratings in a sample (of one person on several scales or several persons on one scale) to the maximum possible value of this sum. Also included in this package are programs for calculating the right-tail probability of the obtained values of R and H and the population means and standard deviations of R and H values based on different numbers of rating categories and number of raters. Program E-6 will also compute the difference between R or H coefficients in two samples and the associated probability.

SUMMARY

In designing a rating scale or a checklist, a great deal can be done at the outset to make certain that the instrument is well-constructed. Clear, correct wording of items, complete and understandable directions, and a neat, attractive format or layout of the instrument can help to ensure the collection of useful assessment data. Before attempting to standardize a psychometric instrument on a representative sample, initial item tryouts should be conducted with small samples to detect any mistakes or other problems in instrument design or administration procedure. Empirical analysis of the statistical characteristics of each item, including determination of the proportion of respondents who selected each option and some measure of the internal and/or external validity of the item, is useful in judging whether the item should be retained as it is, revised, or discarded.

More sophisticated procedures, such as item response theory, may be used to analyze and calibrate items. In addition, item scores may be transformed or converted to appropriate units and a decision made to assign different numerical weights to different items or composites.

Once initial tryouts have been conducted and the composition of the instrument improved by item analysis, we are ready to standardize it on a sample of individuals who are representative of the (target) population for which the instrument is intended. A variety of sampling procedures—sampling from lists, simple random sampling, stratified random sampling, cluster sampling—may be employed in this process. In standardizing a psychometric instrument, stratified random sampling, in which the target population is divided into demographic or other relevant strata and a proportional sample is selected from each stratum, is more likely than other procedures to yield an unbiased sample. Scores obtained by the standardization sample may be converted to percentile ranks, standard scores, or other types of norms to provide a frame of reference for interpretion purposes.

The reliability of scores on a psychometric instrument is concerned with the extent to which the instrument measures consistently, that is, how free the scores are from errors of measurement. Classical test theory defines reliability as the ratio of the true variance of scores to their observed variance. Reliability coefficients, which range from .00 to 1.00, vary not only with the instrument and the sample, but also with the conditions under which the instrument is administered. The standard error of measurement, an index of error used to establish a range of values within which a person's true score on a psycho metric instrument is likely to fall, varies inversely with the reliability coefficient.

Various procedures—test-retest, parallel forms, internal consistency—are used in estimating reliability. All these procedures have drawbacks and in some cases have been superseded by more advanced statistical techniques, among which are item response theory and generalizability theory.

QUESTIONS AND ACTIVITIES

1. Define each of the following terms used in this chapter. Consult Appendix A and/or a dictionary if you need help.

base rate	equating
cluster sample	equipercentile method
coefficient alpha	error variance
coefficient of equivalence	generalizability theory
coefficient of stability	internal consistency
derived score	interrater (interscorer) reliability

item analysis
item-response (character-
   istic) curve
item sampling
Kuder-Richardson
   formulas
linear transformation
normalized scores
normal distribution
norms
norms group
odd-even reliability
parallel forms
percentile band
percentile norms
percentile rank
point-biserial coefficient
random sample

rank-biserial correlation
reliability
reliability coefficient
representative sample
score weighting
Spearman-Brown formula
split-half reliability
standard error of measurement
standard scores
standardization
standardization sample
stratified random sample
T-scores
target population
test-retest reliability
transformations
true score
z-score

2. Consider the following table of the responses of 10 people to a ten-item checklist; 1 indicates endorsement (checked) and 0 non-endorsement (not checked) responses. For each item, find the proportion of respondents who checked it and the point-biserial correlation between scores on the item and total scores on the ten-item composite. Which items should be retained, and which ones need to be revised or discarded?

Item	A	B	C	D	E	F	G	H	I	J
					Examinee					
1	1	1	0	1	1	0	1	0	1	0
2	1	0	0	0	0	1	0	0	0	1
3	1	1	1	1	1	0	1	0	0	0
4	1	1	1	0	0	1	0	1	0	0
5	1	0	1	1	0	0	0	0	0	0
6	1	1	1	0	1	1	1	0	0	0
7	1	0	1	1	0	0	1	1	0	1
8	1	1	1	0	1	1	0	0	1	0
9	1	1	0	1	1	1	0	1	0	0
10	1	1	1	1	1	0	0	0	1	0
Total Scores	10	7	7	6	6	5	4	3	3	2

3. Find the percentile ranks, z-score and T-score norms corresponding to the interval midpoints of the following frequency distribution of supervisory ratings (X) and rated job satisfaction (Y) by 90 employees of a chemical manufacturing plant, where $\overline{X} = 38.17$, $\overline{Y} = 17.93$, $s_x = 6.64$, and $s_y = 4.87$.

Supervisory Ratings		Job Satisfaction	
Interval	Frequency	Interval	Frequency
54–56	2	30–31	2
51–53	3	28–29	1
48–50	4	26–27	0
45–47	4	24–25	4
42–44	10	22–23	12
39–41	20	20–21	17
36–38	16	18–19	19
33–35	15	16–17	8
30–32	5	14–15	11
27–29	9	12–13	6
24–26	2	10–11	5
		8–9	2
		6–7	3

4. Calculate both of the Kuder-Richardson reliability coefficients of the scores on the ten-item composite in question 2. The mean and variance of the scores are 5.30 and 5.21, respectively.

5. Compute the standard error of measurement of a rating scale having a standard deviation of 8 and a parallel-forms reliability coefficient of .82. Use the obtained value of the standard error of measurement to find the 95% confidence interval for the true scores corresponding to obtained scores of 25, 35, and 45.

6. What coefficients and computer programs should be used to determine the reliability of a checklist? Of a rating scale?

7. What are some of the problems that might be encountered in attempting to apply classical or contemporary test theory to rating scales and checklists?

4

Validity and Statistical Methods for Research

Reliability and standardization are means to an end rather than ends in themselves. Both contribute to the ultimate goal of assessment—to make valid judgments or decisions, but they do not ensure the realization of that goal. Thus, a rating scale or checklist may be carefully designed, reliable, and standardized, and still not measure the variable or construct that it was designed to measure. For example, ratings on job performance may be more indicative of the likability or popularity of ratees than of the actual behaviors that contribute to doing the job well. Similarly, behavioral ratings following treatment or institutionalization may reflect ratees' pretense of improvement rather than bona fide changes in behavior.

Reliability is not a sufficient condition for validity, but it is a necessary one. Technically speaking, the validity of a psychometric instrument can be no higher than the square root of its parallel forms reliability. Both reliability and validity are affected by unsystematic errors of measurement, but systematic errors of measurement—consistent bias in scores—affect only validity. Compared with reliability, validity is also affected by the situation in which it is determined. For example, a particular rating scale may be a good predictor or criterion measure of performance in a training program but not of actual on-the-job behavior. Rather than posing the question "Is this instrument valid?" it is more appropriate to ask "For what purposes and under what conditions is the instrument valid?" Validity is relative rather than being a matter of accuracy and utility of measurement in a general sense. Validity also has value implications, in that users of a psychometric instrument should be aware of any social and personal consequences of using it. Even though using the instrument results in short-term gains in efficiency of performance or production, if the long-term consequences of its use are unfavorable for a particular group or section of the population it may warrant a less positive evaluation.

TYPES OF VALIDITY

There are three types of validity: content, criterion-related, and construct.

Content Validity

Perhaps the simplest or most straightforward method of obtaining evidence for the validity of a psychometric instrument is to examine its content. This so-called *content validity* approach is more than a simple matter of superficial appearance, or "face validity." It involves a careful, systematic analysis of the content of the instrument by experts who are familiar with the variables or constructs purportedly measured by it. A content validity analysis is an important first step and an appropriate one with all psychometric measures, but particularly so in the case of achievement tests. The manual of a carefully designed academic achievement test contains a comprehensive outline or table of specifications that spells out precisely what variables the test is designed to measure and which items are included under each variable. A similar approach may be used with a rating scale or checklist, in particular one that measures multiple variables. From an examination of the detailed outline or table of specifications for a test or other psychometric instrument, experts should be able to make sound judgments as to whether the content indicates that the instrument is measuring what it is supposed to measure.

The items on rating scales and checklists designed to assist in clinical diagnosis usually refer to symptoms or signs of those disorders, so one might think it would be easy to establish the content validity of such instruments. Unfortunately, the diagnostic criteria for many disorders are not always clear, and a symptom checklist or rating scale often has only a modest correlation with immediate and long-term behavioral criteria.

Content analysis is facilitated by careful definitions of the variables which the instrument is intended to measure and the relationships or interactions among those variables. In addition, the design of a particular instrument may be based on a theory of behavior, cognition, or personality. Consequently, it is important to understand the assumptions, concepts, and workings of that theory before attempting to determine whether the instrument is content-valid. The Adjective Check List, the Edwards Personality Preference Schedule, and the Thematic Apperception Test, for example, are all based—at least in part—on Henry Murray's need-press theory of personality. For this reason, one should have a good knowledge of that theory before attempting to determining the content validity of these instruments.

V Index

Some years ago I devised a convenient index of content validity, including a test of its statistical significance (Aiken, 1980). Assume that N raters inspect a single item or questionnaire and judge its content validity on a c-category scale ranging from lo to $lo + c - 1$, where lo indicates the lowest degree of content validity. Then an overall index of content validity may be defined as

$$V = \Sigma n_i |i - lo| /[N(c - 1)], \qquad (4.1)$$

where i varies from $lo + 1$ to $lo + c - 1$. The maximum value of V is 1.00, and the minimum value is .00. To illustrate, let the content validity ratings, on a scale of 1 to 5, assigned by five individuals to an item on a rating scale be 3, 3, 4, 4, and 5. Then $V = (0|2 - 1| + 2|3 - 1| + 2|4 - 1| + 1|5 - 1|)/[5(5 - 1)] = 14/20 = .70$. Assuming that the probability of a single rating falling in the ith category is $1/c$, the multinomial formula can be used to find the probability of a particular combination of ratings occurring at random. Then probabilities associated with the several combinations of responses yielding the same V value may be summed to obtain the discrete probability associated with that value of V. The discrete probabilities of all values of V equal to or greater than the value under consideration may be combined to yield the significance level for V. Tables for determining the statistical significance of V computed on c categories and n raters (where $n \leq 25$) may be found in Aiken (1985b).

When N is large, the probability under the standard normal distribution to the right of

$$z = [N(c - 1)(2V - 1) - 1]/\sqrt{N(c - 1)(c + 1)/3} \qquad (4.2)$$

is a good approximation to the exact probability. For example, if 25 people rate an instrument's validity on a five-point scale and the results yield a V index of .70, $z = [25(4)(.4) - 1]/\sqrt{25(4)(6)/3} = 2.76$. The right-tail probability for this value of z is less than .01, leading to the conclusion that the instrument in question has a significant degree of content validity. Program E-6 can be used to compute the value of V for a set of ratings and the right-tail probability in small or large samples associated with that value. The program can also compute the difference between V coefficients in two samples and the associated probability.

Criterion-Related Validity

Because it is based on reasoning, content validity may also be referred to as *rational* validity. The reasoning process in determining the content validity of a psychometric instrument stems from a knowledge of the variables or constructs to be measured and perhaps some theoretical conceptions involving them. In contrast, *criterion-related validity* may be characterized as *empirical*, in that it is based on demonstrated facts or data. While content validation is concerned with what is reasonable or what makes sense according to knowledge and theory pertaining to the domain of interest, empirical validity is a "show me" process of determining an instrument's validity by comparing item or composite scores with performance on a criterion of what the instrument was designed to measure.

Criterion-related validity has traditionally been divided into two types—concurrent (or congruent) and predictive validity—depending on when the criterion measures become available. If those measures are obtained at or about the same time as scores on the instrument being validated the concern is with *concurrent validity.* But when the criterion measures do not become available until sometime in the future, perhaps months later, then a study of the *predictive validity* of the instrument is being conducted. These two types of criterion-related validity are not exclusive. For example, one may decide to compare performance ratings of employees given by coworkers with ratings assigned by supervisors during the same time frame (concurrent), and to compare ratings by coworkers with a direct measure of job performance obtained a few weeks or months later (predictive validity). Either comparison may or may not provide evidence for the validity of coworker ratings as indicators of job performance.

Responses to rating scales and checklists are used extensively in studies of the criterion-related validity of psychometric measures and in a variety of contexts. Developmental research, performance evaluations, and the assessment of behavioral changes produced by therapeutic or other intervention procedures are only some of the situations in which ratings and checklist responses provide information on initial and subsequent status. In predictive validity studies, responses to rating scales and checklists may serve as the predictor variables, criterion variables, or both. In concurrent validity studies, such responses may also serve as either type of variable.

Quite common in investigations of concurrent validation is the *method of contrasting groups.* In this method, two groups of people in different diagnostic, occupational, or other relevant categories are compared in terms of their performance on a rating scale, a checklist, or some other type of psychological assessment instrument. This was the method used in validating the Minnesota Multiphasic Personality Inventory (MMPI), the most popular of all paper-and-pencil measures of personality. The concurrent validity of MMPI items in diagnosing psychiatric patients correctly was determined by the accuracy with which they assigned mental patients to the same diagnostic categories as those assigned by psychiatrists employing observational and interview techniques.

Even more common than concurrent validation studies are investigations of the predictive validity of cognitive and affective instruments. Many of these investigations are conducted in educational and employment contexts, with the resulting data being subjected to a variety of statistical procedures. Among these are correlation and regression procedures. An illustration follows.

Computing the Pearson r

Consider the 90 pairs of numbers in the X and Y columns of Table 4.1; where X is a composite student rating of the personality of an instructor mid-way through a college course and Y is a composite end-of-term

TABLE 4.1. Composite Ratings of Instructor (X) and Course (Y) by Student

Student	X	Y	X^2	Y^2	XY
1	26	6	676	36	156
2	28	10	784	100	280
3	40	28	1600	784	1120
4	37	14	1369	196	518
5	35	14	1225	196	490
6	33	12	1089	144	396
7	33	21	1089	441	693
8	37	20	1369	400	740
9	29	18	841	324	522
10	42	21	1764	441	882
11	38	22	1444	484	836
12	35	19	1225	361	665
13	38	18	1444	324	684
14	39	23	1521	529	897
15	39	21	1521	441	819
16	28	19	784	361	532
17	29	12	841	144	348
18	28	9	784	81	252
19	39	15	1521	225	585
20	40	22	1600	484	880
21	36	22	1296	484	792
22	45	25	2025	625	1125
23	33	15	1089	225	495
24	37	15	1369	225	555
25	29	18	841	324	522
26	35	11	1225	121	385
27	36	16	1296	256	576
28	31	16	961	256	496
29	52	30	2704	900	1560
30	34	18	1156	324	612
31	24	11	576	121	264
32	41	21	1681	441	861
33	41	21	1681	441	861
34	33	10	1089	100	330
35	40	16	1600	256	640
36	33	16	1089	256	528
37	39	21	1521	441	819
38	42	19	1764	361	798
39	37	15	1369	225	555
40	34	13	1156	169	442
41	51	23	2601	529	1173
42	48	24	2304	576	1152
43	54	21	2916	441	1134
44	49	20	2401	400	980
45	38	20	1444	400	760

TABLE 4.1. *(Continued)*

Student	X	Y	X²	Y²	XY
46	55	22	3025	484	1210
47	42	19	1764	361	798
48	47	19	2209	361	893
49	46	22	2116	484	1012
50	53	24	2809	576	1272
51	31	19	961	361	589
52	38	5	1444	25	190
53	40	19	1600	361	760
54	27	12	729	144	324
55	35	15	1225	225	525
56	47	20	2209	400	940
57	39	23	1521	529	897
58	40	17	1600	289	680
59	42	13	1764	169	546
60	42	20	1764	400	840
61	37	18	1369	324	666
62	42	20	1764	400	840
63	43	18	1849	324	774
64	41	19	1681	361	779
65	39	16	1521	256	624
66	44	24	1936	576	1056
67	31	15	961	225	465
68	36	15	1296	225	540
69	34	21	1156	441	714
70	36	18	1296	324	648
71	40	20	1600	400	800
72	39	23	1521	529	897
73	31	23	961	529	713
74	36	10	1296	100	360
75	28	20	784	400	560
76	41	18	4681	324	738
77	40	17	1600	289	680
78	32	19	1024	361	608
79	36	18	1296	324	648
80	28	14	784	196	392
81	39	13	1521	169	507
82	50	7	2500	49	350
83	43	8	1849	64	344
84	34	19	1156	361	646
85	34	14	1156	196	476
86	37	22	1369	484	814
87	35	23	1225	529	805
88	50	21	2500	441	1050
89	41	17	1681	289	697
90	42	30	1764	900	1260
Sums	3428	1610	134482	30952	62637

student evaluation of the course. The 11 items on the personality rating instrument are listed in Figure 2.1. The items included in the course evaluation are the ratings on six five-point scales of the extent to which a sample of students considered the course to have been helpful, informative, interesting, motivating, stimulating, and valuable.

The Pearson product-moment correlation coefficient between the X and Y variables may be computed with

$$r = [n\Sigma XY - (\Sigma X)(\Sigma Y)]/\sqrt{[n\Sigma X^2 - (\Sigma X)^2][n\Sigma Y^2 - (\Sigma Y)^2]} \quad (4.3)$$

The intermediate computations are the number (n) of X, Y pairs, the sum of the X scores (ΣX), the sum of the Y scores (ΣY), the sum of the squares of the X scores (ΣX^2), the sum of the squares of the Y scores (ΣY^2), and the sum of the cross-products of the X and Y scores (ΣXY). Substituting the appropriate values (see last row of Table 4.1) in formula 4.3 yields

$$r = \frac{90(62,637) - (3428)(1610)}{\sqrt{[90(134482) - (3428)^2][90(30952) - (1610)^2]}} = .4529.$$

The value $r = .4529$ indicates that the correlation between composite midterm student ratings of the instructor's personality and end-of-term evaluations of the course is positive and moderate. Thus, to a moderate extent, students who assigned higher ratings to the instructor's personality at midterm tended to assign higher evaluations to the course as a whole at term's end than students who gave lower ratings to the instructor's personality. This result is not particularly surprising, but it may be interpreted as some evidence for the predictive validity of midterm instructor personality ratings.

Simple Linear Regression

As emphasized in Chapter 1, correlation does not imply causation but it does imply prediction. Larger values of r—either positive or negative—indicate greater predictability of variable Y from variable X (or X from Y). The prediction process is made more explicit by constructing a linear regression equation. This is the equation of the straight line that best fits through the cluster of $X - Y$ points, in that the sum of the squared vertical distances of the points from the line is smaller than for any other line than could be passed through those points. A simple linear regression equation has the form $Y_{pred} = a + bX$, where a is the predicted value of Y when $X = 0$ and b is the slope of the line. Both the value of r and the regression equation may be determined by program C-5.

The a and b constants in a simple linear regression equation are computed by

$$b = [n\Sigma XY - (\Sigma X)(\Sigma Y)]/[n\Sigma X^2 - (\Sigma X)^2] \qquad (4.4)$$

$$a = (\Sigma Y - b\Sigma X)/n \qquad (4.5)$$

Substituting the appropriate column totals from Table 4.1 into these formulas yields $b = [90(62,637) - 3,428(1,610)]/[90(134,482) - (3,428)^2]$ $= .3358$ and $a = [(1,610 - .3358(3,428)]/90 = 5.0986$. Entering any value of X within its range, say 35, into the resulting *regression equation* yields $Y_{pred} = 5.0986 + .3358(35) = 16.85$, or approximately 17. The predicted Y value of 16.85 is the approximate mean of the Y ratings assigned by those students whose X rating was 35. Some students with X ratings of 35 assigned Y ratings below 17, while others assigned Y ratings above 17.

Standard Error of Estimate

A useful index of the accuracy of predicting Y from X with a simple linear regression equation is the *standard error of estimate* (s_{est}), computed as

$$s_{est} = s_y\sqrt{1 - r^2} \qquad (4.6)$$

Using this statistic, one can determine an interval within which an actual Y score associated with a particular X score is likely to fall. To illustrate, the standard error of estimate for predicting end-of-course ratings (Y) from midterm instructor personality ratings (X) is $s_{est} = 4.89\sqrt{1 - .4529^2} = 4.36$. Now assume that the overall rating assigned by a certain student to the instructor's personality is 35. As noted above, the predicted Y value for an X of 35 is 16.85. Therefore, we can say that the chances are 68 out of 100 that this student is one of a group of students having X values of 35 whose actual Y values fell between $16.85 - 4.36 = 12.49$ and $16.85 + 4.36 = 21.21$. As suggested by this example, a person's actual Y score may be quite different from his or her predicted Y score. This is especially likely when the correlation between X and Y is low to moderate. The smaller the correlation coefficient, the larger the standard error of estimate and hence the less accurate the prediction of Y from X.

Coefficient of Determination

A useful index of the accuracy of prediction can be derived by squaring the correlation coefficient. The resulting statistic (r^2), referred to as the *coefficient of determination,* is the proportion of variance in the predicted (criterion) variable that can be accounted for (explained) by variance in the predictor variable. For the example, $r^2 = (.4529)^2 = .2051$, so approximately 21% of the variance in end-of-course ratings can be accounted for by variability in midterm ratings of the instructor's personality. The fact that this leaves $100 - 21 = 79\%$ of the variability in end-of-course ratings—known as the *coefficient of alienation*—remaining indicates that nearly four-fifths of this variability was unaccounted for by midterm ratings of the instructor's personality.

Multiple Linear Regression

In the above example, only 21% of the variance in the criterion variable (*Y*) is accounted for by variation in the predictor variable (*X*). One possible way of improving the predictability of *Y* from *X* is to include more independent variables in the regression equation. The computations involved in determining a *multiple regression equation* from scores on multiple predictors and a single criterion variable are complex, but can be carried out quickly by commercially available packages of computer programs such as SPSS/PC + , SAS, SYSTAT, and the like. Furthermore, program C-6 can be used to determine the multiple regression equation for 2 or 3 independent variables. There is, however, no guarantee that the inclusion of other independent variables into a regression equation will improve the accuracy of prediction. Predictive accuracy is higher when the independent (*X*) variables have low correlations with each other and high correlations with the dependent (*Y*) variable. It is also important to realize that a multiple regression approach assumes that each independent variable is linearly related to all other variables in the multiple regression equation and that scores on the dependent variable have a normal (bell-shaped) distribution.

Criterion Contamination

The criterion-related validity of a psychometric instrument is limited not only by the reliabilities of the predictor and criterion variables but also by the validity of the criterion itself as a measure of the particular variable of interest. Sometimes the criterion is *contaminated,* in other words made less valid, by the particular method in which scores on the criterion variable are determined. For example, a clinical psychologist who knows from other information that several patients have already been diagnosed as psychotic may see psychotic signs in their responses to a projective technique. If so, then the method of contrasting groups, in which the scores of psychotics are compared with those of normals, will yield false evidence for the validity of the instrument. Such contamination of the criterion (psychotic vs. normal) can be controlled by *blind analysis*, that is, by making available to the clinician no information about the patients other than their responses to the psycho metric instrument before attempting to make a diagnosis.[1] Many clinicians maintain, however, that blind analysis is unnatural in that it is not how psychometric instruments are actually used in practice. Clinical psychologists typically possess a great deal of additional information about a client or patient and attempt to find consistencies or congruences among the various kinds of information before making a diagnosis or recommendation for treatment.

Base Rate

Another factor that influences the magnitude of criterion-related validity coefficients, and hence the identification or prediction of certain behaviors, is the base rate of those behaviors in the target population. A *base rate* is the proportion of people in the population who manifest the characteristic or behavior of interest. An instrument designed to predict a particular type of behavior is most effective when the base rate is 50% and least effective when it is very high or very low. Thus, characteristics or behaviors such as psychoticism, brain damage, or suicide, which have low base rates in the general population, are more difficult to assess or diagnose, and hence to predict, that those with somewhat higher base rates (e.g., neuroticism, sexual deviation, spouse or child abuse).

Construct Validity

Predictive validity is of primary interest in situations involving occupational or educational selection and placement. Ability tests of various kinds, and sometimes personality and interest tests, are used for this purpose. Of greater concern with respect to personality tests, however, is construct validity. The *construct validity* of a psychological assessment instrument concerns the extent to which the instrument is an accurate measure of a particular *construct*, or psychological variable. Construct validity is not determined by one method or one investigation. It involves a network of investigations and procedures designed to discover whether an assessment instrument designed to measure a particular variable does so effectively. The last half of this chapter describes various types of research designs and statistical methods for obtaining information pertaining to the construct validity of psychometric assessment instruments.

Evidence for Construct Validity

Evidence for the construct validity of a psychometric assessment instrument is obtained from:

1. Experts' judgments of the extent to which the content of the instrument pertains to the construct of interest.
2. Analysis of the internal consistency of the instrument.
3. Studies of the relationships—in both artificially contrived and naturally occurring groups—between measures of responses to the instrument and measures of performance on other variables on which the groups differ.
4. Correlations of the instrument under investigation with other instruments and variables with which the former is expected to have certain relationships, and factor analyses of these intercorrelations.
5. Questioning individuals in detail about their responses to the instrument in order to clarify what specific mental processes were involved in the decision to make those responses.

As noted in this list, various kinds of information contribute to the establishment of the construct validity of a psychometric instrument. These involve such procedures as a rational or statistical analysis (e.g., factor analysis) of the variables assessed by the instrument and studies of the ability of the instrument to predict behavior in situations in which the construct is known to operate. For example, if, in a situation in which anxiety is known to affect performance, people who make high scores on an anxiety rating scale behave in a predictably different manner from those who make low scores, this provides evidence for the construct validity of the scale.

Convergent and Discriminant Validation

To possess construct validity, an assessment instrument should have high correlations with other measures of (or methods of measuring) the same construct (*convergent validity*) and low correlations with measures of different constructs (*discriminant validity*). Information pertaining to the convergent and discriminant validity of a psychometric instrument can be obtained by comparing correlations between measures of (1) the same construct using the same method, (2) different constructs using the same method, (3) the same construct using different methods, and (4) different constructs using different methods. Evidence for the construct validity of the instrument is provided by this *multitrait-multimethod approach* (Campbell & Fiske, 1959) whenever correlations between the same construct measured by the same and different methods are significantly higher than correlations between different constructs measured by the same or different methods. These results are not always obtained in practice: Sometimes correlations between different constructs measured by the same method are higher than correlations between the same construct measured by different methods. In this case, the method (paper-and-pencil inventory, projective technique, rating scale, checklist, interview, etc.) is more important in determining whatever is measured than the construct or trait one is attempting to assess.

STATISTICAL METHODS FOR RESEARCH

Research is necessary to determine whether or not a particular psychometric instrument is a valid measure of the construct(s) it was designed to measure. Research must also be conducted to determine how generally useful the instrument is, under what circumstances and with what kinds of persons it is most useful, and what further questions, ideas, and investigations it may prompt.

The discussion in Chapter 1 emphasized that statistical methods are not essential to research. The results of observations of people or phenomena and of interviewing are, more often than not, evaluated without using statistics. Many social scientists prefer qualitative rather than quantitative methodology, and the conclusions stemming from the former may be no less accurate than those provided by statistics and other quantitative techniques. However, the careful design of research studies and evaluation of the results is facilitated by a set of procedures that assist in narrowing down explanations of a phenomenon to a few possibilities. By controlling—either through manipulation or statistically—for extraneous variables and by stating conclusions in terms of probabilities, one may not be absolutely certain that those conclusions are correct but the degree of certainty is higher than it was before the investigation was conducted.

One aspect of statistical reasoning that is often confusing is the matter of indirect proof or Fisherian inference. Instead of stating what one wants to provide and then proving it directly, the method of indirect proof is employed. This means that we begin by hypothesizing the opposite of what we want to prove—the *null hypothesis*—and then determine by statistical methods whether the probability of the null hypothesis being true is small enough to warrant the conclusion that it is not true. Refutation of the null hypothesis leads to the converse assertion that the alternative or scientific hypothesis—the one we wanted to prove all along—is true. This sometimes confusing and seemingly convoluted procedure is scientifically sound.

Understanding how indirect proof works is not the only problem confronting the researcher. There are difficulties and things to look out for at every stage of research—in planning and implementing the investigation, and in analyzing, interpreting, and reporting the results. Table 4.2, which is a list of observations and recommendations pertaining to research in the behavioral sciences, was prepared to alert beginning researchers to some of these problems and pitfalls. For further discussion of the items on this list, see Aiken (1994b).

TABLE 4.2.   Three Dozen Observations and Recommendations Concerning Research and Statistics

Planning
1. Some people are simply not cut out to do research.
2. Many good (and bad) research ideas have been thought of before.
3. All worthwhile research hasn't been conducted during the past ten years.
4. A research investigation should begin with a question.
5. If there is more than one way to do or say something, always choose the simplest way.
6. Garbage in, garbage out.
7. Much scientific research is trivial.

TABLE 4.2. *(Continued)*

Planning (continued)

8. Researchers shouldn't wait until the data are collected to consult a statistician.
9. The best-laid plans of researchers often go wrong.

Implementation

1. The shotgun approach is usually messy.
2. Be aware of and beware of confounded variables.
3. In making measurements, stay off the ceiling and the floor.
4. The sample of subjects you select is probably not representative.
5. Laboratory research isn't necessarily more controlled, and field research isn't necessarily more real.
6. Not all social science research consists of surveys.
7. Most research in the behavioral sciences is basically correlational.
8. Watch out for the jingle and jangle fallacies in selecting psychometric instrument.
9. Some people can't seem to tell the difference between an independent and a dependent groups design.

Analysis

1. There is more to research than collecting and analyzing data.
2. Don't rely on a fancy statistical procedure to correct errors in design and implementation.
3. Don't use cannons to shoot flies.
4. Pay attention to power and sample size.
5. Minds may be changed, but not statistical significance levels.
6. Correlations and chi-squares are chronically abused and misused.

Interpretation

1. Absence of evidence is not evidence of absence.
2. Don't argue with the facts if they're actually factual.
3. All kinds of effects can get in the way of clear interpretation of results.
4. Research results are seldom conclusive.
5. Causation implies correlation, but correlation doesn't imply causation.
6. Interactions are usually more interesting than main effects.
7. Statistical significance isn't equivalent to practical significance.

Report Writing

1. Always keep your "dear reader" in mind.
2. Strive for well-integrated paragraphs and papers.
3. It's easy to overlook your own mistakes.
4. Good computer software doesn't guarantee good writing.
5. Don't be in a hurry to stop working on a research report.

Source: Adapted from Aiken (1994b). Reprinted with permission.

Internal and External Validity

The concept of *validity* is not only a quality of assessment instruments; it is also relevant in describing the methodology and results of research investigations. Campbell and Stanley (1966) distinguish between internal validity and external validity as properties of research designs. *Internal validity* is similar to reliability, in that it refers to the relative freedom of a research design from measurement errors caused by unwanted, extraneous variables. Random assignment of subjects to the various conditions or groups constituting the independent variable in an experiment helps control for the effects of extraneous variables, thus permitting a clearer identification of the influence of independent variables on dependent variables. *External validity* is concerned with the generalizability of the results of a research study to situations beyond that in which the study was conducted. The findings of an experiment or other research investigation are more likely to be externally valid when the samples of individuals, objects, or events on which the investigation is conducted are selected in such a way that they are representative of the population to which the results are to be generalized. Although experiments usually entail greater control over extraneous variables—either by random assignment or matching of the subjects in the several groups—than correlational or field studies, the findings of experiments conducted in highly controlled situations such as in a laboratory may be less generalizable to "real-life" situations than those from field or correlational studies.

Statistical Decision Errors and Power

Random selection of subjects from a designated population and random assignment of the sampled subjects to various research conditions or groups does not guarantee external and internal validity, but it does permit the application of a formal statistical reasoning process. Using the method of indirect proof discussed earlier, it can be concluded that, if the null hypothesis is true, the probability will be such and such of obtaining results at least as extreme as those actually observed. If the probability is small enough, say 5 out of 100, a decision will be made to reject the null hypothesis and accept the alternative hypothesis of a real difference between the inferred and hypothesized parameters. We may be wrong in drawing this conclusion: The null hypothesis may actually be true, in which case a *Type I error* has been committed. On the other hand, if we decide not to reject the null hypothesis and it is false, we have committed a *Type II error*.

In deciding whether or not to reject the null hypothesis, the researcher must also make a judgment as to the relative seriousness of these two types of errors: Is it more serious to reject a true null hypothesis or to retain a false null hypothesis? The answer depends on the situation as well as monetary, human welfare and other implications of making the two types of errors.

Obviously, we should like to minimize both kinds of errors, but, unfortunately, when one decreases the other increases. The probability of a Type I error, which is referred to as the level of significance or α (alpha), can be and should be set by the researcher at the very beginning of the investigation and adhered to. If the researcher decides to use a more conservative value of α, say .01 instead of .05, the likelihood of a Type I error will be decreased but the probability of a Type II error—referred to as β (beta)—will be increased. Unlike α, β is not under the direct control of the researcher, but it can be decreased by employing a larger sample size and by using a more powerful statistical technique. The *power (P)* of a statistical test—the probability of rejecting the null hypothesis when it is false—is equal to $1 - \beta$. Consequently, an increase in power makes a Type II error less likely. Programs F-5, F-6, and F-7 are based on the relationship between power and sample size, and may be used to compute required sample size for a given power in certain kinds of statistical tests.

Parametric and Nonparametric Tests

In deciding to employ a more powerful statistical test, we must be aware of the fact that the assumptions underlying such a test are more stringent than those for a less-powerful procedure. Thus, *parametric tests*, in which a parameter such as a population mean or variance is being estimated, entail making more assumptions than nonparametric, distribution-free techniques. It is assumed in both parametric and nonparametric procedures that the sample on which the research was conducted was selected at random from the population(s) of interest. When using parametric procedures it is also assumed that: (1) the population(s) of measurements of the people, objects, or events of interest are normally distributed; (2) the population variances of the measurements are equal; and that (3) the measurements are made on an interval or ratio scale. Unlike parametric tests, nonparametric statistical tests involve no assumptions concerning the nature of the population distribution. Depending on the particular technique, the measurements of the people, objects, or events analyzed by a nonparametric test may be at a nominal or an ordinal level. Unfortunately, we pay for the reduced number of assumptions and the lower level of measurement in a nonparametric procedure with an increase in β and a decrease in power. In general, parametric tests are more powerful than their nonparametric counterparts but often not greatly so.

Description and Inference

The concepts and procedures just discussed are concerned with *inferential statistics,* that is, making probabilistic inferences about populations on the basis of sample observations. In analyzing a set of data in a sample, however, it is wise to begin by summarizing the findings by means of frequency distributions, measures of central tendency, variability, and other *descriptive statistics.* In correlational studies, scattergram plots of the paired data sets should be inspected for nonlinear relationships between the independent and dependent variables and non-normality of the dependent variable. These preliminary analyses provide greater familiarity with the data, assistance in interpreting the results of inferential analyses, and often suggest ideas for further, unplanned analyses. However, as implied by Figure 4.1, our primary interest is in the results of inferential analysis.

Relationships and Differences

Statistical procedures can be designated as descriptive or inferential. As shown in Figure 4.1, inferential statistics may be further divided into parametric and nonparametric methods. Both methods may involve the computation of measures of relationship (association, correlation) and measures of differences between distributions. In the case of parametric tests, the significance of differences between population parameters may be determined on one or more samples. Differences between population means or other parameters may be analyzed by conducting tests of hypotheses or by determining confidence intervals for the parameters. Nonparametric tests for one or more samples are also available, but the interest in this case is in comparing distributions as a whole rather than means or variances. As outlined in Table 4.3, various measures of relationships and differences may be computed on data at a nominal,

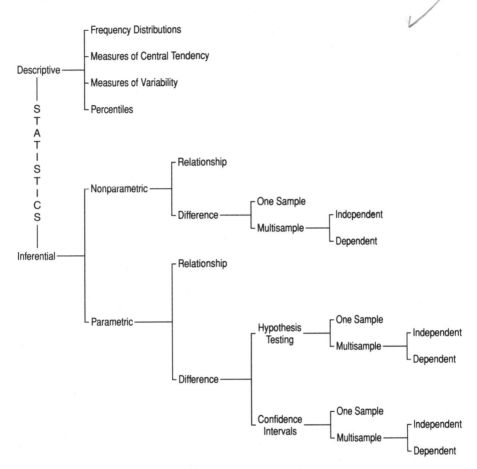

Figure 4.1.   A general outline of statistical procedures.

ordinal, or interval/ratio level. Testing the statistical significance of such measurements at the nominal and ordinal level involves nonparametric procedures, whereas parametric procedures are employed when the data are measures on an interval or ratio scale.

Data obtained from checklists and rating scales qualify as nominal and ordinal measurements, respectively, so nonparametric methods are more applicable than parametric ones in the analysis of such data. However, Pearson r, analysis of variance, and other parametric techniques are often used in analyzing ratings. Because these statistical procedures are fairly robust—that is, affected very little by minor violations in the assumptions underlying them—there is usually no

TABLE 4.3.   Representative Statistical Measures of
Relationship and Difference

Level of Measurement	Measures of	
	Relationship	Difference
Interval/Ratio	Product-Moment r	z- and t-tests
	Part Correlation	Analysis of Variance
	Partial Correlation	Independent Groups
	Multiple Correlation	Repeated Measures
		Mixed Designs
		Analysis of Covariance
Ordinal	Gamma (G)	Mann-Whitney U Test
	Somer's d	Kruskal-Wallis H Test
	Kendall's tau	Sign Test
	Spearman's rho	Wilcoxon Signed Ranks Test
		Friedman's Two-Way ANOVA
Nominal	Phi Coefficient	Chi Square Tests
	Contingency Coefficient	Fisher Exact Probability Test
	Cramer's V	McNemar Test of Changes
	Lambda	Cochran Q Test

great harm in using interval-level procedures with ordinal-level data. Nevertheless, it is wise to check the shape of the frequency distributions, the linearity of $X - Y$ plots, and the variances of samples of ratings before applying a parametric procedure to rating scale data. If the distribution is markedly asymmetrical, the $X - Y$ plots manifestly nonlinear, and/or the variances of ratings in the several groups significantly different, one is probably on more solid ground in using a nonparametric procedure.

Nominal-Level Relationships

Relationships between responses to checklist items and other dichotomous variables can be determined by computing a phi coefficient. The formula for phi (ϕ) is

$$\phi = \sqrt{\chi^2/N} \qquad (4.7)$$

where χ^2 is the value of χ^2 computed from cell frequencies in a 2×2 contingency table and N is the total of the cell frequencies. To illustrate, consider the following 2×2 table of frequencies from the

General Social Survey. The question asked of the respondents was "Would you oppose a law that would require a person to obtain a permit before he or she could buy a gun?"

		Gender		
		Male	Female	Total
Gun Law?	Favor	614	937	1551
	Oppose	251	155	406
	Total	865	1092	1957

The value of χ^2 for this table was found by program G-2 to be 64.50, so $\phi = \sqrt{64.50/1957} = .182$. This is a rather small coefficient, but, as found by comparing a χ^2 of 64.50 with that required for significance at the .01 level (6.64) with one degree of freedom, it is statistically significant. To interpret the significant relationship between sex and attitude toward gun control, we note that 86% of the females but only 71% of the males were in favor of the gun law.

Another nominal measure of relationship—λ (lambda)—is based on the concept of proportional reduction in error (PRE) occurring when one variable (the independent) is taken into account in predicting category membership on the other (dependent) variable. For example, assume that, out of 50 women and 50 men who were asked whether women have the right to an abortion, 20 men and 40 women said Yes and the remainder said No. Using program C-3, it is found that lambda for these data is .25. This means that taking gender into account leads to a 25% reduction in the error of predicting attitude toward abortion.

When a nominal variable has more than two categories, other measures of association must be employed. Consider, for example, the following 2 × 3 contingency table of data from the General Social Survey:

		Race			
		White	Black	Other	Total
Capital	Favor	1932	196	87	2215
Punishment	Oppose	406	150	24	580
	Total	2338	346	111	2795

A χ^2 based measure of association between the row and column variables of the table is the contingency coefficient, defined as

$$C = \sqrt{\chi^2/(N + \chi^2)} \tag{4.8}$$

Since $\chi^2 = 123.83$ for these data, $C = \sqrt{123.83/(2795 + 123.83)} = .202$. With 2 degrees of freedom, the observed χ^2, and hence the contingency coefficient, is significant at the .01 level. To interpret this significant value of C, we note that 83% of the White respondents, 57% of the Black respondents, and 78% of the respondents belonging to other races were in favor of capital punishment.

Because the upper limit of C varies with the dimensions of the contingency table, another statistic—Cramer's V—is preferred as a measure of relationship between nominal variables in contingency tables larger than 2 × 2. The formula for computing Cramer's V is

$$V = \sqrt{\chi^2/(Nm)} \tag{4.9}$$

where m is 1 less than the smaller number of row and column categories. For the above data, $V = \sqrt{123.83/(2795 \times 1)} = .210$ (see program C-3). Because χ^2 is statistically significant, so is V.

Ordinal Relationships

A choice of several different coefficients is also available for analyzing relationships among variables measured on ordinal scales. Four of these—gamma, Somer's d, Kendall's tau-c, and Spearman's rho—may be computed with program C-3. The first three coefficients usually lead to the same conclusion, although gamma is the most popular. Like lambda for nominal data, gamma is a "PRE" statistic, in that it can be viewed as a proportional reduction in the error of predicting the dependent variable when the independent variable is included. Somer's d, however, is preferable when the independent and dependent variables can be clearly differentiated. Kendall's tau-c usually provides more information than gamma and Somer's d, but it is limited to square contingency tables (Healey, 1993).

The oldest of the four ordinal coefficients computed by program C-3 is Spearman's rank-order coefficient ρ (rho). Because the maximum value of rho depends on the number of rows and columns in the table, this coefficient is not really appropriate for determining relationships in contingency tables. In addition, the statistical significance test for rho "piggy-backs" on the significance test for the Pearson r rather than being a true probability test like the one for Kendall's tau. Traditionally, rho has been used as a "shortcut" Pearson r when the pairs of $X - Y$ values are ranks or have been converted to ranks.

To illustrate the procedure for determining the above four coefficients, consider the following ordered contingency table of data from the General Social Survey:

	Education		
Health Status	High School Dropout	High School	Junior College and Up
Excellent	60	163	404
Good	161	305	465
Poor	153	141	142
Total	374	609	1011

For these data, gamma is .367, Somer's d is .234, Kendall's tau-c is .219, and Spearman's rho is .258. Because the value of χ^2 is 149.21, which, with four degrees of freedom, is highly significant, we can conclude that there is a significant positive relationship between education and reported health status. Computation of the row percentages in the above table reveals that 40% percent of the respondents with at least some college education, 27% of those with a high school education, and 16% of high school dropouts reported their health status as Excellent.

Interval/Ratio Relationships

The most commonly used measure of relationship with data on an interval or ratio scale is the Pearson product-moment coefficient (r). In addition to interval-level measurements, the test of significance and interpretation of r are based on the assumptions of a linear relationship between the X and Y variables, a normal distribution of the Y (predicted or dependent variable) marginal frequencies, and homogeneous variances among the Y values for each value of X. These are fairly rigorous assumptions and should not be easily overlooked.

As noted previously, the addition of other independent variables to the regression equation for predicting Y may improve the accuracy of prediction, as reflected in the multiple correlation coefficient (R).

The other two types of correlation coefficients listed in the top row of Table 4.3—part and partial correlation coefficients—are sometimes used to "statistically" (rather than "experimentally") control for extraneous variables. A part correlation coefficient is an index of the relationship between X and Y when the correlation between an extraneous or control variable (Z) has been removed from one of the variables. A partial correlation coefficient, on the other hand, is an index of the relationship between X and Y when the correlation of both variables with Z has been removed. For example, part correlation could be used to determine the relationship between scores on a vocational aptitude test and subsequent performance on a job after removing the overlap between initial job performance and final job performance. In this case, the independent variable consists of scores on the aptitude test, the dependent variable is the score on the subsequent measure of job performance, and the control variable is the initial score of the job performance measure.

As an illustration of the use of partial correlation, consider the relationship between aptitude and job performance after statistically controlling for the effects of chronological age on both aptitude and job performance measures. In this situation, chronological age is the control (extraneous) variable. Other, somewhat more complex procedures for controlling several extraneous variables include second- and third-order partials, double part correlation (see Aiken, 1981), and analysis of covariance.

Ratings are frequently used as criterion measures in prediction studies involving the use of correlational procedures such as Pearson r, multiple correlations, and part and partial correlation. The choice of whether to use these interval-level procedures with what are basically ordinal-level data depends on the investigator and how serious the violation of the assumptions underlying interval-level statistics is viewed as being in a particular research context. Although parametric procedures are fairly robust, a decision to ignore the assumptions on which they are based should not be made lightly.

Nominal-Level Difference Tests

As indicated in Figure 4.1, the statistical analysis of differences may involve one or more samples. Two or more samples may be *independent*—as when subjects are assigned at random to treatments or conditions, or *dependent*—as when measurements under two or more conditions are taken from the same individuals or matched groups. In any case, analyzing sample differences basically entails determining the probability that an observed sample or samples of values could have occurred by chance. As noted previously, in nonparametric tests no assumptions are made concerning the nature of the population distribution of responses or differences. Nonparametric tests focus on direct or indirect ways of determining the probability of selecting a given sample at random.

All statistical tests of hypotheses on nominal-level data begin with a set of observations in two or more categories, as in responses to checklist items. A statistical test of these data consists of a binomial (two categories) or χ^2 goodness of fit test of the hypothesis of equal category frequencies. Consider, for example, the hypothesis that the number of people who agree that the lot of the average man is getting worse is equal to the number disagreeing with that statement. Selecting a random sample of, say, 20 individuals from the Social Survey Data, we find that 14 agreed and 6 disagreed that the lot of the average man is getting worse. To test the null hypothesis that the proportion agreeing is .5, we use program G-1 and find that the right-tail probability that the null hypothesis is true is .0577.[2] This probability is not small enough to warrant rejection of the null hypothesis that the number of people who agreed is equal to the number who disagreed with the statement.

The binomial procedure is appropriate for analyzing dichotomous data in small samples. When the sample size is fairly large, it is simpler to use the χ^2 goodness of fit test. For example, in a sample of 1438 respondents to the General Social Survey, 819 agreed that the lot of the average man is getting worse. From program G-2, we find that the computed value of χ^2 (with Yates' correction) is 27.54. With 1 degree of freedom, this value is significant beyond the .01 level, leading to the conclusion that significantly more than half of the responding sample agreed with the statement.

When the sample sizes are large, χ^2 may also be used to compare frequencies in k (two or more) independent groups. To illustrate, compare the percentages of respondents in four religious groups—Protestant, Catholic, Jewish, Other—who agreed with the statement that it should be possible for a pregnant woman to obtain an abortion if she is not married and does not want to marry the man. These percentages are:

Catholic = 46   Protestant = 43
Jewish = 100   None = 65

should't this
be "other"?
AMS

The value of χ^2, computed by program G-2, is 32.46, which, with 3 degrees of freedom, is significant beyond the .01 level. It is concluded that the percentage agreeing with the proposition was not the same for all four groups.

When two independent samples are to be compared on a dichotomous criterion and the same sizes are small, a Fisher exact probability test may be conducted by using program G-4. This program computes the right-tail probability, which should be doubled in the case of a nondirectional (two-tailed) test.

When two or more samples of nominal-level data are dependent (correlated), as when they are matched on a relevant variable or the same individuals are exposed to all conditions, the Cochran Q test is an appropriate measure of differences among the distributions of dichotomous responses to the various conditions. When there are only two dependent comparison groups, as in before and after designs for determining the effect of some condition occurring between the before and after measurements, the McNemar test for the significance of changes is appropriate. Program G-3 computes the χ^2's for both the Cochran Q and McNemar tests. The resulting values can be evaluated by comparing them with the critical value of χ^2 with degrees of freedom equal to one less than the number of conditions. Consider, for example, the following responses (agree = 1, disagree = 0) of a random sample of 15 American adults to the question "Do you agree that the federal government has too much power?" Responses to the question were obtained from the same individuals both before and after they heard a speech by a conservative congressman.

Person	Before	After	Person	Before	After
1	1	1	9	1	0
2	0	1	10	0	1
3	1	0	11	0	1
4	0	0	12	1	1
5	1	1	13	0	1
6	0	1	14	1	1
7	0	1	15	0	0
8	1	1			

The value of Q is 2.00, and McNemar's χ^2 (with Yates' correction) is 1.12 in this case; with 1 degree of freedom, neither value is statistically significant. Therefore, it cannot be concluded that the speech had an effect on the frequency of agreement with the proposition.

Ordinal-Level Difference Tests

As we go up the measurement ladder from nominal to interval scale, the statistical tests become more powerful. One of the most powerful tests at the ordinal level is the Mann-Whitney U Test. This test, which requires computing a special statistic (U) based on the sum of ranks in two independent samples, is an ordinal-level counterpart of the independent groups t test. Program G-7 can used to compute the value of U, but a special table, which is included in most elementary statistics textbooks, is needed to determine the significance of U in small samples. For large samples, a test of the significance of U may be determined by

$$z = (U - n_1 n_2/2)/\sqrt{n_1 n_2 (n_1 + n_2 + 1)/12} \qquad (4.10)$$

and referring the result to a normal probability table or by computing the corresponding probability with Program D-1.

Just as the Mann-Whitney U test is an ordinal-level counterpart of the t test for independent groups, the sign test and the Wilcoxon test are ordinal-level counterparts of the t test for dependent groups. The sign test uses information only on the direction of the difference (greater than, less than) between paired scores in two matched or repeated measures groups, but the Wilcoxon test takes both the magnitude and direction of those differences into account. Consequently, the Wilcoxon test, though less powerful than the t test and the Mann-Whitney U test, is more powerful than the sign test. The computations for the sign test, which revolve around the determination of the binomial probability of an obtained set of greater-thans (+ 's) and less-thans (− 's), can be performed by program G-8. The value of the T statistic in the Wilcoxon test can be determined by program G-9, but a table of critical values of T (included in most elementary statistics texts) must be consulted to determine its significance.[3]

When the paired samples are large, an approximation to the normal deviate may be computed for both the sign and Wilcoxon statistics. For the sign test, $z = [2(X + C) - n]/\sqrt{n}$, where X is the number of positive signs, n is the number of pairs, and $C = .5$ if $2X < n$ or $−.5$ if $2X > n$. For the Wilcoxon statistic (T)

$$z = [4T - n(n + 1)]/\sqrt{n(n + 1)(2n + 1)/24} \qquad (4.11)$$

To illustrate the computations for the Mann-Whitney, sign, and Wilcoxon tests, consider the data in Table 4.4. An educational psychologist

TABLE 4.4.   Before and After Scores of a Sample of Men and Women on the Mathematics Attitude Scale

| | Attitude toward Mathematics | | | |
| | Females | | Males | |
Subject	Before Film	After Film	Before Film	After Film
1	65	66	75	77
2	81	80	89	88
3	24	32	32	37
4	39	43	47	50
5	68	66	76	79
6	68	70	71	70
7	41	45	44	48
8	78	75	82	85
9	75	77	84	90
10	23	30	27	30
11	49	51	59	64
12	29	33	37	39
13	83	80	86	87
14	33	38	42	40
15	57	61	65	68

was interested in the effects of a motion picture film concerned with career opportunities for high school graduates having good mathematics training. Fifteen randomly selected women students and fifteen randomly selected men students completed a 24-item inventory of attitudes toward mathematics (see program J-1) both before and after viewing the film. Their scores are given in Table 4.4. By using a Mann-Whitney U test, we can compare the attitudes of women with those of men before the film and then make a second comparison of the attitudes of the two sexes after the film. Using program G-7, the first comparison yields a U of 88 and the second comparison a U of 87.5. Because neither value of U is less than or equal to the critical value of U (64) in a two-tailed test at the .05 level when both samples contain 15 observations, the obtained U values are not significant. We cannot conclude that the males' attitudes toward mathematics were different from those of the females, either before or after the film. Sign and Wilcoxon tests of the differences between the before and after scores for each sex group were also conducted. The sign test for females yielded 11 +'s and 4 −'s and a right-tail binomial probability of .0593, which is not statistically significant. The corresponding sign-test values for the males were 12 +'s and 3 −'s and a right-tail probability of .0176, which is statistically significant. The Wilcoxon before-and-after comparison for females yielded a sum of positive ranks of 21, a sum of negative ranks of 99, and a T of 21. The Wilcoxon before-and-after comparison for males yielded a sum of positive ranks of 9, a sum of negative ranks of 111, and a T of 9. Because both T values are less than the critical value of $T = 25$ in a .05-level two-tailed test, it can be concluded that, for both sexes, the results of the Wilcoxon test indicate that the attitude scores after viewing the film were higher (more favorable) than before viewing the film.

A test of significance of the differences in ranks among k independent samples may be conducted with the Kruskal-Wallis H statistic. H is a χ^2 value and can be evaluated by comparing it with the critical value of χ^2 with $k - 1$ degrees of freedom. Finally, the Friedman two-way analysis of variance by ranks is appropriate for evaluating the differences in ranks in k dependent groups. The statistic computed in the Friedman test is also a χ^2 and, like the Kruskal-Wallis H, can be evaluated by comparison with the critical value of χ^2 with $k - 1$ degrees of freedom. Program G-6 makes the computations for the Kruskal-Wallis test, and program G-5 for the Friedman test.

Interval-Level Difference Tests

The most powerful of all statistical tests assume measurement on at least an interval scale. The simplest of these tests are designed to test the null hypothesis that the mean of the population from which the sample was selected is equal to a specified value, say μ, against a one- or two-tailed alternative hypothesis that the mean of the population is not equal to μ. If, in addition to interval-level measurement, we can meet the assumption of normality of the population distribution, and if the population standard deviation is known and the sample size large, then a normal curve z ratio may be computed to test the null hypothesis. If the population standard deviation must be estimated from the sample standard deviation, then the t ratio should be used. Tests of hypotheses of differences between parameters can also be made from data in two samples. If the samples are dependent, a correlated groups t test may be conducted; otherwise, a t ratio for independent groups is computed. In general, a correlated group's t test is somewhat more powerful than an independent groups t test, but is not always the proper choice when carryover effects and other sources of contamination are present.

The most elementary analysis of variance (ANOVA) design—the randomized groups design—is a generalization on the t test for independent groups. The F ratio statistic computed in this design is a nondirectional (two-tailed) test of the equality of k population means, where k is the number of groups. F is a ratio of the variance due to differences among the group (treatment) means (between groups variance) to the variance due to differences between the scores in each group and the group mean (within groups variance). The randomized groups ANOVA is the parametric counterpart of the Kruskal-Wallis H test, and the repeated measures (within subjects) ANOVA is the counterpart of the Friedman analysis of variance by ranks. In a repeated measures design, rather than being randomly assign to one condition (as in the randomized groups design), every subject is exposed to all k conditions and hence acts as his or her own control.

Analysis of variance procedures are not limited to one independent variable or even to one dependent variable. Designs in which there are two or more independent variables are known as factorial designs. Many factorial designs are mixed, in that they contain at least one between-subjects and at least one within-subjects variable. Designs may also involve nesting, in which case the conditions of one independent variable are nested within another independent variable or factor. To control for order and sequence effects when the same individual is exposed to more than one condition, Latin squares and even more elaborate designs may be employed. In addition to univariate ANOVA designs, an analysis of covariance, which controls for a third variable (covariate) while assessing the effects of the independent variable on the dependent variable, and multivariate analyses of variance and covariance involving several dependent variables may be conducted.

Programs for computing t and F ratios are not included in the package accompanying this book, but many of the programs in category F (Sample Selection and Assignment) can assist in setting up analysis of variance designs. In addition to the programs for sample selection and assignment (programs F-1 through F-4), programs F-7 through F-10 are directly relevant to the construction of ANOVA designs.

Although all parametric statistical procedures are basically concerned with the estimation of population parameters, the estimation process is only implicit in analysis of variance. It becomes more explicit when confidence limits for a parameter or for the difference(s) between two or more parameters are constructed. In a very real sense, determination of a confidence interval for a population parameter yields a more general result than hypothesis testing, in that the latter is concerned with a specified value of the parameter. However, once a confidence interval for a population parameter has been determined, any null hypothesis in which the stated parameter falls outside the interval can be rejected. As with F tests, all tests of hypotheses based on confidence intervals for parameters are nondirectional.

SUMMARY

A psychometric instrument can be reliable without being valid, but it cannot be valid without being reliable. Validity is basically concerned with the extent to which an instrument or procedure does what it was designed to do—measures what it was designed to measure. Like reliability, validity depends to a great extent on the situation or context: An instrument may be a more valid measure of a particular construct in one context than in another.

Traditionally, three types of validity, or rather three sources of evidence pertaining to validity, have been identified: content, criterion-related, and construct. Content validity is concerned with the extent to which the appearance and composition of an instrument are what an expert would expect them to be. Criterion-related validity, which is subdivided into concurrent (congruent) and predictive validity, is concerned with the accuracy with which an instrument classifies respondents in the same way as another measure obtained during the same time frame (concurrent validity) or sometime in the future (predictive validity). The determination of criterion-related validity involves correlational and regression analysis. The standard error of estimate, criterion contamination, and the base rate of the criterion variable are also important considerations in evaluating the predictive validity of an instrument.

Construct validity is a more general concept that encompasses both content and criterion-related validity information. It is the extent to which scores on a psychometric instrument designed to measure a certain characteristic or construct are related to measures of behavior in situations in which the construct is a significant determinant of behavior. In other words, do high and low scorers on the instrument behave in ways they are expected to behave according to theory or logical reasoning? Evidence for construct validity is obtained by means of various experimental and nonexperimental procedures, among which are convergent and discriminant validation studies and the associated multitrait-multimethod matrix.

Research involving quantification of variables is not the only kind of research, but statistical methodology does provide a systematic way of designing, implementing, and evaluating research investigations. Applications of statistics in research should be undertaken with an awareness of the distinctions between statistical description and statistical inference, independent and dependent variables, true experiments and pseudo-experiments, internal and external validity, samples and populations, statistics and parameters, sample selection and assignment, random and matched samples, null and alternative hypotheses, directional (one-tail) and nondirectional (two-tail) hypotheses, parametric and nonparametric techniques, experimental and statistical control, Type I and Type II errors, measures of relationship and difference, as well as the concepts of power, levels of measurement, and the assumptions underlying the applications of certain statistical procedures.

Although nominal- and ordinal-level procedures are usually more appropriate than interval- or ratio-measures of relationship for analyzing responses to rating scales and checklists, Pearson r, t tests, and analysis of variance are often used in analyzing ratings. The computer diskette accompanying this text contains programs for conducting the most popular nonparametric tests of correlation and differences in addition to sample selection and assignment.

QUESTIONS AND ACTIVITIES

1. Define each of the following terms used in this chapter. Consult Appendix A and/or a dictionary if you need help.

alpha	coefficient of determination
analysis of variance	concurrent validity
analysis of covariance	construct validity
base rate	content validity
beta	contingency coefficient
blind analysis	convergent validity
chi square	criterion-related validity
Cochran test	descriptive statistics
coefficient of alienation	discriminant validity

external validity
Friedman analysis of
   variance by ranks
gamma
inferential statistics
internal validity
Kendall's tau
Kruskal-Wallis *H* Test
lambda
linear regression equation
Mann-Whitney *U* Test
McNemar test
method of contrasting
   groups
multiple regression
   equation
multitrait-multimethod
   approach
nonparametric statistics

null hypothesis
one-tail test
parametric statistics
parametric tests
part correlation
partial correlation
phi coefficient
 power
predictive validity
sign test
significance level
Spearman's rho
standard error of estimate
t test
two-tail test
Type I error
Type II error
Wilcoxon test

2. What is the standard error of estimate in predicting composite performance ratings having a standard deviation of 5.4 from a vocational aptitude test having a correlation of .60 with the performance ratings? Interpret the result. Between what two values on the performance rating composite are you 68% certain that the score of an employee with a predicted performance rating of 70 will fall?

3. Using the data in Table 4.4, find gamma, Somer's *d*, Kendall's tau-*c*, Spearman's rho, and the Pearson product-moment correlation between: (1) the scores of females before and after the film, (2) the scores of males before and after the film. Use the appropriate computer programs in the package accompanying the text to make the computations. Interpret the obtained coefficients.

4. Find the median of the *X* scores and the median of the *Y* scores in Table 4.1. Then set of a 2 × 2 contingency table containing in the four cells: (1) the frequency of scores below the medians of both *X* and *Y*, (2) the frequency of scores below the median on *X* and above the median on *Y*, (3) the frequency of scores above the median on *X* and below the median on *Y*, (4) the frequency

of scores above the median on both variables. From the contingency table, compute and interpret the values of the phi coefficient and lambda.

5. The following are the composite ratings of 54 females and 36 males of the 90 instructor personality ratings in Table 4.1. Using the appropriate computer programs, conduct a Mann-Whitney U test and a Kruskal-Wallis H test of the differences in the ratings assigned by females and males. Interpret the results.

Females ($n = 54$)

```
26  40  35  33  33  37  38  38  39  28  29  28  39  36  45  29
35  36  31  34  40  33  37  51  54  49  38  55  42  47  46  53
38  35  47  39  42  42  43  39  34  36  40  36  41  40  50  43
34  34  35  50  41  42
```

Males ($n = 36$)

```
28  37  29  42  35  39  40  33  37  52  24  41  41  33  39  42
34  48  31  40  27  40  37  42  41  44  31  36  39  31  28  32
36  28  39  37
```

6. Design a study to compare job performance ratings of three groups of employees by supervisors, peers, and the employees themselves (self-ratings). What are the independent and dependent variables in your study? What are some possible extraneous or confounded variables? What statistical procedures are appropriate for analyzing the data?

7. What are the appropriate statistical tests to conduct for the following purposes?
   a. To find the correlations among items on a checklist of supervisory practices?
   b. To find the correlations among items on a scale of behavior ratings?
   c. To determine the significance of the differences in rated improvement under three types of psychotherapy?
   d. To determine the significance of differences in rated athletic performance at four two-week intervals during training?
   e. To determine the presence or absence of certain behaviors in five groups of individuals?
   f. To determine the presence or absence of certain behaviors in a group of people at five different times?

5

Assessment in Business and Industry

Ratings of people, products, organizations, and environments are commonplace in business and industrial settings. In the "people" category, the popular press has featured articles on ratings of air pilots, executives, manufacturers, merchants, sales personnel, and women managers. With respect to civil service personnel and governmental officials, ratings of military officers, police officers, congressmen, senators, and even the president are made and reported.

In the "product" or "thing" category, numerous articles on ratings of computer/video games and other toys, bonds (corporate, industrial, municipal, revenue, state and local, treasury), money market funds, mortgage insurance, and even commercial paper are to be found. For example, municipal bonds are rated by Moody's Investor Service as "Aaa, Aa, A, Baa, Ba, B, Caa, Ca, C," depending on their relative investment qualities.

In the organizational and businesses environment spheres, ratings are provided for insurance companies and other organizations, as well as business climate, cities and towns, quality of life, suburbs, and retirement climate. Many business organizations hire statisticians to keep track of such ratings and compare them with the ratings of competitors or competing products.

More widely known to the general public than other evaluations in business and industry are those made in the entertainment and sports fields. These include ratings of motion pictures, television programs, radio programs, sports teams, and the entertainers or principals themselves. Some of these evaluations, such as the Nielsen ratings of television programs, are commissioned by producers to provide estimates of the share of the audience that particular programs capture at a given time. Nielsen ratings, which are obtained by means of boxes (Audimeters) attached to selected television sets to provide a record of the channels being watched, are viewed as indexes to the success or failure of television programming. Other entertainment ratings, such as the listings of motion pictures and television programs in the printed media, are ostensibly there to provide information to potential viewers. The rating system for motion pictures is G, PG, PG-13, R, and NC-17 (see Table 5.1). Some listings rate movies shown on television as *, **, ***, **** or some other variation.

In this chapter we concentrate on ratings of people at work and human factors on the job. We begin with a discussion of the selection and classification of personnel, following which the topics of employee

TABLE 5.1. Motion Picture Ratings

G. **General Audiences.** All ages admitted. The film contains nothing which would, in the opinion of the rating board, be offensive to parents whose younger children view the film.

PG. **Parental Guidance suggested.** Parents may consider some material in the film unsuitable for their children, but the parent must make the decision.

PG-13. **Parents are strongly cautioned.** This is a sterner warning to parents to determine for themselves whether they consider some material in the film unsuitable for children, and younger children in particular.

R. **Restricted**. Children under 17 are not admitted unless accompanied by a parent or adult guardian. The film definitely contains adult material. Parents are strong urged to find out more about the film before allowing their children to accompany them.

NC-17. **Children under 17 not admitted.** Clearly an adult film, although not necessarily obscene or pornographic. This can mean that the film contains strong violence, sex, aberrational behavior, drug abuse, or other material which parents consider off-limits for viewing by their children.

Source: From Consumers' Guide to Product Grades and Terms by T. L. Gall and S. B. Gall, 1993. Detroit: Gale Research Inc.

performance appraisal and human factors and the work environment will be discussed at some length. Finally, a topic that has occasioned alarms of "hidden persuaders" and "big brotherism" in the past—that of consumer behavior—will be considered.

PERSONNEL SELECTION AND CLASSIFICATION

The first and most extensive of the many applications of psychology to the world of work was in the selection, placement, and training of personnel. *Personnel psychology*, as it is called, is a branch of industrial/organizational psychology that has its roots in the research of Walter Dill Scott, Hugo Munsterberg, and other psychologists during the first decade of this century. Munsterberg's studies of the selection of streetcar motormen in Boston were perhaps the first systematic studies in personnel psychology. However, they were not the first attempt to provide a rigorous procedure for selecting employees. Thousands of years before, the Mandarin Chinese had administered a series of oral examinations every three years to applicants and employees of the government to determine their skills and abilities and whether they were suitable for employment or advancement. These examinations, and the employee-selection system which they represented, served as a model for similar programs in Great Britain and Germany during the latter part of the 19th century.

Pioneer personnel psychologists such as Scott and Munsterberg were, like the industrial engineers Frederick Taylor and Frank Gilbreth, motivated primarily by the goal of greater productivity—a motive that led them to advocate a two-sided approach to improving industrial efficiency. One side consisted of the analysis and redesign of jobs and equipment; the other side emphasized selection of the most able employees. Employee satisfaction or happiness played little part in the research and proposals of these men: Their aim was simply to make industrial production more efficient by means of employee selection and training combined with the redesign of tools, machinery, and work procedures. Proponents of this *scientific management* approach to industrial production maintained that both employers and employees would benefit by matching people to jobs. People would be selected for and placed on jobs they could perform most effectively, and hence they would be more productive and thereby earn higher wages. By the same token, selecting more competent workers and placing them on jobs for which they were best suited would benefit employers by making production more efficient and increasing the profit margin.

Although today personnel psychologists are concerned more with job satisfaction and employee attitudes than their predecessors, the emphasis is still on work efficiency. Activities such as job analysis, job evaluation, and the recruitment, selection, classification, development, and performance appraisal of employees are all important. Many individuals who work in business, industry, and other organizational settings are specialists in one or more of these areas. For example, a job analyst obtains information by means of interviews, questionnaires such as the Job Analysis Questionnaire or the Work Elements Inventory, and by careful observation of the activities or components involved in performing a specific job. A detailed description of the job, including title, activities and procedures, working conditions and physical environment, social environment, and conditions of employment is then prepared (Cascio, 1991).[1] A thorough job description leads to a listing of the job specifications—the knowledge, skills, abilities, and personality characteristics that are considered necessary for performing the job. After the job has been analyzed and described and the job specifications prepared, job evaluators examine these materials carefully and make a *job evaluation*—a formulation concerning what the job is worth to the organization in monetary terms.[2] Information obtained from a job analysis is also important in designing tests and other assessment instruments to predict how well employees will perform on the job and to measure their performance.

Personnel selection is concerned with selecting, from a group of applicants, those who can best perform certain tasks. Many different methods may be used to select a specified number of people from a larger pool of applicants or candidates. Random selection—although it seldom produces the most capable employees—may be a fair approach under certain circumstances, as when everyone in the job pool can perform the tasks fairly well. Selecting employees according to political, familial, or other connections or sources of influence is still widely practiced. Another personnel selection method involves giving a job tryout to anyone who wants it but retaining only those who prove themselves capable of performing effectively. This "sink-or-swim" strategy may be democratic, but it can also be costly to the organization and the employees. The most scientific, but by no means the uniformly dominant approach to personnel selection, is to use psychological tests and other psychometrically evaluated procedures to screen, select, classify, and place employees. A quota system in which a certain percentage of applicants in a given demographic group is selected has been the practice under affirmative action guidelines in recent years. Under the Uniform Guidelines on Employee Selection (Equal Employment Opportunity Commission, 1978), employers are required to adopt selection techniques having the least adverse impact. The legal definition of *adverse impact* follows the *four-fifths rule,* according to which a condition of adverse impact exists if one ethnic or gender group has a selection rate that is less than four-fifths (80%) that of any other applicant group.

The decision to select a particular applicant on the basis of education and training, job experience, and aptitude is not always made as soon as these kinds of information become available. In many organizations, the names of applicants who meet the position requirements are placed on a list and selections are made when openings occur. And in certain organizations, such as the federal government, applicants are placed on a register list but not ranked or assigned a numerical score until there are job openings. In this *deferred rating system,* when jobs become available the best-qualified applicants are placed at the top of the list and referred for employment consideration by the department or agency in which openings exist.

Cutoff Scores

Almost all organizations use some form of screening procedure for rejecting applicants who are clearly unsuitable. If the screening instrument is a psychological test, applicants who score below a specified minimum are rejected, while those who score at or above the minimum are accepted. The minimum acceptable score may be established rationally or statistically. An illustration of the rational determination of a cutting score is when a designated authority decides from personal observation and reasoning that individuals who made below a particular score will not be able to perform the job well.

A more systematic and scientific approach to personnel selection is to apply statistical procedures to set a cutoff score on a predictor (selection) variable corresponding to the lower boundary of acceptable performance on the criterion variable(s). When setting the cutoff score on the selection instrument, a comparison is made between scores on the selection variable and the job performance measure. Then, by using simple or multiple linear regression procedures or by frequency comparisons in an expectancy table, the score on the selection variable corresponding to the lowest acceptable performance on the criterion is determined. This becomes the cutoff score on the selection or predictor variable.

A number of factors should be considered in deciding where to set the minimum acceptable score on the criterion and the corresponding cutoff score on the selection variable(s). Among these are the nature of the labor market, the consequences of selection errors, and the validity of the selection instrument or procedure. For example, if the labor market is "tight," there will be relatively few applicants and so the selection ratio—the percentage of applicants who are actually selected for a job or training program—must be set high and the cutoff score on the selection variable set relatively low if a sufficient number of applicants are to be hired. But when the labor market is "open," there will be many applicants, and hence the selection ratio will be low and the cutoff score on the selection variable relatively high. Understandably, how high or low the selection ratio should be in either a tight or an open labor market also depends on the qualifications of the applicant group. Even in a wide open labor market, when the cutoff score is high but all applicants are functionally illiterate, none of them will be found suitable for certain jobs! In this case, if the jobs are to be filled it will be necessary to establish a program of education and training for those who are hired.

The expected proportion of applicants who can perform a job successfully varies with the base rate, the selection ratio, and the validity of the selection instrument or procedure. In general, selection is most accurate when the base rate is around .50, that is, when 50% of the applicants possess the requisite qualifications for success on the job. As shown in Figure 5.1 for a base rate of .60, the proportion of applicants expected to succeed on a job varies directly with the validity of the selection instrument or procedure but inversely with the selection ratio. For this reason, when the selection ratio is fairly small, even a selection instrument with low validity can result in a substantial improvement over the base rate in the selection of applicants who will be successful.

False Positives and False Negatives

By setting the selection ratio close to 50%, the number of correct predictions will be maximized and the combination of *false positive errors*— errors made when success is predicted but failure occurs—and *false*

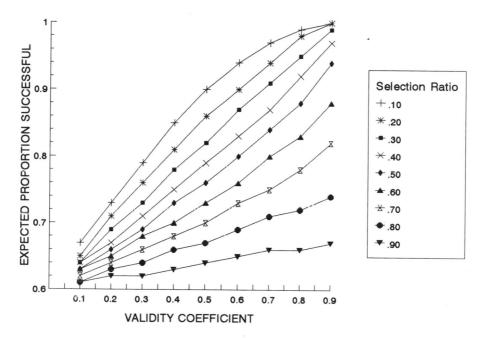

Figure 5.1. Plot of Taylor-Russell table for base rate of .60. Based on data from Taylor and Russell, 1939.

negative errors—errors made when failure is predicted but success occurs—will be minimized. In general, it is desirable to minimize both types of errors, but when one type of error decreases the other increases. Lowering the cutoff score on a selection test leads to a decrease in the number of false negative errors but an increase in false positive errors. On the other hand, raising the cutoff score leads to a decrease in false positives errors but an increase in false negative errors (see Figure 5.2).

The decision as to where the cutoff score(s) on the predictor variable(s) should be set depends to some extent on the relative seriousness of the two types of errors. Is it worse to reject someone who would have succeeded or to accept someone who fails? The answer depends on the situation and the criterion. In selecting college students, for example, false negative errors are probably more serious than false positive errors. In other words, it is considered more serious to reject a student who would have succeeded in college than to accept a student who fails. Even students who fail presumably realize some benefit from attending college, but those who are rejected are deprived of the

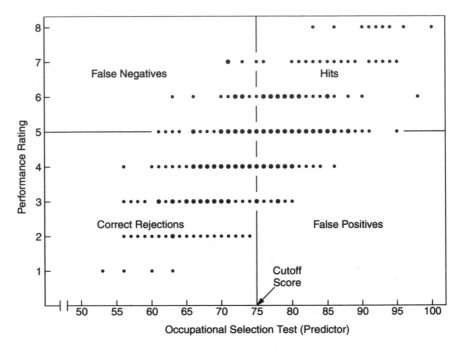

Figure 5.2.   Effects of predictor cutoff scores on errors, hits, and correct rejections. The light dots represent one case, and the bold dots represent two or more cases.

opportunity to obtain any benefit at all from the college experience. In selecting employees for dangerous jobs, however, false positive errors are more serious than false negative ones. Thus, no amount of benefit an employee may have received from being hired can compensate for a fatal accident.[3]

Classification and Placement

Initial screening is usually followed by *classification*, or assignment of those who have been selected to one of several occupational categories. In the past few decades, the emphasis in staffing positions in business and industry has shifted somewhat from selecting only the "cream of the crop" to classifying and placing people on jobs best suited to their abilities and needs. A consequence of this change in employment of the labor force has been a greater focus on tests and other classification procedures for matching particular patterns of abilities and personal characteristics to specific jobs.

Classification decisions may involve grouping people on the basis of their scores on more than one psychometric instrument, including not only tests of ability but measures of personality, attitudes, work habits, and the like. Screening and classification are frequently followed by *placement* of those who have been selected at a particular level of a certain job or program.

The process of personnel selection usually consists of a sequence of stages entailing a series of yes-no decisions based on information obtained from application blanks, letters of recommendation, telephone calls, personal interviews, observations, and psychological assessment instruments. The purpose of collecting such information is identical to that of any other application of behavioral science: to make better predictions of future behavior on the basis of past and present behavior. The more reliable and valid the information is, the greater the likelihood that accurate predictions of on-the-job or in-the-program behavior will be made and hence the sounder will be the selection decisions. The reliability and validity of psychological assessment instruments and procedures for making selection decisions cannot be determined merely by inspecting the assessment materials. Reliability and validity must be evaluated empirically, which is one of the primary tasks of the personnel psychologist.

An Expectancy Table

When tests and other assessment instruments are used for selection purposes, it is helpful but not essential to determine the predictor-criterion correlation and the regression equation linking predicted criterion scores to test scores. For example, the correlation coefficient and regression equation for the data in Table 5.2 are .689 and $Y' = .11608(X) - 4.11008$, respectively.

Correlational methods are applicable to the construction of theoretical-expectancy tables, but an empirical *expectancy table* can be constructed without computing a correlation coefficient or any other statistic except frequencies and percentages. Assume, for example, that Table 5.3 was constructed from a joint frequency distribution of the scores of 250 job applicants on an Occupational Selection Test (OST) and the ratings given to the applicants by their work supervisors 6 months after being hired. The OST score intervals are listed on the left

TABLE 5.2. OST Scores (X) and Performance Ratings (Y)

X	Y	X	Y	X	Y	X	Y	X	Y	X	Y	X	Y
98	6	96	8	100	8	91	5	95	5	91	7	92	7
93	7	94	7	95	7	91	8	92	8	93	8	94	8
86	4	86	5	87	5	88	5	89	5	90	5	86	5
86	5	88	5	86	6	88	6	90	6	86	7	87	7
88	7	89	7	86	8	90	8	81	4	82	4	83	4
84	4	81	5	82	5	83	5	84	5	85	5	81	5
82	5	83	5	84	5	85	5	81	6	82	6	83	6
84	6	85	6	81	6	85	6	81	7	82	7	83	7
84	7	85	7	83	8	76	3	77	3	78	3	79	3
80	3	78	3	76	4	77	4	78	4	79	4	80	4
76	4	77	4	78	4	79	4	80	4	76	4	80	4
76	5	77	5	78	5	79	5	80	5	76	5	77	5
78	5	79	5	80	5	76	5	77	5	78	5	79	5
80	5	78	5	76	6	77	6	78	6	79	6	80	6
76	6	77	6	78	6	79	6	80	6	76	6	78	6
80	6	76	7	80	7	71	2	72	2	73	2	74	2
71	3	72	3	73	3	74	3	75	3	71	3	75	3
71	4	72	4	73	4	74	4	75	4	71	4	72	4
73	4	74	4	75	4	71	4	72	4	73	4	74	4
75	4	71	4	72	4	73	4	74	4	75	4	71	4
72	4	73	4	74	4	75	4	71	5	72	5	73	5
74	5	75	5	71	5	72	5	73	5	74	5	75	5
71	5	72	5	73	5	74	5	75	5	71	5	72	5
73	5	74	5	75	5	73	5	71	6	72	6	73	6
74	6	75	6	71	7	73	7	75	7	66	2	67	2
68	2	69	2	70	2	66	3	67	3	68	3	69	3
70	3	66	3	67	3	68	3	69	3	70	3	66	4
67	4	68	4	69	4	70	4	66	4	67	4	68	4
69	4	70	4	66	4	67	4	68	4	69	4	66	5
67	5	68	5	69	5	70	5	66	5	70	5	66	6
70	6	63	1	61	2	62	2	63	2	64	2	65	2
63	2	61	3	62	3	63	3	64	3	65	3	61	3
63	3	65	3	61	4	62	4	63	4	64	4	65	4
61	5	62	5	63	5	64	5	63	6	56	1	60	1
56	2	57	2	58	2	59	2	60	2	56	3	57	3
58	3	59	3	56	4	60	4	53	1				

side of the table, and the supervisory ratings (on a scale of 1 to 8) are listed across the top. The unitalicized frequencies in the lower part of the cells in the table are the numbers of employees who obtained OST scores within a specified five-point range and the rating indicated at the top of a given column. For example, 10 employees whose OST scores

TABLE 5.3. An Empirical Expectancy Table

Occupational Selection Test Score	Performance Rating							
	1	2	3	4	5	6	7	8
96–100						(100) 1		(67) 2
91–95					(100) 2		(82) 5	(36) 4
86–90				(100) 1	(94) 8	(50) 3	(33) 4	(11) 2
81–85				(100) 4	(85) 10	(48) 7	(22) 5	(4) 1
76–80			(100) 6	(88) 12	(63) 16	(31) 13	(4) 2	
71–75		(100) 4	(94) 7	(83) 25	(45) 21	(12) 5	(5) 3	
66–70		(100) 5	(87) 10	(61) 14	(24) 7	(5) 2		
61–65	(100) 1	(96) 6	(72) 8	(40) 5	(20) 4	(4) 1		
56–60	(100) 2	(85) 5	(46) 4	(15) 2				
51–55	(100) 1							

were between 81 and 85 received a rating of 5 by their supervisors, whereas 14 employees whose OST scores fell between 66 and 70 received a rating of 4.

The italic numbers in parentheses in Table 5.3 are the percentages of employees whose OST scores fell in a specified interval and whose ratings equaled the rating in those cells or higher. Thus, 85% of employees whose OST scores fell in the interval 81–85 received ratings of 5 or higher, and 61% of those having OST scores between 66 and 70 had ratings of 4 or higher.

To illustrate how this kind of information is applied in employee selection, assume that Frank, one of a group of job applicants similar to those on whom Table 5.3 was constructed, makes a score of 68 on the Occupational Selection Test. Then it can be estimated that Frank's chances of receiving a rating of 4 or higher on job performance by his supervisor six months after beginning the job are 61 out of 100, but his chances of obtaining a rating of 6 or higher are only 5 out of 100. If a performance rating of 4 or higher is considered acceptable, Frank will be hired.

PERFORMANCE APPRAISAL

A necessary but frequently distasteful part of a supervisor's or manager's job is evaluating the performance of subordinates. Some type of *performance appraisal* has been in use for thousands of years. In the United States, a formal system for appraising the performance of military personnel was established in 1813 and for evaluating civilian personnel in the federal government in 1842 (Grant, 1987). The Civil Rights Act of 1964 led to numerous legal challenges to performance appraisal of programs in the private and public sectors. Because of difficulties in defending selection programs against these legal challenges, the administration of psychological tests and other standardized assessment procedures was discontinued by some organizations. In many cases, however, the legal challenges had the effect of promoting research on performance appraisal systems that had never been adequately validated.

Accurate performance appraisals serve a number of functions, including the provision of information for personnel decisions, feedback to employees, planning of training and employee counseling programs, and other matters concerned with the operation and development of an organization. With respect to behavioral prediction, the results of performance appraisals also serve as criteria for selection and placement procedures and as predictors of subsequent performance by employees. Employee selection and placement are not the only personnel decisions that depend on performance appraisals. Promotions, job transfers, pay increases, training, disciplining, and other matters related to the reward/punishment system of an organization are affected by the results of formal and informal procedures for evaluating employee performance.

Depending on the job, both objective and subjective methods may be used to evaluate employees. Some of the most common objective performance criteria are direct measures of productivity (e.g., volume or dollar amount of sales, quantity and quality of materials produced, number of errors or mistakes made), as well as less direct indicators of performance such as tardiness, absences, accidents, interpersonal altercations, and turnover. These behavioral measures are, however, not available for evaluating performance on many jobs or positions in business and industry. For example, what are the direct measures of production or services rendered by managers or executives? Appraisal of supervisory and other jobs concerned with managing people in organizations entails reliance on more subjective criteria.

Ratings of Performance

All subjective criteria are based on human judgment—on the ability of the evaluator to use logical observation and reasoning to make decisions concerning the effectiveness of people. Information on which the subjective judgments for performance appraisal depend may be obtained not only from watching and listening to a person but also from what other people say and how they react to the person. Judgments about people may involve "absolute" standards of what the appraiser considers effective performance as well as relative comparisons of the person with other people and even the appraiser himself.

Rather than recording their observations and judgments of others in writing or electronically, people generally store the information in their heads, where it consciously or unconsciously affects their future dealings with others. In organizational settings committed to employee evaluation, however, sooner or later the results of formal and information appraisals of employees are recorded in essay form and/or marked on a rating scale or behavioral checklist. Subjective as they are and depending on human judgment as they do, ratings (sometimes referred to as *efficiency ratings* or *merit ratings*) are by far the most popular method of appraising employee performance. Indeed, they are often the only available criteria for validating methods of selecting and placing employees on certain jobs or training programs and for other personnel actions such as promotions, transfers, and pay increases.

All of the various types of rating scales discussed in Chapter 2— graphic, numerical, forced-choice, mixed standard, behaviorally anchored, behavior observation—are used by different organizations. In constructing these scales, information from job analyses and job descriptions is rephrased to be as objective as possible and still provide sufficient information concerning performance. Because the majority of jobs are multifaceted, involving many duties and requiring a number of abilities, the associated performance rating scales should measure those multiple facets. As seen in the "tongue-in-cheek" behaviorally anchored scale in Figure 5.3, a typical rating scale may measure not

	Performance Degrees				
Performance Factors	Far Exceeds Job Requirements	Exceeds Job Requirements	Meets Job Requirements	Needs Some Improvement	Does Not Meet Minimum Requirements
Quality	Leaps tall buildings with a single bound	Must take running start to leap over buildings	Can only leap over a short building or medium with no spires	Crashes into buildings when attempting to jump over them	Cannot recognize buildings at all, much less jump
Timeliness	Is faster than a speeding bullet	Is as fast as a speeding bullet	Not quite as fast as a speeding bullet	Would you believe a slow bullet	Wounds self with bullets when attempting to shoot gun
Initiative	Is stronger than a locomotive	Is stronger than a bull elephant	Is stronger than a bull	Shoots the bull	Smells like a bull
Adaptability	Walks on water consistently	Walks on water in emergencies	Washes with water	Drinks water	Passes water in emergencies
Communication	Talks with God	Talks with the angels	Talks to himself	Argues with himself	Loses those arguments

Figure 5.3. Tongue-in-cheek behaviorally anchored rating scale for employee appraisal. Adapted from *The Industrial-Organizational Psychologist*, *17*(4), p. 22, and used with permission.

only the quality and quantity of work output, but also such factors as speed or promptness, dependability, cooperativeness, motivation, inventiveness, and relationships with coworkers. An instrument consisting of ten or so performance dimensions to be rated on scales containing 4 to 8 categories is usually satisfactory, but some rating forms consist of many more scales than this. Space should also be reserved for written comments, which many evaluators view as the most useful if not the most objective, part of the rating form.

Depending on the particular type and level of job, employees may be rated by many different people in an organization—by coworkers, immediate supervisors, middle- and upper-level managers, and even themselves. Of these, the most common, and usually the most valid source, is the immediate supervisor. This is the person who is responsible for direct oversight of the employee's work and hence has the most opportunity to observe and evaluate him.

Postappraisal Interviews

Ideally, performance appraisal is an ongoing, continuous process rather than an occasional chore. In the interest of time and efficiency, however, most organizations schedule appraisals of employees at periodic intervals. Shortly after the ratings have been made, or perhaps for the purpose of making the ratings themselves, an interview is held with the employee. In the case of a post-appraisal interview, the results of performance evaluation are communicated to and discussed with the employee. Such interviews are necessary not only to provide employees with appropriate, realistic feedback on their performance, but also to provide them with an opportunity to ask questions, discuss how they might improve, and express their feelings and aspirations concerning the job. Unfortunately, a performance appraisal interview is rarely a pleasant experience for any participant. The human ego is a fragile thing, and negative feedback often leads to resentment, denial, and excuses—even when the appraiser makes an effort to be tactful, supportive, encouraging, and generally helpful and understanding. In a survey of General Electric employees conducted over three decades, the majority of employees who were questioned reported that they were even more uncertain about the status of their job performance following a post-appraisal interview than before (Schultz & Schultz, 1994).

The goals of an appraisal interview are more likely to be met when the interviewer is perceived as fair and as an attentive listener who is specific and encourages the interviewee to participate in the appraisal process. As noted by Cascio (1991), in the most effective performance appraisal system, the supervisor (or whoever is communicating the results to the employee) engages in certain activities before, during, and after the actual appraisal interview to make the experience a more pleasant and productive one. An outline of these activities is given in Figure 5.4.

Training Raters

It is not easy to make reliable and valid judgments of people under any circumstances, and particularly when the behaviors or characteristics

Before Performance Appraisal

Communicate frequently with subordinates about their performance.
Get training in performance appraisal.
Judge your own performance first before judging others.
Encourage subordinates to prepare for appraisal interviews.

During Performance Appraisal

Warm up and encourage subordinate participation.
Judge performance, not personality and mannerisms.
Be specific.
Be an active listener.
Avoid destructive criticism.
Set mutually agreeable goals for future improvement.

After Performance Appraisal

Communicate frequently with subordinates about their performance.
Periodically assess progress toward goals.
Make organizational rewards contingent on performance.

Figure 5.4. Supervisory activities before, during, and after performance appraisal. Adapted from *Applied Psychology in Personnel Management* (4th ed.), by W. F. Cascio, 1991, p. 102. Englewood Cliffs, NJ: Prentice-Hall. Adapted by permission of Prentice-Hall.

are poorly defined or highly subjective. Not only are personal biases likely to affect ratings, but raters frequently are not sufficiently familiar with the ratee to make accurate judgments. Training can help make ratings more objective, by being aware of the various kinds of errors that can occur in rating, becoming more familiar with the persons and traits being rated, and recognizing the multidimensionality of jobs and the situation specificity of much behavior. Raters should also be encouraged to become more familiar with the ratee's behavior, but to omit items on the rating form that they feel unqualified to judge.

Lectures, practice in making ratings, group discussion of rating procedures, and feedback on one's performance all play a role in effective rater training programs. Trainees are encouraged to be active participants rather than passive listeners, attending to feedback and striving to base their ratings on more representative samples of ratee behavior, improving their observational skills, using rating scales properly, and arriving at good judgments and reasonable conclusions from observational and interview data.

With regard to errors in rating, raters can be taught to be less lenient, to avoid the halo effect, and to make ratings more variable. Unfortunately, such training does not necessarily improve the accuracy of ratings. For example, a preoccupation with avoiding the leniency error and with the need to make ratings more variable may actually result in a disservice to a group of employees who are all highly effective on their jobs. In recent years, the training of raters has focused not only on the awareness and avoidance of rating errors but also on basing ratings on objective observations of ratees in multiple situations, on several occasions, and on a number of behavioral variables. Raters should be thoroughly familiar with the particular job and the context in which it is performed, in addition to the behavior and characteristics of the ratee which influence his or her job performance.

There are other techniques that might be expected to improve the validity of ratings. Certainly combining the ratings given by several individuals will tend to even out the response biases of individual raters. For this and certain statistical reasons, such group ratings tend to be more reliable than individual ratings. It also makes sense that careful attention to the design of rating scales, for example, defining the points clearly with precise behavioral descriptions of the characteristics to be rated, might improve the validity of ratings. But the simple conclusion from the results of extensive research in laboratory and field settings is that one rating format is about as good as another. Thus, a behaviorally anchored scale (BARS) or a behavioral observation scale (BOS) is not generally superior to a simple graphic or numerical scale.

Cleveland and Murphy (1992) have emphasized the social and communicative features (ratee with rater, rater with the organization, etc.) rather than the traditional measurement functions of performance appraisals. They view appraisal from a dynamic, organizational perspective in which raters and ratees are active participants in the rating process—participants who frequently have varied and conflicting goals.

Pulakos (1991) also sees the organizational context as important in performance appraisal. The purpose(s) of performance appraisal, time constraints and opportunities for raters to observe ratees' behavior, pressures on raters by politicians and unions,[4] the extent to which raters are required to make and justify their ratings, and other organizational factors all influence ratings of job performance.

Judgments of other people are never made in a vacuum. There are always political, social, and economic factors to consider in making and using performance appraisals. Above and beyond the actual use of appraisal information, the very process of appraisal can contribute to organizational goals. For these reasons—many of which have little or nothing to do with the validity and practical utility of ratings, executives in business and industrial organizations continue to be in favor of periodic performance appraisals and ratings.

HUMAN FACTORS AND THE WORK ENVIRONMENT

Research oriented toward discovering ways of improving industrial productivity and simultaneously enhancing job satisfaction has increased steadily during this century. Beginning with industrial engineering and time-and-motion studies in the first three decades and influenced by the Hawthorne studies of the 1930s (Roethlisberger & Dickson, 1939), research in industrial psychology has progressed toward a greater consideration of the role of attitudes, morale, and other human needs and goals. Major developments in the field of *engineering psychology (human engineering)* took place during World War II with military research on the design of sensory displays and control systems. These explorations and experiments continued after the war under different names, including *ergonomics, operations research,* and, more recently, *organizational behavior* and *systems research and design.* Although much of the research on the role of human factors in job performance began in psychology, a truly interdisciplinary field, including many of the behavioral and social sciences as well as engineering, was created. Studies of the effects of human factors on performance have dealt with the design of physical equipment, facilities, and the work environment to make them more congruent with human needs and abilities. Evaluation of the effectiveness of various modifications of materials and people explored in these studies has involved both objective performance measures and more subjective measures, such as ratings of design features and inventories of attitudes and work satisfaction. Since the 1940s, much of the research on human factors has been directed toward analyzing man-machine systems—an analysis based on a recognition of the complementarity of humans and machines in the performance of jobs in both the military and civilian sectors.

Organizational Behavior

Most of the findings of the engineering psychologists that resulted in improvements in designing machines so they could be operated more efficiently and safely by humans was eventually absorbed into engineering proper. Many behavioral scientists continued to specialize in engineering psychology, but the interests of industrial psychology expanded in the direction of research on entire systems or organizations. Although still focusing on human factors, *organizational psychology* is broader, encompassing all structural and dynamic factors that contribute to organizational functioning.

As noted in the discussion of performance appraisal, tangible criteria of productivity and job satisfaction are often unavailable. Consequently, observations, interviews, checklists, rating scales, attitude inventories, and other subjective psychometric and sociometric measures must be used. A survey of the attitudes of employees toward their immediate supervisors and management in general, as well as toward working conditions, benefits, and other physical and social features of the work environment, may assist in identifying problem areas and provide clues to causal factors.

Work Environment

Many management problems concerning employees are directly related to the work environment (Moos & Billings, 1991). For example, the rapid pace of many jobs and the constant interaction with other people on the job add to the level of stress experienced by workers. The creation of a more positive work environment, both physical and sociopsychological, leads not only to a reduction in stress but also increases employee morale, productivity, and innovation and reduces turnover.

A number of standardized paper-and-pencil instruments are available for measuring job attitudes and features of the work environment. Examples are the Organizational Climate Index (from Evaluation Research Associates), the Organizational Climate Questionnaire (Litwin & Stringer, 1968), the Job Descriptive Index (Smith, Kendall, & Hulin, 1969), the Organization Health Survey (by P. T. Kehoe & W. J. Reddin,

Organizational Tests, Ltd. Canada), and the Work Environment Scale (Moos, 1986).

The Work Environment Scale (WES) is available from Consulting Psychologists Press in three forms (Real, Ideal, Expectations) designed to measure the work environment, compare what is with what might be, and thereby monitor and improve work settings. The 90 items on each form of the WES can be answered in 15 to 20 minutes and then scored on 10 subscales grouped into three domains: Relation ships (Involvement, Peer Cohesion, Supervisory Support), Personal Growth (Autonomy, Task-Orientation, Work Pressure), and System Maintenance and Change (Clarity, Control, Innovation, Physical Comfort). It was standardized on over 3,000 employees. Moos maintained that an analysis of work environments in terms of these three domains can lead to the formulation of criteria for an ideal environment and optimal methods for instituting environmental changes.

As illustrated in Figure 5.5, standard scores on the 10 subscales of the WES may be plotted as a profile for purposes of analysis and comparison. Such profiles are useful in describing, evaluating, and improving work environments. As shown in the figure, however, assessments of the climate of an organization may vary significantly with the employees or groups doing the assessments. In a review of the WES, Kanungo (1985) concluded that it is a convenient, easy, quick, and reliable method of assessing different types of work environments.

An Analysis of General Social Survey Data

Surveys involving psychometric measures of attitudes and opinions toward work and the job environment are not limited to on-the-job situations. Large scale surveys by the Gallup and Roper organizations, as well as other pollsters, are a continuing part of public opinion research that yields practical benefits. As an illustration, consider the General Social Surveys conducted for the National Opinion Research Center (Davis & Smith, 1994). This annual survey entails asking hundreds of socially, politically, psychologically, and economically relevant questions of several thousand Americans. Many of the questions, which cover a wide range of personal information and opinions, are of the checklist or rating scale variety.

Using the database for the 1994 General Social Surveys (Davis & Smith, 1994), I determined the frequencies of responses to the following

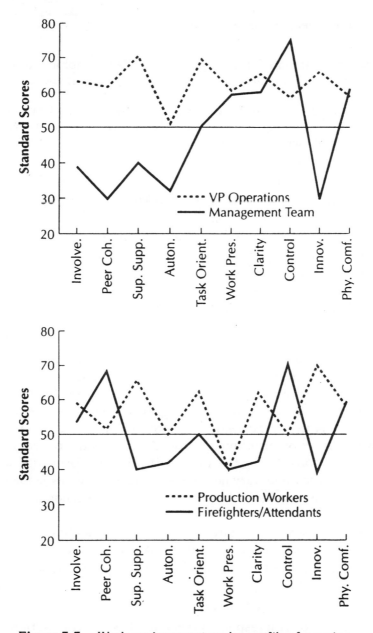

Figure 5.5. Work environment scales profiles for a vice-president of operations and his management team. From "Understanding and Improving Work Climates" by R. H. Moos and A. G. Billings. In *Applying Psychology to Business: The Handbook for Managers and Resource Professionals*, pp. 552–562, 1991. Lexington, MA: D. C. Heath. Reprinted by permission.

item and crosstabulated them against the demographic variables of marital status, race, income, socioeconomic status, and sex:

Which one thing on this list would you most prefer in a job? What comes next? Which is third most important? Which is fourth most important? Which is fifth most important?

A. High income.

B. No danger of being fired.

C. Working hours are short, lots of free time.

D. Chances for advancement.

E. Work important and gives a feeling of accomplishment.

The rating (rank) scale for these items was: 1 = Most important, 2 = Second, 3 = Third, 4 = Fourth, 5 = Fifth.

On this scale, the medians for the five items were: A = 2.55, B = 3.62, C = 4.66, D = 2.50, E = 1.55. Thus, the most important job factor to the respondents as a group was "Work important and gives a feeling of accomplishment." The second most important factor was "Chances for advancement," followed closely by "High income."

It would be a mistake to conclude that these results hold for all respondents or all demographic subgroups. Over 80% of the respondent sample were White, so the overall findings may be more characteristic of Whites than of other ethnic groups. As the results of crosstabulations of the response to the five items with the five demographic variables indicate, the ranks vary not only with race of the respondents but also with income, marital status, gender, and socioeconomic status:

1. The socioeconomic status of the respondents has a significant negative relationship with the ranks of items A, B, and C and a significant positive relationship with items D and E.

2. Compared with Blacks, Whites gave a lower rank to item A and a higher rank to item E.

3. Compared with respondents having lower incomes, those with higher incomes gave a higher rank to item E.

4. Women respondents gave a higher rank than men to item E.

5. Whites gave a higher rank than Blacks to item D.

6. Married respondents gave a higher ranking than nonmarrieds to item B.

In sum, compared with other demographic groups, Blacks and people of lower socioeconomic status (SES) gave higher ranks to item A; married respondents gave a higher rank to item B than unmarried respondents; respondents of lower SES gave a higher rank to item C than respondents of higher SES status; Whites and people of higher SES gave higher ranks than their counterparts to item D; women, Whites, those with higher incomes, and those with higher SES gave higher ranks than other groups to item E. These findings are not particularly surprising and certainly not independent of each other. Because socioeconomic status (SES) is significantly related to income and race, correlates of SES would be expected to be related to these two variables as well. Thus, the general results of surveys of work-related attitudes, opinions, and experiences do not necessarily apply to specific groups or individuals.

CONSUMER BEHAVIOR

Demographic features of target populations (chronological age, socio-economic status, gender, ethnicity, etc.) are taken into account in marketing decisions. To determine the success or likely future success of a product or service, particular subgroups have been targeted by means of questionnaires and field testing. Although less prominently, the personal characteristics of potential consumers have also been considered in advertising and selling certain products and services. Motivation research studies, in particular, have revealed that the reasons for making purchases are often complex and even unconscious—a finding that stimulated the interest of certain "Madison Avenue" psychologists after World War II and led directly to a new field of investigation and application—consumer psychology.

Consumer psychology is concerned with identifying attitudes, interests, opinions, values, personality traits, and lifestyles associated with preferences for and purchases of certain products and services. Checklists, rating scales, and attitude inventories have been used extensively in gauging consumer reactions to products and services, and particularly purchasing decisions concerning them.

An important focus of consumer psychology is *psychographics*, which attempts to describe the characteristic patterns of temperament, cognition, and behavior that differentiate between diverse human components of the marketplace. The results of psychographic research may contribute to the segmentation of a particular market according to the personality characteristics and behaviors of consumers and the preparation of advertising, packaging, and promotional materials that will appeal to and motivate identifiable segments of the market. Two popular approaches in psychographic studies are AIO inventories and VALS (values and lifestyles).

AIO Inventories

An *AIO inventory* consists of statements of the activities, interests, and opinions to be administered to specific groups of people. Illustrative of this approach are the following items on an AIO inventory administered to a sample of young men (18–24 years old) who both drank and drove (Lastovika, Murray, Joachimsthaler, Bhalla, & Scheurich, 1987):

> It seems like no matter what my friends and I do on a weekend, we almost always end up at a bar getting smashed.
>
> A party wouldn't be a party without some liquor.
>
> I've been drunk at least five times this month.
>
> Being drunk is fun.
>
> The chances of an accident or losing a driver's license from drinking and driving are low.
>
> Drinking helps me to have fun and do better with girls.
>
> A few drinks will have no noticeable effect on my coordination and self-control.

An AIO inventory is usually designed with a particular product and market in mind, and responses to a well-designed inventory can differentiate a particular segment of the market from another segment.

VALS™ 2

VALS™ 2 (Business Intelligence Center in Menlo Park, CA) is based on the dimensional concepts of self-orientation and resources. Consumers are viewed as being motivated by one of three *self-orientations:* principle, status, and action. Principle-oriented consumers are guided in their choices by abstract, idealized criteria, rather than by feelings, events, or the behaviors or opinions of other people. *Status-oriented* consumers are interested in products and services that indicate success to their peers, and *action-oriented* consumers are motivated toward social or physical activity, variety, and risk-taking.

The *resources* dimension of the VALS 2 system refers to the psychological, physical, demographic, and material means and capacities available to consumers. Such resources include education, income, self-confidence, health, eagerness to buy, and energy level. Resources, which are on a continuum from minimal to abundant, generally decrease in old age, when depression, financial reverses, and physical or psychological impairment are more likely to occur.

The three self-orientations and the minimal to abundant resources dimensions define eight segments of adult behavior and decision making (Figure 5.6). Each segment, which contains approximately

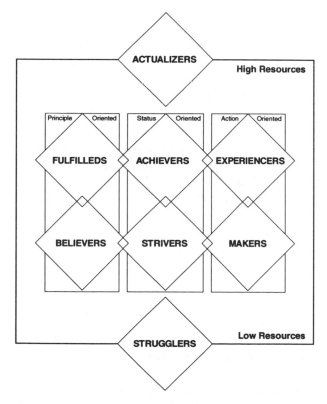

Figure 5.6. VALS™ 2 Network. From SRI International, VALS™ 2. © 1995 SRI International. All rights reserved. Unauthorized reproduction prohibited.

the same proportion of the population as any other segment, is a viable marketing target. At the top of the VALS 2 hierarchy are *Actualizers*, who have abundant resources and who represent a combination of the principle-, status-, and action-orientations. The two segments with a principle-orientation are *Fulfilleds* and *Believers*, but the former have more abundant resources than the latter. The two primarily status-oriented segments are *Achievers* and *Strivers*, the former having more resources than the latter. The two primarily action-oriented segments are *Experiencers* and *Makers*, the former with more abundant resources than the latter. At the bottom of the VALS 2 network are *Strugglers*, who have minimal resources, constricted and difficult lives, and are cautious consumers.

SUMMARY

Personnel psychology is concerned with the selection of capable, motivated, and efficient workers and with job satisfaction and attitudes toward the work situation. The analysis and evaluation of jobs, and the recruitment, selection, classification, training, and performance appraisal of workers all constitute part of personnel psychology.

The various methods of selecting employees include random selection, recommendations and influence, open selection, psychological assessment, and the use of nontest criteria. Combinations of these methods, as well as the use of quotas, may also be employed. Statistical procedures are applied in personnel selection to establish cutoff scores on selection (predictor) variables, below which applicants are not hired. False positive errors occur when applicants scoring above cutoff cannot perform the job satisfactorily; false negative errors occur when rejected applicants could have performed the job satisfactorily if they had been hired. Cutoff scores on the selection variables are set higher in an open labor market than a tight labor market and when false positive errors are considered more serious than false negative errors. Cutoff scores are set lower in a tight labor market and when false negative errors are more serious than false positive ones.

Expectancy tables for forecasting performance criteria from scores on selection variables may be either empirical or theoretical. Table 5.3 is an empirical expectancy table. A theoretical expectancy table for the same data may be constructed from the linear regression equation determined from the data given in Table 5.2.

Performance appraisal, which is a necessary but rarely a pleasant experience, may be based on objective and/or subjective criteria. Objective criteria include direct measures of the quantity and quality of goods or services produced, as well as absenteeism, tardiness, accidents, and the like. Subjective criteria consist primarily of ratings or other subjective evaluations of employees on a variety of factors. Information obtained from performance appraisals is shared and discussed with employees in postappraisal interviews, typically by the immediate supervisor.

Raters can be trained to avoid errors, but this does not necessarily make the ratings more accurate or valid. The validity of ratings can be improved by observing ratees in multiple situations and rating them on several behaviorally variables and on several occasions. Thorough familiarity with the ratee's job and the context in which it is performed can also contribute to the validity of ratings.

Research on rating forms or scales has not revealed any one format to be superior to all others. More significant than rating scale format in determining ratings in performance appraisals are the social and political purposes served by performance appraisals in an organizational context.

Research on human factors and organizational climate has used rating scales and checklists as measures of both independent and dependent variables. Beginning with studies of equipment design by industrial engineers and engineering psychologists in the military and civilian sectors, human factors research expanded to include entire man-machine systems and studies of organizational structure and dynamics. The results of studies of work environments, as conducted by Rudolf Moos and other investigators using rating scales and inventories, underscore the importance of organizational climate for productivity and employees' sense of well-being.

Consumer research has employed a variety of psychometric instruments and procedures to identify and analyze the determinants of purchasing behavior. One interest of consumer psychologists is psychographics, which involves the design and administration of instruments such an AIO inventory and VALS 2 for purposes of identifying market segments and applying that knowledge to both advertising and selling.

QUESTIONS AND ACTIVITIES

1. Define each of the following terms used in this chapter. Consult Appendix A and/or a dictionary if you need help.

Achievers	Makers
action-oriented	man-machine systems
Actualizers	market segmentation
adverse impact	merit ratings
AIO inventories	operations research
Believers	organizational behavior
classification	organizational psychology
consumer behavior	performance appraisal
cutoff scores	personnel psychology
deferred rating system	personnel selection
efficiency ratings	placement
expectancy table	principle-oriented
Experiencers	psychographics
false positive errors	scientific management
false negative errors	self-orientations
four-fifths rule	status-oriented
Fulfilleds	Strivers
human factors	Strugglers
human engineering	systems research
job evaluation	VALS 2

2. How are checklists and rating scales used in job analysis and performance appraisal? Would they be expected to yield different results from observations and interviews?

3. Given that the correlation coefficient for the data in Table 5.2 is .689, how accurately can Performance Ratings be predicted from OST scores?

4. Assuming that an acceptable, or "passing," rating on the performance criterion for the data in Table 5.3 is 5, where should the cutoff score on the Occupational Selection Test (OST) be set? If a rating of 5 or above is acceptable, how many false positive and false negative errors will occur if the cutoff score on the OST is set at 75? What effect will lowering the OST cutoff score to 70 have on the number of false positive and false negative errors? What effect will raising it to 80 have?

5. Describe several roles that industrial/organizational psychologists perform in business and industry.

6. What special abilities or other characteristics do humans possess that make them more effective than machines in: (a) space flight, (b) modern warfare, (c) high technology production, (d) obtaining information? What special characteristics or abilities do machines possess that make them more effective than machines in the same contexts? How could humans and machines be made to work together in these situations to take advantage of the superior abilities of each?

7. Describe the VALS 2 psychographics system of segmenting markets according to consumer characteristics.

8. Would segmenting a potential market by demographic variables such as age, sex, ethnicity, and socioeconomic status yield different segments than segmenting the market by personality variables and attitudes? In what way?

9. Rating scales have been used extensively in investigations of ethnic and gender differences in attitudes and beliefs concerning a host of social issues. Many of these differences have been examined from responses to large social surveys such as those conducted by the Gallup and Roper organizations. For example, the General Social Survey, which is conducted annually by the Roper Center for Public Opinion Research for the National Opinion Research Center, asks large samples of Americans to evaluate on a scale ranging from 1 (hardworking) to 7 (lazy) how they would rate Asians, Blacks, Hispanics, and Whites in general. In the 1994 survey, the following percentages of Whites, Blacks, other races, males, and female gave ratings of 1 or 2 to the respective ethnic and gender groups on this item. Analyze these data, separately by race and sex, with a chi square test of independence (program G-2) and interpret the results.

| | Group Rated | | | |
Respondents	Asians	Blacks	Hispanics	Whites
Whites	31	6	10	26
Blacks	58	39	18	27
Other races	44	5	25	24
Males	38	10	12	25
Females	33	10	11	27

6

Educational and Developmental Assessment

Although educational institutions are organizations in which people perform services and produce results, they are not businesses or industries in the same sense as most profit-making organizations. Still, the results of schooling and the people who are responsible for ensuring that its functions are performed well must, like the personnel, procedures, and products of businesses, be appraised periodically. In addition, though perhaps less energetically than most businesses, schools use the results of these evaluations to improve the quality and quantity of their products and services and the efficiency with which they are provided.

This chapter focuses principally on evaluations of people, procedures, products, and contexts in educational institutions. The people who are involved with schools consist not only of the students, teachers, and administrators who spend a good portion of the weekdays within the walls of these institutions but also with the officials, parents, and extramural service persons who interact with and influence the operation of schools. The contributions made by all these groups to the effective functioning of schools can be, and are to some extent, assessed, but systematic evaluations are typically carried out only on instructional personnel and students.

It is reasonable to conclude that the effectiveness of any educational activity depends primarily on the abilities, attitudes, and habits of students and teachers, but the materials and programs, as well as the non-instructional personnel who administer them, are also important in the educational enterprise. Consequently, in addition to teachers and students we shall discuss evaluations of educational programs, materials, and environments in which instruction and learning take place.

To complete this chapter and provide a transition to the next one, we shall consider procedures for evaluating the development of children and, in particular, "special" children. As used here, "special children" refers to children who, because of biological or environmental mishap, have special needs and require special programs and materials in order to attain maximum benefit from their educational experiences.

EVALUATING STUDENT PERFORMANCE

Educational evaluation has traditionally been *summative*, in that an achievement test of some kind is administered at the end of an instructional unit or course to determine whether students have attained specified educational objectives. A more dynamic, and realistic, approach—that of *formative evaluation*—is based on the notion that evaluation and instruction should be integrated. In formative evaluation, testing and other procedures for assessing educational achievement take place continuously while instruction is going on. Each student's progress is monitored throughout the learning process, serving as feedback to guide review and subsequent instruction.

Most common of all instruments for evaluating student performance in school classrooms are objective, teacher-made tests (true-false, multiple-choice, short answer, etc.) or standardized tests marketed by commercial organizations. Well-designed objective tests provide an efficient and fairly comprehensive way of assessing student achievement in school subjects and, to some extent, determining the effectiveness of instructional programs. In this section we shall focus on educational evaluations involving the use of checklists, rating scales, and rankings. The construction, administration, scoring, and analysis of educational tests is considered at length in other sources (e.g., Aiken, 1994a).

Scoring Ranking Items

The simplest method of scoring an objective test is to give 1 point for each correct response and 0 points for each incorrect response or omission. An exception occurs in the case of rearrangement or ranking items, which, because of the large number of different orders in which a group of items can be arranged, presents a special problem. For example, putting an item in second place when it actually belongs in first place is not as serious a mistake as putting the same item in fourth place.

The following formula can be used for scoring ranking items:

$$S = c[1 - 2\Sigma d/(c^2 - k)] \tag{6.1}$$

In this formula, c = the number of things ranked, the d's are the absolute values of the differences between the ranks assigned by the examinee and the keyed ranks, and $k = 0$ if c is even and 1 if c is odd. To illustrate the use of this formula, assume that five states are to be arranged in rank order according to population by assigning a rank of 1 to the state with the largest population, 2 the next largest state, and so on. The names of the five states are given in the first column of Table 6.1, the keyed ranks in the second column, and the ranks assigned by a hypothetical person in the third column. In the fourth column are listed the absolute values of the differences between the correct rank and the keyed rank for each state. The sum of the absolute values of the differences between the ranks assigned by our hypothetical person and the keyed ranks is 6 and the sum of the squared differences is 28. Substituting $c = 5$, $\Sigma d = 6$, and $j = 1$ in Formula 6.1 yields $5[1 - 2(6)/(5^2 - 1)] = 2.5 \approx 3$. Program A-8 of the computer diskette accompanying this book can be used to facilitate the scoring of ranking or rearrangement items by this procedure.

TABLE 6.1.   Scoring an Illustrative Rearrangement Item

State	Correct (Keyed) Rank	Ranking by Examinee	Absolute Value of Difference
Florida	4	5	1
Texas	3	4	1
New York	2	1	1
Pennsylvania	5	3	2
California	1	2	1
Sum			6

Scoring Essay Examinations

Also quite popular in schools are essay tests and themes or term papers, with oral and performance tests being third or fourth in frequency of administration. Unlike objective tests, which can be scored objectively by a clerk or an electronic scoring machine in which the answers have been recorded, scoring procedures for essay, oral, and performance tests are fairly subjective.

The scoring of essay items can be made more objective by structuring the task clearly so different examinees interpret the item in much the same way. In addition, by making the scoring process as structured and as objective as possible, a person's score depends less on noncontent, impressionistic factors and more on the level of knowledge and understanding demonstrated. Scoring on the basis of neatness rather than quality of the answers, being overly general (*leniency error*), and awarding a high score on an item simply because an examinee makes high scores on other items (*halo effect*) are among the mistakes that can affect scores on essay items.

A number of things can be done to make the scores on essay tests and papers more objective and reliable. To begin, the scorer must decide whether to score the answer (paper) as a whole or to assign separate numerical weights to different components. Whole (*global* or *holistic*) scoring is common, but it is perhaps more meaningful to use an analytic scoring procedure in which a specified number of points is assigned to each item of information or skill included in the response. An example of analytic scoring for style is to give separate ratings on capitalization, division of words, documentation, grammar, punctuation, references, spelling, and vocabulary.

The maximum number of points allocated to an essay item is determined not only by the teacher's judgment of the importance of the item, but also by the assigned length of the answer. When the directions specify a half-page answer, the item should be weighted less than when a whole page answer is required.

Whatever scoring weights are assigned to specific questions and answers, it is advisable for the test designer to prepare ideal answers to the questions before the test is administered. Prior to scoring the test papers, the names of examinees should be blocked out so the responses can be scored anonymously. Other recommendations are to score all answers to a question before going on the next one, score all answers to a given item during a single scoring period, evaluate content and organization (style) separately, have the papers scored by more than one person, and make written comments on the papers.

Scoring Oral Examinations

Although errors are more likely to occur in scoring responses to oral than to objective questions, special forms for rating performance can improve the objectivity of scoring oral tests (see Figure 6.1). Careful attention to the design of questions, construction of model answers to questions before administering the test, using multiple raters or scorers, and training examiners to avoid favoritism and other rater biases can also decrease errors in scoring oral tests. If the time allotted to scoring is not critical, the accuracy with which oral tests are scored can

---

Directions: For each of the questions listed below, rate the oral report on a scale of 1 to 10, 1 being very low and 10 being very high. Write the appropriate number (1 to 10) in the marginal dash.

____ 1. What is the level of the student's knowledge of the subject matter in the report?
____ 2. How well was the report organized?
____ 3. How effective was the introduction to the report in capturing your attention?
____ 4. How clearly and distinctly did the student speak?
____ 5. How interesting was the topic?
____ 6. How effectively used were audiovisual materials (films, posters, chalkboard, etc.)?
____ 7. To what extent did the student look at the class during the report rather than looking at his or her notes?
____ 8. How effectively did the student use gestures, body postures, and other nonverbal messages to communicate?
____ 9. To what extent did the student refer to research or other primary sources in presenting the report?
____ 10. How would you rate the closing (summary of major points, presentation of thought questions, etc.) of the report?

Comments:

Figure 6.1. A form for evaluating oral reports.

be improved by electronically recording examinees' responses for later playback and (re)evaluation (see Aiken, 1983a).

In addition to information and organization, oral responses may be rated on personal qualities, style, and manner of speaking (loudness, pitch, rate, enunciation, pronunciation, word usages, etc.). The categories employed by examiners in rating students' responses should cite specific, observed behaviors rather than nebulous concepts such as "creative potential," "character," "general ability," or "interpersonal effectiveness."

Performance Evaluation

In planning a test to measure how well a person has learned a particular skill, it is useful to construct a detailed list of the behaviors that are indicative of a range of proficiency in that skill. Decisions should be made beforehand concerning the range of (numerical) ratings or weights to be given to each aspect of the performance, and what deductions (if any) will be made for mistakes, slowness, and sloppiness. In those instances where the performance is not only a process but also results in a visible or tangible end-product, a product scale may be devised beforehand. An example of a *product scale*, which consists of a series of sample products representing various degrees of quality, is the handwriting scale in Figure 6.2.

A performance test should focus mainly on the product or end-result of performing a skill, but the way in which it is performed (the process) is also important. For example, what counts most in playing golf is how many strokes it takes the player to get the ball in the hole. However, all golf instructors recognize the importance of style. On performance tests involving a tangible finished product, not only the quantity and quality of that product but also how efficiently it was made should be noted.

Both the products and processes of performance are typically evaluated subjectively, primarily by observation, combined with a written or electronic record and a checklist or rating scale. In particular, careful observation, as free as possible of bias, is critical to the accurate evaluation of performance. Structured performance tests, in which every examinee is tested under the same conditions, are usually more objective than unstructured tests. In the latter, students are observed and evaluated surreptitiously during class, in the hall, or on the school grounds. But even when the utmost care is taken, performance tests are

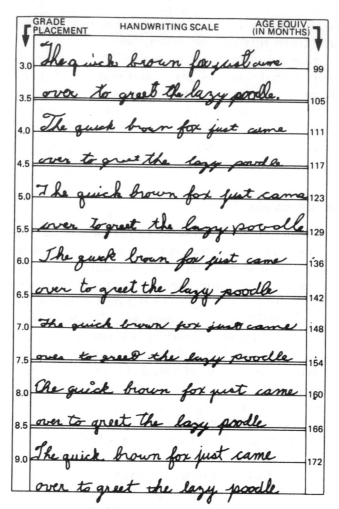

Figure 6.2. Handwriting scale for the California achievement tests. Copyright © 1957 by California Test Bureau. Used by permission of CTB/McGraw-Hill.

less objective, and consequently less reliable, than written tests. In addition, performance tests take more time than written tests and often require expensive equipment and other time-consuming arrangements.

Finally, performance evaluations may involve groups as well as individuals. The educational progress of a school class as a whole may be reported by the teacher on a *whole-group checklist* and used for designing review sessions and/or making curriculum modifications. Performance evaluations may also be made of the behavior of individuals *within* groups. For example, either a checklist or a rating scale may be devised to record the evaluator's judgment of the extent to which each participant in group work:

shares information

contributes ideas

listens to others

follows instructions

shows initiative in solving group problems

gives consideration to the viewpoints of others

accepts and carries out group-determined assignments (Kubiszyn & Borich, 1990)

Score Evaluation and Grading

Perhaps the most feared and certainly the most talked-about rating scale in educational contexts is the scale on which students are graded. In the case of teacher-made tests, the evaluation and interpretation of tests or other educational performances usually implies the assignment of letter grades or marks (A, B, C, D, F, and variations). Grade assignment is a fairly subjective process, depending not only on the score(s) attained by a particular student, but also on the expectations of the evaluator and the scores of other students. Some teachers grade strictly on the curve, whereas others grade in terms of a fixed performance standard or criterion. The majority, however, probably employ a combination of curve and fixed-standard grading. In one curve-grading procedure, the *Cajori method*, As are assigned to the top 7% of test papers, Bs to the next 24%, Cs to the next 38%, Ds to the next 24%, and Fs to the lowest 7%. A disadvantage of this method is its failure to consider that tests vary in difficulty and that the overall ability level of students in different classes is not the same. An alternative curve-grading procedure establishes letter-grade boundaries on classroom tests when the ability level of the class, the class's test performance relative to that of other classes, and the test scores themselves are all taken into account (Aiken, 1983b). Program A-9 on the computer diskette accompanying this book may be used to assign grades to a group of individuals by means of this modified Cajori procedure.

EVALUATING TEACHER PERFORMANCE

Because teachers are in a central position to influence the educational accomplishments of students, it is little wonder that political leaders, parents, and others who are concerned with educational quality should focus on teacher competency. Teachers are not the only factor in the educational mix, but whenever a discussion of the effectiveness of formal education arises the question of teacher competency comes into the conversation.

Because of continuing public concern over the failure of public schools to educate students adequately, particular attention has been directed toward responsibility or *accountability* for student learning. Proponents of accountability in education believe that the evaluation of instructional effectiveness should be based on student attainment of certain educational competencies or objectives. Many supporters of accountability and competency-based instruction also advocate *performance contracting*—making teachers' salaries contingent upon the extent to which their students attain specific educational competencies. Those who are opposed to strict accountability and the associated notion of performance contracting maintain, however, that it is unfair to tie the livelihoods of teachers to students' attainment of educational competencies. They point out that teachers are typically not permitted to select their students, and in any case have only limited control over them. Many forces and influences are at work in the lives of children, including family and peer support for education and as many hours spent watching television as are spent in school.

Testing Teachers and Prospective Teachers

Whatever the causes of the state of public education in the United States may be, increasing public concern during the 1970s and 1980s led to the inauguration of formal statewide minimum competency testing programs in the public schools. In addition to requiring that students attain a specified minimum score on a basic skills test in order to graduate from high school, almost all states established some form of teacher evaluation system. Most states now require that college students who are planning to enter teacher education programs make a passing score on a specific test before being accepted into such programs. Although testing of in-service teachers is less popular, a handful of states also use tests for recertification (certificate renewal) and the allocation of merit pay. Teacher-competency tests such as the

National Teacher Examinations, the Pre-Professional Skills Test, and the California Basic Educational Skills Test measure a combination of basic skills, subject-area knowledge, and professional pedagogical knowledge and skills. Measures of on-the-job (teaching) performance are also important, though less objective.

Several states have implemented formal observation and rating systems for beginning teachers. In these states, beginning teachers are given assistance in teaching for a trial period, after which a recommendation is made to state officials as to whether the candidate should be granted regular certification.

Dissatisfaction with traditional teacher-competency tests, as seen in legal disputes in several states (e.g., *Georgia Association of Educators* v. *Nix*, 1976; *United States* v. *South Carolina*, 1977), stimulated efforts to devise more realistic and generally acceptable measures of teacher capabilities and performance. Some authorities maintain that a combination of tests employing computer technology, portfolios with documentation of teaching performance, and standardized paper-and-pencil tests should be used to evaluate both prospective (pre-service) candidates for teaching programs and positions as well as experienced (in-service) teachers for recertification, promotion, merit pay, and tenure. Observations and interviews, and associated checklists and rating scales, would also be used to evaluate performance and impressions.

Student Evaluations of Teachers

It can be argued that, because they have more opportunities to observe teachers "on the job," students are in a better position than school administrators, peers, parents, or others to evaluate teachers. Be that as it may, student evaluations of teachers are not very common or popular below the college level. In higher education, however, teacher and course evaluations have become a regular part of the course activities. Questionnaires such as the one in Figure 6.3 are administered at midterm and/or at the end of almost every course.[1] These questionnaires consist of a combination of rating scales, checklists, and free-response (open-ended) items concerning the behaviors and characteristics of teachers, the nature (difficulty, interest level, etc.) of the course, and the materials, assignments, and evaluations (tests, papers, reports, projects, etc.). The objective portions of the questionnaires are usually machine-scored and compared with norms and a report of the results is transmitted to the teacher in a (hopefully) timely fashion.[2]

College Course and Instructor Evaluation

The Seaver College faculty believes that constructive student evaluations of courses and instructors can assist in improving the quality of instruction. Your frank, thoughtful evaluation of this course and instructor will be appreciated.

Part I. Fill in the appropriate number to the right of each statement to indicate how descriptive that statement is of the course or instructor. Fill in any number from 1 (Not at all descriptive) to 5 (Very descriptive). Fill in NA if the statement is not applicable to the course.

	Not At All Descriptive		Very Descriptive	Not Applicable
1. The course is well organized. Comment:	1 2 3 4 5			NA
2. The course objectives have been defined and met. Comment:	1 2 3 4 5			NA
3. The textbook and other reading assignments are appropriate in content. Comment:	1 2 3 4 5			NA
4. The papers, reports, and/or other written or oral assignments are reasonable and fair. Comment:	1 2 3 4 5			NA
5. The tests and other evaluations are appropriate and fair. Comment:	1 2 3 4 5			NA
6. The instructor shows interest and enthusiasm for the course. Comment:	1 2 3 4 5			NA
7. The instructor has been available when needed outside of class during posted office hours. Comment:	1 2 3 4 5			NA
8. The instructor has provided quality advising during office hours. Comment:	1 2 3 4 5			NA
9. The instructor is prepared for class and makes good use of class time. Comment:	1 2 3 4 5			NA
10. Lecture and course material is clearly explained. Comment:	1 2 3 4 5			NA
11. The workload in the course is demanding. Comment:	1 2 3 4 5			NA
12. The course material is challenging. Comment:	1 2 3 4 5			NA
13. Overall, the instructor is an excellent teacher. Comment:	1 2 3 4 5			NA
14. Overall, this is an excellent course. Comment:	1 2 3 4 5			NA

Course: _____

Instructor: _____

Grade in course: _____

Date: _____

Figure 6.3.   College course and instructor evaluation form.

In combination with their research accomplishments (as evinced by grants and scholarly publications) and service to the institution and the wider community, ratings by students, peers, and administrators are used in hiring, rank, tenure, promotion, and merit pay decisions concerning college and university faculty. Low ratings on teaching effectiveness may also be a reason for nonrenewal of the teaching contract or appointment of a nontenured faculty member. Firing a tenured faculty member is, however, extremely difficult. To do so, the institution must prove incompetence or moral turpitude or must demonstrate that the program in which the faculty member is serving is being discontinued for financial reasons.

Ratings given on teacher and course evaluation forms are fairly reliable (Morrow, 1977; Smith, 1979), moderately related to students' grades and course difficulty, and higher for teachers with more teaching experience (Driscoll & Goodwin, 1979; Gillmore, Kane, & Naccarato, 1978). Evidence for the validation of student ratings of teaching effectiveness has also been found in a number of studies (Aleamoni, 1978; Kulik & McKeachie, 1975; Marsh, 1977; Rotem & Glasman, 1979).

Ideally, teacher and course evaluation questionnaires should identify areas in which improvement is needed and in which teachers are no longer effective and not likely to become so. Furthermore, as with performance appraisals in business and industry, postappraisal interviews of teachers with their immediate supervisors (department heads, principals, deans) should be conducted in an informative, understanding, and helpful manner. The administration of teacher and course evaluation questionnaires is often supplemented with classroom observations by fellow teachers and by department heads. The results of these classroom observations are summarized in narrative form and ratings of both teacher and student behaviors are made on a series of bipolar or graphic scales.

Do course and teacher evaluations improve the quality of instruction and the quality and quantity of student learning? Unfortunately, not always. Sometimes the evaluation forms are returned to the teachers long after the course is over and too late to be helpful in modifying the present course or even in planning the one for next term. Although ratings are more objective than free-response items, busy administrators and committees often interpret small differences in average teacher ratings as significant without taking into account the standard error of measurement or even being aware of the concept. Small, insignificant differences in ratings are often used by committees and administrators to justify decisions concerning rank, tenure, promotion, and pay increases for faculty. Furthermore, it is usually left up to the evaluated teacher how he or she will make use of the information on the forms. In theory, schools and colleges should provide assistance to teachers who make poor ratings in improving the quality of their instruction. However, funds are seldom available for this service, leaving the teacher who receives a poor evaluation to discard the evaluation information and/or seek job security by collective union action. Regarding student responses to teacher and course evaluations, after filling out the evaluation forms every term on every one of their teachers for several terms running, students may become so uninterested in the process or so convinced of its ineffectiveness in improving teaching that they make their ratings and answer the free-response questions in an uncaring, slipshod manner.

One interesting use of teacher ratings involves discrepancy evaluation—comparing self-ratings with supervisory ratings. This is the method employed with the Teacher Evaluation Rating Scale (TeachERS)(J. E. Ysseldyke, S. J. Samuels, & S. L. Christenson, Pro-Ed). Each of the six areas (Instructional Planning, Instructional Management, Teaching Procedures, Monitoring Procedures, Personal Qualities, Professionalism) assessed by TeachERS has 2 to 5 components, yielding a total of 20 components. Ratings of each of the 20 components are made by the teacher and his or her supervisor on five-point Likert scales, and a discrepancy score is determined by subtracting the teacher's self-rating from the supervisor's rating. Planning for improvement in each of the six areas starts with the discrepancy score. Unfortunately, the reliability and validity data for TeachERS are skimpy to nonexistent, and it has received mixed reviews (Gresham, 1992; Wheeler, 1992).

EVALUATING OTHER FEATURES OF THE EDUCATIONAL CONTEXT

Less frequently and less formally, but nevertheless conducted, are evaluations on the administrators, materials, and environments of educational institutions. Evaluations of administrators by school teachers and college faculty are becoming more commonplace, and a number of rating forms for this process have been devised. Instructional materials, such as books and films, may also be evaluated on rating scales and checklists. For example, state committees charged with the responsibility for approving textbooks for the public schools employ checklists to make certain that the books cover the agreed-upon educational material and rating scales to evaluate competing volumes. In addition to providing a narrative description and evaluation, reviewers of college textbooks may rate them on a scale such as 1 to 100 (see Figure 6.4).

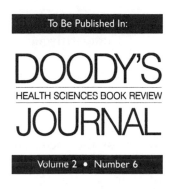

To Be Published In:

DOODY'S
HEALTH SCIENCES BOOK REVIEW
JOURNAL

Volume 2 • Number 6

Aiken / Aging: An Introduction to Gerontology

Author: Aiken, Lewis R., PhD

Bibliographic Data: Sage Pubs, 1995. ISBN: 0-8039-5445-X, LCCN: 94-3377, LC: HQ1064.U5A638, Textbook, 13 chpt, 469 pp, Appendix(es) Included, Glossary Included, 7" x 10", Hard Cover, $55.00.

Doody's Notes: Primary Audience: Undergraduate Sociology Students. Secondary Audience: Undergraduate Psychology Students. This book contains black-and-white illustrations.

Reviewer's Expert Opinion: Description: This is a basic textbook of human gerontology that comprehensively covers aging and the aged, with a special emphasis on the psychology of aging. Purpose: The purpose is to review what is known about aging and older adulthood, the methods by which this information is obtained, and to provide practical guidelines for dealing with the problems of an aged population. The author meets these goals very well. Audience: This book is written for undergraduate and graduate students. Even geriatricians in training will find this a lucid exposition of human gerontology. Features: This book's well-organized chapters are clearly illustrated. There are boxes that highlight concepts and a list of further readings in addition to well-cited references. At the end of each chapter, there are questions and exercises. Assessment: This textbook is a welcome addition to the field. It is very well written and organized. Both teachers and students will enjoy using this textbook. Rating: 98

Reviewer: David O. Staats, MD (Univ of Illinois at Chicago Coll of Medicine)

Figure 6.4. A brief review and rating of a textbook. All reviews © 1995, Doody Publishing, Inc., the foremost publisher of timely, independent reviews of medical books.

Evaluating Educational Environments

To evaluate the psychosocial environment of a classroom or school, instruments such as the Learning Environment Inventory, My Class Inventory, the Classroom Environment Scale, the University Residence Environment Scale, the Effective School Battery, and the Classroom Environmental Index can be administered to students. These instruments were designed to measure aspects of the school or college learning environment that influence students' acquisition of knowledge and skills.

Learning Environment Inventory (LEI)

The LEI (Fraser, Anderson, & Walberg, 1982) was designed to elicit secondary school students' perceptions of the classroom environment. It consists of the following 15 scales, each with seven items to be answered "strongly disagree, disagree, agree, or strongly agree."

Cohesiveness	Friction	Democracy
Diversity	Goal Direction	Cliqueness
Formality	Favoritism	Satisfaction

| Speed | Difficulty | Disorganization |
| Material Environment | Apathy | Competitiveness |

My Class Inventory is a simplified version of the LEI designed for children between 8 and 12 years of age.

Classroom Environment Scale (CES)

The CES (Moos & Trickett, 1987) is designed to assess the social climate in junior and senior high school classrooms and is administered to junior and senior high school students in regular, vocational, and alternative school settings. It consists of 90 true-false items grouped into nine subscales:

1. Involvement
2. Affiliation
3. Teacher Support
4. Task Orientation
5. Competition
6. Order and Organization
7. Rule Clarity
8. Teacher Control
9. Innovation

Subscales 1 to 3 are "Relationship" variables, subscales 4 to 5 are "Personal Growth" variables, and subscales 6 to 9 are "System Maintenance and Change" variables.

There are four forms of the CES: (1) R—perception of *current* classroom environment by teachers and students; (2) S—a shortened version of Form R for total classroom, not individual student, diagnosis; (3) I—students' conceptions of the *ideal* classroom environment; and (4) E—what prospective class members expect the classroom environment to be like. The CES was standardized on 382 classes in public and vocational schools, and the test-retest reliability of the profiles of scores on the nine subscales are quite acceptable (over .90) over short time intervals (Moos & Trickett, 1987).

University Residence Environment Scale

Another instrument designed by Moos (1988) to assess educational environments is the University Residence Environment Scale (URES).

The social climates or environments assessed by the URES are university student living groups—dormitories, fraternities, sororities, and student cooperatives. The scale consists of 100 items that can be scored on ten subscales: Involvement and Emotional Support are "Relationship" subscales; Independence, Traditional Social Orientation, Competition, Academic Achievement, and Intellectuality are "Personal Growth" subscales; Order and Organization, Student Influence, and Innovation are "System Maintenance and Change" subscales. The test-retest reliabilities are in the .60s and .70s, and the profile stability coefficients average over .90 over one month. Norms for the URES are based on 168 university living groups from 16 colleges and university throughout the United States.

Effective School Battery (ESB)

The ESB (G. D. Gottfredson; Psychological Assessment Resources) is designed to provide a detailed picture of the school environment from the responses of secondary school students and teachers. The Teacher Survey consists of 115 items (12 parts) that can be answered in 30 minutes; a 118-item (4 parts) Student Survey can be answered in 50 minutes. Student and teacher perceptions of school safety, staff morale, administrative leadership, fairness and clarity of school rules, respect for students, classroom orderliness, academic climate, school rewards, and 26 other aspects of school effectiveness are assessed by the ESB.

Evaluating Educational Programs

In addition to assessing student and teacher competencies, tests are often used to evaluate the effectiveness of educational programs, projects, materials, and curricula. Much of the evaluation that goes on in schools is informal, but such procedures lack adequate reliability and validity and hence are of limited value in educational decision making and planning.

Difficulties in measuring change and other technical problems in determining the effectiveness of educational and psychological programs led to the creation of a new professional specialty—*program evaluation* during the 1960s. The goal of program evaluation is to make judgments concerning the utility or value of educational, psychosocial, and other social intervention programs. Before beginning the evaluation of a program, however, a number of who, what, where, when and how questions must be answered: Who will conduct the evaluation, who will be evaluated and where, when, and how? Decisions must also be made concerning how and when the results will be reported and how the political, ethical, and interpersonal issues will be resolved (Worthen, Borg, & White, 1993).

Like all scientific enterprises, formal program evaluation, starts with a question such as:

1. Is student achievement in mathematics classes any different when relevant films are shown as compared with spending an equivalent amount of class time working problems? Do students' attitudes toward mathematics improve more with one instructional method than another?

2. What are the effects of requiring two full years rather than one year of foreign language study on students' knowledge of and interest in other countries and cultures?

3. What are the advantages and disadvantages of increasing the length of the school day by one hour?

4. Is mainstreaming of special students more or less effective than ability grouping in enabling them to reach their cognitive potential?

5. What are the desirable and undesirable effects of distributing birth control information and protective devices to students at school?

Most educational evaluations are conducted by *internal evaluators*—teachers, school administrators, and other personnel—rather than by *external evaluators* who have no vested interest in the institution. Which type of evaluator is better—internal or external—cannot be answered unequivocally. Internal evaluators tend to know more about the particular educational institution, whereas external evaluators are usually less influenced by the political and social climate of the institution and consequently more objective in evaluating the program. In any event, procedures for evaluating educational outcomes should not be designed unilaterally by specialists in psychometrics and research, but in collaboration with educators, human service personnel, health personnel, and other interested professionals. The contributions of measurement specialists, however, are the important ones of recommending and/or designing instruments to evaluate program outcomes. Such evaluation instruments may include standardized tests, rating scales, attitude inventories, checklists, measures of personality and adjustment, and other psychometric devices.

Various models for program evaluation have been proposed, including the CIPP (context, input, process, product) model, discrepancy evaluation, and adversary evaluation. Numerous books and articles have been written on these and other models, but only a brief description of one approach will be given here.

A comprehensive model proposed by Rossi and Freeman (1993) characterizes the overall process of program evaluation in terms of four successive stages: planning, monitoring, impact assessment, and economic efficiency assessment. During the first, or *program planning*, stage, the extent of the problem (for example, drug dealing and use in the schools), the goals, and the target population of the program are identified. After the goals and target population have been specified, a decision is made as to whether the program can be properly implemented. Once a decision has been made to proceed with the program, the *program monitoring* stage begins. During this stage, implementation or operation of the program is continuously monitored to see whether it is providing the designed resources and services to the target population.

At the third, or *impact assessment*, stage, the actual outcomes of the program are evaluated to see if the goals have been met. Various statistical and nonstatistical procedures are applied to determine whether the outcomes are significant and in the predicted direction. Other unintended or unexpected outcomes are also evaluated at the impact-assessment stage, but, even when statistically significant, they may not be of sufficient practical significance. Consequently, it is the purpose of the fourth stage—*economic efficiency assessment*—to determine whether the results of a program are worth the costs incurred in implementing it. This is a matter of cost-benefit analysis, in which the costs of the program are weighed against its potential benefits to the individual and society. For example, even if the program works, it may be that the monetary and other resources required to implement it could be used more effectively elsewhere. When the results of a cost-benefit analysis favor the program, it is a signal to go ahead and put the program in place. But even after the program has been initiated, its effectiveness should be evaluated and reviewed periodically.

Although the various models of program evaluation differ in their details, they all attempt to determine the goals, resources, procedures, and management of a program in order to judge its merit. Indicative of the level of interest in these efforts and public support for them is the existence of centers for research and development in educational evaluation and other types of program evaluation at prominent American universities. The findings of studies conducted at these centers provide a more rational basis for answering questions concerning the processes and outcomes of various types of social programs.

Evaluating Colleges and Universities

Every year millions of students and their parents must decide to which colleges the students should submit applications and which offers of admission to accept. Detailed information on the characteristics and quality of colleges and universities is sought to facilitate those decisions. As stated by R. Miles Uhrig, Director of Admissions at Tufts University, "The public wants *anything* that will rate and compare colleges" (Carmody, 1987, p. 19). A number of organizations (e.g., Gale Research Inc. and *U.S. News & World Report*) are dedicated to providing this information.

The methodology employed in the *Educational Rankings Annual* of Gale Research (Hattendorf, 1995) includes: rankings on institutional reputation based on the opinions of administrators and senior faculty; analysis of citations of the research, writings, and other creative products of institutional scholars; the number of papers and books published by faculty; statistics on endowments, library facilities, selective admissions rates, and other data that are presumed to be indicative of institutional quality.

The most eagerly awaited and widely quoted annual rankings of colleges and universities in the United States are those published yearly in a late September or early October issue of *U.S. News & World Report*. As seen in the column headings in Table 6.2, these rankings are in terms of academic reputation, student selectivity, faculty resources, financial resources, graduation rate, and alumni satisfaction. An overall score based on the rankings in these six areas is also calculated for each institution. For purposes of ranking, the hundreds of American colleges and universities are grouped into five categories: national universities, national liberal arts colleges, regional colleges and universities, regional liberal arts colleges, and specialized institutions. The rankings of the institutions in each group are summarized in tabular form similar to those in Table 6.2 for the top 25 national universities in 1994.

A number of university administrators and faculty have expressed concern that some institutions are "fudging," "cooking," or "massaging" the statistics they provide to *U.S. News and World Report* and publishers of college and university guidebooks. An alternative

TABLE 6.2. The Top 25 National Universities in the United States in 1995

Rank	University	Overall Score	Academic Reputation	Student Selectivity	Faculty Resources	Financial Resources	Graduation Rate Rank	Alumni Satisfaction
1	Harvard University	100.0	1	1	1	5	2	3
2	Princeton University	98.8	4	3	5	14	2	1
2	Yale University	98.8	4	2	10	4	1	6
4	Stanford University	98.1	1	6	3	6	7	38
6	Massachusetts Institute of Technology	98.0	1	4	6	7	10	16
5	Duke University	96.8	8	9	13	11	5	9
7	California Institute of Technology	95.5	8	5	2	1	28	24
7	Dartmouth College	95.5	17	7	18	12	4	7
9	Brown University	95.3	14	7	12	20	6	13
10	Johns Hopkins University	94.6	4	21	15	2	22	10
11	University of Chicago	94.4	8	22	7	9	23	11
11	University of Pennsylvania	94.4	14	14	8	17	17	15
13	Cornell University	94.0	8	11	11	22	12	72
13	Northwestern University	94.0	14	17	4	16	15	49
15	Columbia University	93.8	8	12	14	10	19	57
16	Rice University	93.6	20	10	9	21	18	12
17	Emory University	90.5	32	26	16	15	15	40
18	University of Notre Dame	90.1	36	16	21	53	8	5
19	University of Virginia	89.6	17	18	33	62	9	46
20	Washington University	89.2	26	40	30	3	20	26
21	Georgetown University	88.9	27	15	48	27	11	34
22	Vanderbilt University	88.8	27	30	37	18	32	30
23	Carnegie Mellon University	87.2	20	34	19	18	50	25
24	University of Michigan at Ann Arbor	86.9	8	39	26	42	23	142
25	Tufts University	86.6	49	28	29	31	13	41

Note: Schools with the same numbered rank are tied. Reputational surveys conducted by Market Facts Inc. From *U.S. News & World Report*, September 18, 1995, pp. 126–127. Reprinted by permission.

proposed by Rothkopf (1995) is for each institution to retain an independent accounting firm to examine and certify the accuracy of the information it submits to ranking or rating agencies, as is done with institutional reporting of financial data to the U.S. Office of Education at the end of the year.

SCALES OF DEVELOPMENT AND ADAPTIVE BEHAVIOR

From birth, children are rated on their abilities. A routine procedure for rating newborn babies is the APGAR Scale (see Table 6.3). At one minute after delivery and again five minutes after birth, the newborn infant is given a rating of 0, 1, or 2 on heart rate, respiration, muscle tone, reflexes, and color (Apgar, 1953). The total score ranges from 0 to 10, and 90% of neonates receive a score of 7 or more. When the score is below 7, the baby needs help in breathing; when it is below 4, the baby is in danger and needs immediate life-saving treatment.

A baby does not begin its existence at birth: a great deal of growth and development has already occurred prenatally since the moment of conception. However, it is the postpartum development of children that has been of greatest interest to parents and researchers. This is the period of life when the individual is most frequently evaluated on his or her appearance and behavior, and a period when he or she is presumably most malleable or subject to change.

Systematic studies of human development—the sequence of structural and functional changes that occur as children mature—began

TABLE 6.3. APGAR Scale for Rating Newborn Babies

Sign	Rating		
	0	1	2
Heart rate	Absent	Slow (below 100)	Rapid (over 100)
Respiration	Absent	Irregular, slow	Good, crying
Muscle tone	Limp	Weak, inactive	Strong, active
Reflexes	No response	Grimace	Coughing, sneezing crying
Color	Blue, pale	Body pink, extremities blue	Entirely pink

Source: From "A Proposal for a New Method of Evaluation in the Newborn Infant" by V. Apgar, 1953. *Current Research in Anesthesia and Analgesia, 32,* p. 260.

during the 19th century with the detailed observations and baby biographies of Charles Darwin and other scientists of their own children. During the first part of the 20th century, psychologists and pediatricians devised measures of child development that provided the means for assessing changes in abilities over time. A pioneer in these efforts was Arnold Gesell, whose studies of developmental changes in infancy and early childhood were based on the notion that development follows an orderly maturational sequence. Gesell employed observational, interview, and experimental methods to collect data on the motor, language, and personal-social development and adaptive behavior of children from birth to age six.

Since the 1920s, numerous developmental scales have been published, including the Gesell Developmental Schedules, the Neonatal Behavioral Assessment Scale, and the Bayley Scales of Infant Development.

Bayley-II and FirstSTEP

A recent revision of the last of the above instruments is the Bayley Scales of Infant Development-Second Edition (Bayley-II). In addition to a Mental Scale and a Motor Scale, the Bayley-II contains a Behavior Rating Scale to provide information supplementary to that obtained on the Mental and Motor Scales. The 30-item Behavior Rating Scale is used to rate children (ages 1–42 months) on test taking behavior and provides measures of four functions: Attention/Arousal, Orientation/Engagement, Emotional Regulation, and Motor Quality.

Many other tests of ability, including the time-honored Stanford-Binet Intelligence Scale, are accompanied by rating scales or checklists to evaluate the examinee's behavior during the test. Developmental rating scales and checklists composed of items such as those listed in Table 6.4 assist teachers and parents to monitor the growth and development of their children. By providing a sequential picture of a child's development, a completed checklist can help teachers plan the classroom experiences of their pupils. Criterion-referenced checklists like the one devised by Marsden, Meisels, Steel, and Jablon (1993), as well as Beaty's (1994) and Wortham's (1990) checklists, are good examples. Special-purpose checklists such as the Early Childhood Safety Checklist can also be helpful.

Checklists and ratings are also an integral part of the developmental evaluations provided by more comprehensive instruments such as FirstSTEP. FirstSTEP was designed to assess five developmental

TABLE 6.4. Skills, Behaviors, and Traits Found on Developmental Checklists for Young Children

I. Physical Development
  A. Large Muscle Development
       1. Climbs on climbing equipment
       2. Hops on one foot
       3. Bounces a ball
       4. Catches a ball
       5. Throws a ball
       6. Walks on tip toes
       7. Walks on a balance beam
       8. Jumps from a stool
       9. Skips
       10. Gallops
       11. Claps in time to music
  B. Fine Muscle Development
       1. Fastens buttons
       2. Ties shoelaces
       3. Strings beads
       4. Puts puzzles together
       5. Colors in the lines
       6. Cuts with scissors
       7. Copies letters and shapes
  C. Sensory Development
       1. Recognizes objects drawn on board from across room
       2. Holds book at appropriate distance for reading
       3. Follows pictures in sequence across page with eyes
       4. Responds to oral directions from across the room
  D. General Health
       1. Appears to be well nourished
       2. Remains awake and alert throughout the day
       3. Enters into outdoor play energetically
       4. Attendance records indicate adequate health
II. Language Development
  A. Speech Development
       1. Speaks clearly
       2. Expresses needs adequately
       3. Speaks language of school fluently
       4. Talks about everyday experiences
       5. Answers willingly when spoken to

TABLE 6.4.   *(Continued)*

      6. Modulates voice

      7. Asks questions

   B. Vocabulary Development

      1. Asks about meanings of unfamiliar words

      2. Labels objects and actions correctly

      3. Describes objects in terms of size, shape, color

      4. Uses relationship words appropriately

      5. Uses appropriate category labels

   C. Language Development

      1. Understands language of school

      2. Follows three-part oral directions correctly

      3. Completes sentences with a logical ending

      4. Completes story with a logical ending

      5. Retells a familiar story

      6. Discriminates between words

   D. Written Language

      1. Shows an interest in reading

      2. Attempts to read

      3. Asks about words written around the room

      4. Recognizes own name when written

      5. Attempts to write own name

      6. Dictates a phrase or sentence about an experience

      7. Knows reading progression (left to right, top to bottom)

III. Cognitive Development

   A. Information

      1. Names colors

      2. Names shapes

      3. Names sizes

      4. Knows the five senses

      5. Names body parts

      6. Gives own name

      7. Gives own address

      8. Gives own telephone number

   B. Awareness of Details

      1. Recognizes likenesses and differences of objects

      2. Recognizes likenesses and differences of people

      3. Includes details when drawing a person

(Continued)

TABLE 6.4. *(Continued)*

C. Memory
1. Memorizes names of other children
2. Memorizes songs and rhymes
3. Recites the alphabet
4. Counts to 20

D. Temporal and Spatial Concepts
1. Names days of the week
2. Names seasons of the year
3. Uses today, tomorrow, yesterday correctly
4. Tells time to the hour
5. Tells time to the half-hour
6. Identifies right and left on own body
7. Identifies right and left in space

IV. Social-Emotional Development
A. Intrapersonal Skills
1. Recognizes own property
2. Keeps track of own property
3. Tries new activities
4. Tolerates a reasonable amount of frustration
5. Shows pride
6. Demonstrates responsibility
7. Shows creativity
8. Listens to a story for at least 15 minutes
9. Listens to directions before responding
10. Perseveres for at least 10 minutes on a single task
11. Completes tasks
12. Works alone without distraction
13. Responds positively to change in routine
14. Finds way from school to bus, carpool, or home

B. Interpersonal Skills
1. Plays cooperatively/competitively as appropriate
2. Takes turns
3. Helps children and adults spontaneously
4. Follows adult direction without complaint
5. Leaves parents with little or no reluctance
6. Seeks help when needed
7. Responds appropriately to the emotions of others
8. Shows feelings

TABLE 6.4.   *(Continued)*

      9. Protects self
     10. Takes lead in playing with younger children
     11. Participates in conversations
  C. Hygiene/Self-help
      1. Toilet trained
      2. Dresses self
      3. Tries new food

Source: From "Formal Measures of Early Literacy" by A. C. Stallman and P. D. Pearson. In L. M. Morrow and J. K. Smith (Eds.), *Assessment for Instruction in Early Literacy,* pp. 7–44, 1990. Newton, MA: Allyn & Bacon. Copyright © 1990 by Allyn & Bacon. Reprinted by permission.

domains described in the Individuals with Disabilities Education Act (IDEA, PL-99-457). The first three IDEA domains are Cognition, Communication, and Motor. The fourth domain, assessed by an optional Social-Emotional Rating Scale and a Parent/Teacher Rating Checklist, involves Attention/Activity Levels, Social Interactions, Personal Traits, and Serious Behavior Problems. An optional Adaptive Behavior Checklist is used to assess the fifth IDEA domain, including Activities of Daily Living, Self-Control, Relationships and Interactions, and Functioning in the Community.

Deaf/Blind Children

Few standardized tests are appropriate for measuring the mental abilities of children who are both blind and deaf. Rating scales and checklists like the Callier-Azusa Scale (CAS), which assesses the development of deaf-blind children from birth to nine years in 16 developmental areas (motoric, language, daily living, socialization, etc.), are most often used for this purpose. Items on each of the 16 subtests of the CAS are checked only if "present fully and regularly." When developmental changes related to specific interventions are being evaluated, the CAS is completed by teachers, parents, or other significant persons on two or more occasions.

Other Developmental Checklists and Scales

The above instruments by no means exhaust the list of checklists and scales for assessing a child's developmental status. For example, the School Readiness Checklist and the First Grade Readiness Checklist (both available from Jastak) may be used to assist in determining a child's readiness for school.

There are also many children in school who seem to be developmentally delayed in that they fail to learn and achieve in school as expected, but who have good mental ability, good hearing and vision, and adequate emotional adjustment and motor ability. A useful instrument for identifying such learning-disabled children is the Pupil Rating Scale Revised: Screening for Learning Disabilities (available from The Psychological Corporation). The 24 behaviorally descriptive items, which are rated on five-point scales by the child's teacher, are grouped into five categories: Auditory Comprehension and Memory, Spoken Language, Orientation, Motor Coordination, and Personal-Social Behavior.

Deaf/blind children and others with sensory disorders, as well as those with learning disabilities, fall in the category of "special children." Hyperactive children and autistic children are also "special" in the sense that this term is used. The Conners' Teacher Rating Scale is the instrument of choice in identifying hyperactivity in children. For identifying autistic children, the Behavior Rating Instrument for Autistic & Other Atypical Children (2nd ed.) by B. A. Ruttenberg et al., Stoelting) is recommended. This untimed instrument, can be used with autistic children of all ages and assesses: relationship to an adult, communication, drive for master, vocalization and expressive speech, sound and speech reception, social responsiveness, and psychobiological development.

Finally, as any teacher knows, some children learn more readily through one sensory modality than another. The Learning Channel Preference Checklist (available from Research for Better Schools) may be helpful in identifying the learning style preferences of children. This instrument, which can be used with upper elementary and secondary-school students, is scored on three variables corresponding to three learning "channels": Visual, Auditory, and Haptic.

Adaptive Behavior

Physical disorders are handicaps that can limit effective functioning, but the degree of disability or impairment varies not only with the severity of the particular physical disorder but also with the individual. A person's life may be made more difficult by a physical handicap, but for some people the handicap acts as a challenge that spurs them on to perform at a higher level. Such individuals adapt better than others to a disability, and by compensating (or overcompensating) for the condition they may become even more successful than they might otherwise have been.

In diagnosing mental retardation, the American Association of Mental Deficiency (AAMD) recommends that diagnosticians take into account not only scores on intelligence tests but also academic and vocational attainments, motor skills, and socioemotional maturity. Measures of *adaptive behavior,* which refers to the degree of independent functioning and maintenance of the individual as well as his or her ability to meet cultural demands for personal and social responsibility, are considered essential in diagnosing mental retardation. The concept of adaptive behavior is sometimes viewed as synonymous with *intelligent behavior,* but current practice is to apply the former term to what a person typically does rather than what he or she is capable of doing under optimal conditions. Adults who adapt reasonable well to their environments take reasonable care of their personal needs, perform useful work, and engage in acceptable recreational and other leisure activities. Adaptive behavior in children and adolescents consists of activities that lead to or prepare them for the above activities in adulthood.

Adaptive behavior can be assessed by an informal analysis of a child's history and current behavior or by one of the standardized rating scales and tests listed in Table 6.5. These instruments, the great majority of which can be completed by interviewing a parent, a teacher, or another caregiver who has observed the child closely, cover a wide range of behaviors pertaining to personal and social adjustment.

AAMD Adaptive Behavior Scales

The two instruments in the second edition of this series cover the age range from three years through adulthood. The Adaptive Behavior Scale—Residential and Community, 2nd ed. (ABS-RC:2) evaluates the ability to cope with the social demands of the environment. It was designed to measure adaptivity in institutionalized mentally retarded or developmental disabled adults as well as school children. Among the applications of the ABS-RC:2 are determining strengths and weaknesses among a person's adaptive assets and liabilities, diagnosing developmental disabilities, documenting progress in intervention programs, and measuring adaptive behavior in research studies. Part One of ABS-RC:2 focuses on personal independence (important coping skills for daily living), whereas Part Two deals with social behavior and manifestations of disorders of personality and behavior. Both parts may be completed, in 30 to 40 minutes, by someone who has a personal knowledge

TABLE 6.5. Rating Scales and Checklists for Assessment of
Adaptive Behavior

AAMD Adaptive Behavior Scales—Residential and Community, Second Edition (K. Nihira, H. Leland, & N. Lambert; © 1969, 1974, 1992; ages 3 to adult; PAR.

AAMD Adaptive Behavior Scales—School Edition, Second Edition (N. Lambert, H. Leland, & K. Nihira; © 1969, 1974; 1975, 1992; ages 3 to adult; PAR, Psychological Corporation, & Hawthorne).

Adaptive Behavior Inventory (L. Brown & J. E. Leigh; © 1986; ages 5–18; pro.ed & WPS).

Adaptive Behavior Inventory for Children (J. R. Mercer & J. F. Lewis; © 1982; ages 5–11 years; Psychological Corporation).

Adaptive Behavior Evaluation Scales (S. B. McCarney; ages 6–18; Hawthorne).

Checklist of Adaptive Living Skills (L. E. Morreau & R. H. Bruininks; ages infant to adult; Riverside & DLM).

Children's Adaptive Behavior Scale (R. H. Kicklighter & B. O. Richmond; Stoelting).

Comprehensive Test of Adaptive Behavior (G. L. Adams; © 1984; ages birth to 60 years; Psychological Corporation).

Normative Adaptive Behavior Checklist (G. L. Adams; © 1984; birth to 21 years; Psychological Corporation).

T.M.R. School Competency Scales (S. Levin, F. F. Elzey, P. Thormahlen, & L. F. Cain; ages 5–17; © 1976; CPP).

Vineland Adaptive Behavior Scales (S. S. Sparrow, D. A. Balla, & D. V. Cicchetti; © 1984, 1985; birth to adulthood; AGS).

of the individual being rated or from information obtained by interviewing a close friend or relative. The ABS-RC:2 was standardized on 4,103 developmentally disabled persons. Internal consistency and test-retest reliabilities for Part One and the eight domain scores of Part Two are all over .80.

The AAMD Adaptive Behavior Scale—School, 2nd ed. (ABS-S:2) was designed for children aged 3 to 16 years whose behavior suggests mental retardation, emotional disturbance, or other learning handicaps. The 95-item scale, which is answered by someone with a detailed knowledge of the child's behavior, is divided into two parts covering 21 domains of adaptive behavior grouped into five factors. Personal independence in daily living tasks is evaluated by Part I, and personality and behavior disorders by Part II. The administrative and diagnostic manuals for ABS-S:2 provide percentile norms tables, interpretive information on using the findings for diagnostic and placement purposes, and instructional planning profiles.

Vineland Adaptive Behavior Scales

This 1984 revision of the Vineland Social Maturity Scale comes in three editions: Interview Edition, Survey Form; Interview Edition, Expanded Form; and Classroom Edition. The Survey and Expanded forms assess the adaptive behavior of children from birth to 18 years, 11 months and low-functioning adults. The Classroom Edition is used with children aged 3 years to 12 years, 11 months. Adaptive behavior in four domains—communication, daily living skills, socialization, motor skills—is assessed, with two to three subdomains under each skill. Scores on the four domains are combined to yield an Adaptive Behavior Composite. A fifth domain, Maladaptive Behavior, is assessed by the Survey and Expanded forms of the Vineland.

The Vineland Adaptive Behavior Scales were standardized on a representative national sample of 3,000 children selected according to the 1980 U.S. Census data. Supplementary norms based on samples of mentally retarded, emotionally disturbed, visually handicapped, and hearing-impaired children are also provided. Various types of norms, including standard scores and error bands, percentile ranks, stanines, and age equivalents are provided for each domain. The Expanded Form has the highest reliability and the Classroom Edition the lowest reliability. Computer software (Vineland ASSIST) is available for converting raw scores to norms and for preparing a narrative report of results.

Adaptive Behavior Inventory for Children

Another noteworthy adaptive behavior scale listed in Table 6.5 is the Adaptive Behavior Inventory for Children (ABIC). The ABIC was designed for children aged 5 to 14 years and is available in English or Spanish. The 242 questions concerning the child's behavior are asked in a 45-minute interview with a parent or principal guardian of the child. The inventory is divided into two sections; the first section is applicable to all children, whereas the questions in the second section are graded and administered according to the child's age. The ABIC measures six areas of adaptive behavior: Family, Peers, Community, School, Earner-Consumer, and Self-Maintenance.

The ABIC was standardized on 2,085 children, aged 5 to 12 years and in three ethnic groups, in California public schools. Its reliability appears to be satisfactory, but it has been criticized for failing to take into account the influences of motivational and other non-socioeconomic factors in assessing adaptive behavior. Be that as it may, the ABIC is probably as satisfactory as the AAMD Adaptive Behavior Scales and perhaps even the Vineland Adaptive Behavior Scales as a measure of adaptive behavior in mentally retarded children.

Classroom Behavior and Problems

Just like adults, children have problems, many of which are not readily perceived but must be identified if the child is to function effectively. The use of checklists and scales for clinical purposes is discussed in some detail in Chapter 7, but our interest here is in problems that occur in the schools and affect academic performance. Teachers are among the most important persons in a child's life and are in a unique position to observe their behavior over an extended period of time. Furthermore, teachers have more training in the careful observation of children than most parents and are less likely to be biased in their ratings.[3] Consequently, checklists and rating scales completed by teachers can be useful in identifying factors that influence the child's learning and planning intervention procedures.

A representative list of checklists and rating scales designed specifically for school situations is given in Table 6.6. Several of these instruments will be described in more detail.

Student Referral Checklist

This checklist, which is filled out by teachers, provides a comprehensive review of the problems of school children. The two versions—K–6 and Jr./Sr. High—contain 180 items in 10 areas: Emotions, Self-Concept/Self-Esteem, Peer Relations, School Attitude, Motor Skill/Activity Level, Language and Cognition, Behavior Style, Moral Development, Health and Habits, Addition Problems.

School Behavior Checklist

This instrument is a brief checklist of true-false statements and 11 global judgments describing the child's classroom behavior. Form A1 is for children aged 4 to 6, and Form A2 for children aged 7 to 13. Either form can completed by a teacher in 8 to 10 minutes. Standardized evaluation of the child's classroom behavior can be evaluated in terms of: Need Achievement, Cognitive or Academic Deficit, Aggression, Hostile Isolation, Anxiety, and Extraversion.

TABLE 6.6.   Representative Checklists and Rating Scales for Identifying Problems in School Children

ADD-H: Comprehensive Teacher's Rating Scale, Second Edition (RNA K. Alumna, E. K. Sleator, & R. L. Sprague; MetriTech).

Behavior Dimensions Rating Scale (L. M. Bullock & M. J. Wilson; CPPC).

Behavior Rating Profile (L. Brown & D. D. Hammill; Pro-Ed).

Comprehensive Behavior Rating Scale for Children (R. Neeper, B. B. Lahey, & P. J. Frick; Psychological Corporation)

Conners' Teacher Rating Scale (C. K. Conners; Psychological Corporation).

Devereaux Behavior Rating Scale—School Form (J. A. Naglieri, P. A. LeBuffe, & S. I. Pfeiffer; Psychological Corporation).

Disruptive Behavior Rating Scale (B. T. Erford; Slosson, Stoelting).

Hahnemann Elementary School Behavior Rating Scale (G. Spivack & M. Swift; George Spivak & Marshall Swift).

Hahnemann High School Behavior Rating Scale (G. Spivack & M. Swift; George Spivak & Marshall Swift).

Pre-School Behavior Checklist (J. McGuire & N. Richman; WPS).

School Behavior Checklist (L. C. Miller; WPS).

School Social Skills Rating Scale (L. J. Brown, D. D. Black, & J. C. Downs; Slosson).

Student Referral Checklist (J. A. Schinka; PAR).

Teacher's Report Form (T. M. Achenbach & C. Edelbrock; Thomas M. Achenbach).

Walker Problem Behavior Identification Checklist (H. M. Walker; WPS)

Teacher's Report Form

Designed as a parallel version of the Child Behavior Checklist, the Teacher's Report Form (TRF) is completed by teachers or teacher aides to provide a picture of the problem behaviors, school performance, and adaptive behaviors of elementary school children. The four-page form lists 118 behavior problems or symptoms in the school setting. A three-step response scale (not true, somewhat or sometimes true, very often true) is provided for indicating how often the behavior has occurred in the previous two months. Performance on academic subjects is rated on a five-point scale ("far below grade" through "far above grade"), and four items regarding adaptive behavioral functioning are rated on a seven-point scale ("much less" through "much more"). The TRF was standardized initially on boys aged 6 to 11, but norms for other groups of children have been obtained since then. The teacher's manual for the Second Child Behavior Profile (Edelbrock & Achenbach, 1984) cites reliability and validity data for the TRF, which appear satisfactory for an instrument of this type. For example, the instrument has been shown to discriminate between clinical and nonclinical groups of children, and between children in regular classes versus those in special education. Correlations with observations of children's behaviors are also high (Ebelbrock, 1988).

Devereaux Behavior Rating Scale-School Form

This 40-item rating scale is administered by teachers, parents, or assessment professionals to detect severe emotional disturbances in 5 to 18 year old children. There are two forms: Child (5–12 years), and Adolescent (13–18 years). The scales were designed to identify interpersonal problems, inappropriate behaviors and feelings, depression, and physical symptoms and fears, according to federal criteria. Separate norms by age and sex for both parent and teacher raters are given in the manual.

Conners' Teacher Rating Scales (CTRS)

Perhaps the most widely used rating scale in school settings is the CTRS. It is available in both a 39-item form (CTRS-39) and a 28-item form (CTRS-28), and completed by teachers on children between the ages of 4 and 12 years. CTRS-39 is scored for hyperactivity, conduct problem, emotional overindulgent, anxious-passive, asocial, and day-dream-attendance problems. The norms on CTRS-39, for children aged 4 to 12 years, were obtained in 1969. CTRS-28 can be scored on scales for Conduct Problem, Hyperactivity, and Inattentive-Passivity. Separate norms by gender for children aged 3 to 17 years were obtained on the CTRS-28 in 1978. A fair amount of evidence for the reliability and validity of the CTRS-39 and CTRS-28 scales has been obtained.

SUMMARY

This chapter deals with a variety of topics concerning the use of rating scales and checklists in schools and other educational settings. Evaluation of student performance, including the scoring of ranking items, essays, oral examinations, and performance is discussed first. Numerical scales and weights are used extensively in assigning scores to these criteria of educational achievement.

Quality education demands that not only students but also teachers and administrators be evaluated periodically. Competency testing of in-service teachers is more controversial and less common that testing of education students and candidates for teaching positions. Standardized tests such as the National Teacher Examinations are commonly used as screening devices for pre-service teachers, although test scores may also be used in evaluating teachers for merit pay, recertification, and tenure. Most college and university professors are evaluated by means of student ratings, classroom observations by peers and administrators, and in terms of their research and institutional and community service.

All aspects of the educational environmental are evaluated informally or subjectively by individuals both within and outside the institution. However, rating scales, checklists, and other psychometric instruments are used infrequently in the formal evaluation of the physical and psychosocial components of the educational environment. Textbooks, buildings and grounds, the food service, safety arrangements, and the like may all be rated, but it is not a regular occurrence. In addition, the learning and social environments of an educational institution are accurately evaluated by formal instruments such as the Learning Environment Inventory, the Classroom Environment Scale, and the Effective School Battery. Because it is demanded by public and private funding agencies, the formal evaluation of educational programs and projects is more common. Examples of program evaluation models are CIPP (context, input, process, product) and Rossi and Freeman's four stage model (planning, monitoring, impact assessment, economic efficiency assessment). Colleges and universities are ranked on several criteria by various guidebooks and annually by *U.S. News and World Report.*

Tests and scales for assessing the cognitive, motor, and socioemotional development of children can help identify developmental problems and plan intervention strategies. Two widely used instruments containing rating scales for measuring cognitive and behavioral variables are the Bayley Scales of Infant Development-Second Edition and FirstSTEP. Special rating scales for assessing the abilities of children with sensory handicaps and mentally retarded children are also available. Adaptive behavior scales, which provide information on the level of maturity of a child's behavior, are administered along with tests of general intelligence for diagnosing mental retardation. Among the most popular measures of adaptive behavior are the AAMD Adaptive Behavior Scales, the Vineland Adaptive Behavior Scales, and the Adaptive Behavior Inventory for Children.

Administration of a problem checklist is an efficient method of identifying the multitude of problems that children may have, and the first step in planning treatment or intervention. The discussion of problem checklists and rating scales in this chapter is limited to those instruments that are used in schools to identify school-related problems. Five relevant instruments were described briefly: the School Behavior Checklist, the Student Referral Checklist, the Teacher's Report Form, the Devereaux Elementary School Behavior Rating Scale II, and the Conners' Teacher Rating Scales.

QUESTIONS AND ACTIVITIES

1. Define each of the following terms used in this chapter. Consult Appendix A and/or a dictionary if you need help.

accountability	global (holistic) scoring
adaptive behavior	impact assessment
analytic scoring	intelligent behavior
Cajori method	internal evaluator
classroom climate	performance contracting
cost-benefit analysis	performance evaluation
developmental scales	product scale
economic efficiency	program evaluation
assessment	program monitoring
educational environment	program planning
external evaluator	summative evaluation
formative evaluation	whole-group checklist

2. Construct a checklist or rating scale of teacher behaviors that you consider important for the instructional process. Be certain to phrase the items in terms of objective behaviors, not subjective or abstract characteristics. Now go through and rate each item on a scale of 1 (most important) to 10 (least important) according to how important you believe it to be for a good teacher.

3. Consult the *Reader's Guide,* the *New York Times Index,* and other reference sources for articles in popular magazines and newspapers on minimum competency testing of students and teacher evaluation. Read several of the articles, and then write a paper describing the pros and cons of both kinds of assessment.

4. What are some arguments for and against testing each of the following groups for competency?
   a. high school seniors
   b. college seniors
   c. prospective (pre-service) school teachers
   d. experienced (in-service) school teachers

5. Visit your local school district office and request a meeting with the testing officer or director of research. Ask her (him) for what purposes rating scales and checklists are used in the schools of that district to evaluate students, teachers, administrators, and educational programs.

6. The following are two questions concerning education asked in the 1994 General Social Survey and the corresponding percentages giving the listed response:

   As far as the people running educational institutions in this country are concerned, would you say you have a great deal of confidence, only some confidence, or hardly any confidence at all in them?

Year	Percentage Answering "A great deal"
1987	38%
1990	26%
1994	21%

   Do you think we're spending too much money, too little money or about the right amount of money on education (in this country)?

Year	Percentage Answering "Too little money"
1987	75%
1990	69%
1994	70%

   Interpret these results.

7. Did your mother keep a baby diary on you? If so, consult it, or ask your mother, to determine how many months old you were when you:
   ____ a. Could sit with support (4 months)
   ____ b. Could sit on a lap and grasp an object (5 months)
   ____ c. Could sit in a high chair and grasp a dangling object (6 months)
   ____ d. Could sit alone (7 months)
   ____ e. Could stand with help (8 months)

____ f. Could stand holding furniture (9 months)
____ g. Could creep (10 months)
____ h. Could walk when led (11 months)
____ i. Could pull to stand by furniture (12 months)
____ j. Said your first word (12 months)
____ k. Could climb stair steps (13 months)
____ l. Could stand alone (14 months)
____ m. Could walk alone (15 months)

Compare your data with the norms given in parentheses. If you can't obtained this information on yourself, ask someone you know about the development of her baby.

8. What are the things which a beginning freshman must learn to adapt to in a college environment? Make a list of these things in the form of an Adaptive Checklist for College Life and administer it to several freshmen. Which things on your list posed the greatest problems of adaptation for the respondent? Why?

9. Use computer program C-5 to determine the correlation between each pair of variables in Table 6.2 (academic reputation, student selectivity, faculty resources, financial resources, graduation rate rank, alumni satisfaction). Interpret the results.

10. Administer the following Educational Values Inventory (EVI) to several students of various backgrounds and compute their scores. (*Note:* A computer-based version of the EPI is available as program J-6 on the computer diskette accompanying this book.) Construct and compare the profiles of scores of the students on the six educational values scales. Responses to each item on the EVI are scored on a scale of 1 to 5 from left (U or N) to right (E), respectively. The sum of the scores on items 2, 7, 18, and 21 is the Aesthetic Value score. The sum of the scores on items 1, 8, 13, and 24 is the Leadership Value score. The sum of the scores on items 4, 9, 15, and 23 is the Philosophical Value Score. The sum of the scores on items 5, 12, 16, and 19 is the Social Value score. The sum of the scores on items 6, 11, 17, and 22 is the Scientific Value score. The sum of scores on items 3, 10, 14, and 20 is the Vocational Value score.

Educational Values Inventory

Part I. Each of the items in this section refers to a possible goal or emphasis of higher education. Check the appropriate letter after each of the following statements to indicate how important you believe the corresponding goal should be. Use this key: U = unimportant, S = somewhat important, I = important, V = very important, E = extremely important.

1. Ability to lead or direct other people.   U   S   I   V   E

2. Appreciation of the beautiful and harmonious things in life.   U   S   I   V   E

3. Preparation for a vocation or profession of one's choice.   U   S   I   V   E

4. Gaining insight into the meaning and purpose of life.   U   S   I   V   E

5. Understanding social problems and their possible solutions.   U   S   I   V   E

6. Understanding scientific theories and the laws of nature.   U   S   I   V   E

7. Acquiring the ability to express oneself artistically.   U   S   I   V   E

8. Understanding how to direct others in the accomplishment of some goal.   U   S   I   V   E

9. Development of a personal philosophy of life.   U   S   I   V   E

10. Learning how to succeed in a chosen occupation or field.   U   S   I   V   E

11. Learning about scientific problems and their solutions.   U   S   I   V   E

12. Understanding people of different social classes and cultures.   U   S   I   V   E

Part II. Check the appropriate letter after each of the following items to indicate your estimate of how valuable the particular kinds of college courses are to students in general. Use this key: N = not at all valuable, S = somewhat valuable, V = valuable, Q = quite valuable, E = extremely valuable.

13. Courses concerned with how to direct
and organize people.   N S V Q E

14. Courses in one's chosen vocation or
professional field.   N S V Q E

15. Courses dealing with philosophical
and/or religious ideas.   N S V Q E

16. Courses concerned with understanding
and helping people.   N S V Q E

17. Courses in science and mathematics.   N S V Q E

18. Courses in music, art, and literature.   N S V Q E

Part III. Check the appropriate letter after each of the following items to indicate how much attention you feel should be given to each kind of college course in the education of most college students. Use this key: N = no attention at all, L = little attention, M = a moderate degree of attention, A = above average attention, E = an extensive amount of attention.

19. Courses concerned with how to understand
and be of help to other people.   N L M A E

20. Courses in the vocational or professional
field of your choice.   N L M A E

21. Courses in art, literature, and music.   N L M A E

22. Courses in scientific and mathematical fields. N L M A E

23. Courses concerned with philosophy
and religion.   N L M A E

24. Courses concerned with organizing and
directing people.   N L M A E

7

Personality and Clinical Assessment

The study of personality is concerned with the individuality or uniqueness of the ways in which people typically behave. The behavior pattern or "style" that characterizes a given personality is more or less organized and fairly consistent. During infancy, behavior is highly stimulus-dependent and exploratory, but it becomes governed more by memories and habits as the person matures and gains experience. This relatively consistent repertoire of behaviors—ways of coping with reality to satisfy one's needs—constitutes the personality of the individual.

Psychologists who investigate the structure, dynamics, origins, development, and aberrations of personality typically begin with certain preconceptions about these things. These preconceptions may take the form of theoretical propositions or they may simply be judgments or biases based on limited personal experience. Whatever the sources of their ideas or hypotheses concerning what human personality is and how it works, personality researchers should be aware of the fact that the findings are greatly dependent on the instruments they design or select to assess the variables in which they are interested. Some of the available instruments focus on "normal" personality, whereas others are more concerned with serious behavioral or cognitive disorders. This chapter considers both types of instruments—measures of normal and abnormal behavior—and a number of variables or constructs in each domain.

HISTORY AND THEORIES

Many writers and scientists in ancient times were interested in the origins and nature of individual differences. The ancient Greeks, including dramatists such as Sophocles, Aeschylus, and Euripides and philosophers such as Plato, Aristotle, and Theophrastus, provided interested descriptions of personalities. Several hundred years later, the Roman physician Galen proposed that there was a link between body secretions ("humors") and personality: persons with an excess of yellow bile were characterized as "choleric," those with an excess of black bile were "melancholic," those with an excess of blood were "sanguine," and those with an excess of phlegm were "phlegmatic."

Little empirical study of personality occurred before the 19th century, although many famous writers evinced a keen understanding of individual characteristics and "quirks." Playwrights and novelists such as William Shakespeare and Migel de Cervantes, in particular, were noted for their observations and descriptions of personality "types." Nineteenth-century novelists, such as Charles Dickens, Leo Tolstoy, and Henri Balzac, continued the tradition of character description in their stories, albeit in a deeper, more morose vein in many instances.

Psychoanalysis

The depths of the human psyche that novelists of the late 19th and early 20th centuries attempted to plumb were examined more systematically and scientifically in the researches of the French psychiatrists (Charcot, Janet, etc.) and Sigmund Freud. Freud's psychoanalytic theory was the first comprehensive, dynamic explanation of personality, and his analyses and interpretations have served as a backdrop for almost every other theory of personality since his time. Psychoanalytic theory is based on several propositions—the concept of the unconscious, the idea of psychic determinism and conflict (between id, ego, and superego), and the notion of psychosexual stages in development. To Freud, personality was shaped by an interplay of fantasy and reality—by a compromise between what we desire and what we can acquire or attain. Furthermore, Freud maintained that people are usually not even aware of most of what goes on in their minds: Much of what they do, say, or dream about is determined by events occurring below the level of awareness and therefore beyond conscious control.

Body Type Theories

One conception of personality that was not influenced by psychoanalysis was that body build is related to temperament. As mentioned above, Galen believed that bodily secretions ("humors") were related to personality. Furthermore, writers since Shakespeare time and before had thought of personality as being related to appearance and mannerisms. Another attempt to find a physical basis for personality characteristics is represented by the work of the phrenologists. The 19th-century phrenologists tried to relate both personality and mental disorders to bumps on the skull. Systematic research on personality and body build began, however, with the work of Ernest Kretchsmer on the relationships of the asthenic (tall, thin, lanky, angular) build to withdrawing or introverted tendencies (schizoid temperament) and the pyknic (rotund, stocky) build to emotional instability (cycloid temperament). Kretschmer believed that persons having an asthenic build were more likely to become schizophrenia, while those with a pyknic build were more likely to develop bipolar (manic-depressive) disorder. Another body typologist, the criminologist Cesare Lombroso, believed that criminals were more likely to have certain physical characteristic (large jaws, receding foreheads, and other primitive traits) that place them at a lower stage of development than noncriminals; hence, one might say they were born to be criminals.

William Sheldon and S. S. Stevens (1942; Sheldon, Stevens, & Tucker, 1940) also proposed a typological theory. In their *somatotype* system, human physiques are rated on a scale of 1 to 7 according to the degree of endomorphy (fatness), mesomorphy (muscularity), and ectomorphy (thinness). A 7-1-1 types is an extreme endomorph, a 1-7-1 is an extreme mesomorphy, and a 1-1-7 is an extreme ectomorphy. Each of the three components was determined from measurements taken from photographs of the standing person taken at various angles.

Sheldon and Stevens found that an excess of any of the three components of body build was related to a particular temperament. Continuing their research, they used questionnaires and observations to evaluate people on 20 trait dimensions. These evaluations were then used to rate an individual, on a 7-point scale, on each of three temperament dimensions: viscerotonia, somatotonia, and cerebrotonia. *Viscerontonics* are jolly, sociable, and loving comfort and eating. *Somatotonics* are assertive, dominating, noisy, callous, have a youthful orientation, and love physical adventure and exercise. *Cerebrotonics* are restrained, fast-reacting, introversive, hypersensitive to pain, have difficulty sleeping, and are oriented toward later periods of life.[1] The degree of endomorphy was found to be moderately related to the viscerotonic rating, the degree of mesomorphy moderately related to the somatotonic rating, and the degree of ectomorphy moderately related to the cerebrotonic rating. The somatotype theory of Sheldon and Stevens is interesting, but there are many exceptions to the hypothesized relationships of body build to personality. Consequently, the scientific status of this theory and other body-type theories of personality is not very high.

Trait Theories

Another influential conceptualization of personality is Carl Jung's theory that inclinations in feelings and behavior are describable in terms of four bipolar types: Introversion-Extraversion, Sensing-Intuition, Thinking-Feeling, and Judging Perceptive. This is the theory underlying the development of the Myers-Briggs Type Indicator (Consulting Psychologists Press).

More common than type theories, and more influential in the development of personality assessment instruments than either psychoanalytic or type theories, are trait theories of personality. Trait theorists view human personality as a combination of traits—cognitive, affective, or psychomotor characteristics possessed in different amounts by different people. Two of the most prominent trait theorists were Gordon Allport and Henry Murray.

Allport viewed human personality as a dynamic organization of traits that determines a person's unique adjustment to the environment. Most general of all traits in terms of their influence on behavior across situations are *cardinal traits,* such as Machiavellianism and narcissism. The next most pervasive are *central traits,* such as sociableness and affectionateness, and next are *secondary traits,* such as preferences for types of foods or music. Allport also differentiated among traits in terms of the extent to which they are shared by different people; there are, in order, common traits, individual traits, and personality dispositions.

A second trait theory, which played a greater role in the development of personality assessment instruments than Allport's theory, was Henry Murray's personological theory. Murray maintained that human beings are driven to reduce tensions generated by forces that are internal *(needs)* and external *(press)* to the person. Behavior is a function of both needs, which may be physiogenic or psychogenic, and press, which may be alpha (objective, from the environment) or beta (perceived). Although the assessment instrument for which Murray is best known is the Thematic Apperception Test, in the context of this book, we are more interested in the influence of the theory in the development of the Adjective Check List.

Trait/factor theories of personality have guided the development of many personality scales and inventories. An example of a theory that has been closely tied to instrument development is Hans Eysenck's conceptualization of personality in terms of three basic factors—extraversion-introversion, neuroticism (emotionality), and psychoticism. Currently, there is a great deal of interest in a *five-factor model* of personality. These five factors, which appear to be highly consistent across various groups of people in different situations, are defined by Costa and McCrae (1986) as follows:

- *Neuroticism*—worrying vs. calm, insecure vs. secure, self-pitying vs. self-satisfied;
- *Extraversion*—sociable vs. retiring, fun-loving vs. sober, affectionate vs. reserved;
- *Openness*—imaginative vs. down to earth, preference for variety vs. preference for routine, independent vs. conforming;
- *Agreeableness*—soft-hearted vs. ruthless, trusting vs. suspicious, helpful vs. uncooperative;
- *Conscientiousness*—well-organized vs. disorganized, careful vs. careless, self-disciplined vs. weak willed.

Several standardized measures of these five factors are available (e.g., the NEO-PI-R and the NEO-FFI), but the rating scales in program I-4 of the computer program diskette for this book can be used for a preliminary assessment of personality in terms of the five factors.

Self Theory

The concept of the *self* has played an important role not only in psychology but also in philosophy and religion. Two psychologists who made the self and its experiences the center of their theories of personality were Abraham Maslow and Carl Rogers. Both theories are in the tradition of the philosophical school known as phenomenology, which emphasizes the role of personal experience in determining what is real for the individual. Phenomenologists make a distinction between the real world—that which objectively exists—and the phenomenal world—the world as experienced by the observer. To the self-theorist, a part of the *phenomenal world* of the person becomes differentiated with experience into those things that relate to the person's body, influence, and other qualities concerned with the identity, individuality or ego; this is the *self.* The perceptions, ideas, and beliefs that a person has concerning his or her self constitute the *self-concept.*

To both Maslow and Rogers, the individual strives to attain a state of *self-actualization*—a congruence or state of harmony between the real and ideal selves. The basic direction of a person's existence is toward self-actualization and pleasant relations with other people, but that effort can be inhibited in various ways. Rogers pointed out that most people are not open to or willing to accept the full range of their experiences. In the process of maturing they learn that they are objects of *conditional positive regard* in that their parents and other people accept them only if their behavior conforms to expected standards *(conditions of worth).* As a consequence, the child learns to recognize and accept only a part of his or her experiences and cannot become totally functioning unless unconditional positive regard is received from others.

Although Rogers made little use of psychological tests or scales in his work with patients, a number of psychometric measures of self-concept and self-esteem have been constructed. Among these are the Tennessee Self-Concept Scale, the Piers-Harris Self-Concept Scale, and the Coopersmith Self-Esteem Inventories. Only the first of these instruments will be described here.

The Tennessee Self-Concept Scale (W. H. Fitts, Western Psychological Services) consists of 100 self-descriptive statements to be answered on a five-point scale ranging from "completely false" to "completely true." It is written at a sixth-grade reading level and can be administered in 10 to 20 minutes to individuals aged 12 years and over. There are two forms: a Counseling Form scored on 14 variables and a Clinical and Research Form scored on the same 14 variables plus 15 other scores. The 14 variables are self-criticism, 9 self-esteem scores (identity, self-satisfaction, behavior, physical self, moral-ethical self, personal self, family self, social self, total), and 3 variability-of-response measures. The Tennessee Self-Concept Scale is the most widely administered of all measures of self-concept in counseling and research contexts. Unfortunately, the reliability and validity of the instrument leave much to be desired (Walsh, 1984).

Program I-2 on the computer program diskette accompany this book presents a series of 20 self-descriptive adjectives twice. The respondent begins by ranking the 20 adjectives in terms of how descriptive they are of his or her real self. Then they are ranked a second time in terms of how descriptive they are of his or her ideal self. A percentage agreement score between the real and ideal self rankings is a measure of the congruence between the respondent's real and ideal selves.

The similarity between perceptions of one's "real" and "ideal" selves is not the only possible index of adjustment. For example, even when there is a large discrepancy between the real and ideal selves, one may not be greatly dissatisfied if everyone else is in the "same boat." Happiness is not just a matter of getting what one wants but also whether what one has is equitable with what other people have—the so-called "principle of relative deprivation." With regard to personality, one may not paint a very flattering picture of his or her personality, but it may be easier to bear if other people are perceived to be pretty much like oneself. This degree of "similarity" between the "real" and "other" selves may be assessed by the checklist in program I-3. The respondent indicates whether each of 25 adjectives is descriptive of him (her) personally and whether it is descriptive of people in general in the respondent's chronological age and sex group. Responses are scored in terms of the number of agreements between "self" and "other" response and the percentage of total possible agreements between the "self" and "other" responses.

OBSERVATIONS AND INTERVIEWS

Various procedures are used in the assessment of personality—observations, interviews, checklists, rating scales, personality inventories, and projective techniques. Here we are interested primarily in ratings scales and checklists, but these devices are often used in connection with objective observations and interviews.

As noted in Chapter 1, observations may be controlled or uncontrolled, depending on whether they are prearranged and contrived or simply unplanned observations of ongoing behavior. To be valid, observations should be objective and unobtrusive. However, in *participant observation* the observer is a participant in the observed situation rather than remaining uninvolved on the sidelines. In the type of controlled observation known as *situational testing*, the persons to be observed are placed in a prearranged, realistic situation to see how they cope or solve certain problems.

Checklists and rating scales are frequent accompaniers of controlled observations, serving as efficient, objective methods of recording what is seen and heard. An example of such an instrument for behavioral observations of anxiety is the checklist in Figure 7.1. This checklist can be used repeatedly to assess the effects of a drug or any intervention procedure on the incidence of specific behaviors indicative of anxiety.

An interesting and efficient method for obtaining information on a person's thoughts, feelings, and behaviors is *self-observation*. Here the person keeps a written record of his or her activities and thoughts for later analysis and interpretation. The *content analysis* of a diary, an autobiography, a letter or other records involving self-observations is a complex process but can provide important insights into personality and behavior.

Behavior Modification

Behavior modification constitutes a set of psychotherapeutic procedures based on learning theory and research and designed to change inappropriate behavior to more personally and/or socially acceptable behavior. Among the maladaptive behaviors that have been modified by these procedures are specific fears (or phobias), smoking, overeating, alcoholism, drug addiction, underassertiveness, bedwetting, chronic tension and pain, and sexual inadequacies of various kinds. The behaviors to be modified must be defined precisely and occur with sufficient frequency to be recordable and modifiable. Such behaviors have typically been rather narrowly defined, but behavior therapists of a more cognitive orientation have also been successful in dealing with less specific problems such as a negative self-concept or an identity crisis.

Behavior therapists try to understand behavior by examining not only its antecedents, which include both the social learning history and current environment of the person, but also the results or consequences of the behavior. A basic tenet of this approach is that behavior is controlled by its consequences. This implies that, in designing a procedure for modifying undesirable behavior, both the reinforcing consequences that sustain the behavior and the conditions that precede and trigger it must be identified. The antecedents and consequences of the target behavior may be either overt, objectively observable conditions, or covert mental events.

Behavior Observed   Time Period

	1	2	3	4	5	6	7	8
1. Paces								
2. Sways								
3. Shuffles feet								
4. Knees tremble								
5. Extraneous arm & hand movement (swings, scratches, toys, etc.)								
6. Arms rigid								
7. Hands restrained (in pockets, behind back, clasped)								
8. Hand tremors								
9. No eye contact								
10. Face muscles tense (drawn, tics grimaces)								
11. Face "deadpan"								
12. Face pale								
13. Face flushed (blushes)								
14. Moistens lips								
15. Swallows								
16. Clears throat								
17. Breathes heavily								
18. Perspires (face, hands, armpits)								
19. Voice quivers								
20. Speech blocks or stammers								

Figure 7.1. A behavioral checklist for performance anxiety. Reprinted from *Insight vs. Desensitization in Psychotherapy* by Gordon L. Paul, 1966, p. 109, with the permission of the publishers, Stanford University Press. © 1966 by the Board of Trustees of the Leland Stanford Junior University.

Various procedures, including observations, interviews, checklists, rating scales, and questionnaires completed by the patient and/or a person who is closely connected with the patient, are used to analyze or assess the antecedents and consequences of specific behaviors. The observational procedures include taking note of the frequency and duration of the target behaviors and the particular contingencies (antecedents and consequences) of their occurrence. Such information can be recorded by teachers, parents, nurses, nursing assistants, or anyone who is acquainted with the patient. The diagnoses of psychopathology, for example, can be facilitated by recorded observations made by nurses and psychiatric aids of a patient's behavior on a hospital ward. Rating scales such as the Nurses' Observation Scale for Inpatient Evaluation (NOSIE-30) (Honigfeld & Klett, 1965) and the Ward Behavior Inventory (Burdock, Hardesty, Hakarem, Zubin, & Beck, 1968) are useful devices for assessing patients' aggressive, communicative, and cooperative behaviors as well as other behaviors and appearance.

Several other procedures for behavioral assessment have been proposed (see Ciminero, Calhoun, & Adams, 1986; Haynes, 1990; Haynes & Wilson, 1979; Hersen & Bellack, 1982; Kendall & Korgeski, 1979; Ollendick & Green, 1990). Many questionnaires, checklists, and inventories, some of which are commercially available, may be employed. Examples are the Forms for Behavior Analysis with Children (Research Press). There is, however, no standard, recommended battery of assessment instruments for this purpose.

Self-observation for purposes of behavior analysis and modification involves having patients carry with them at all times materials such as index cards, a notepad, a wrist counter, and a timer. The patients are instructed to use these materials to record occurrences of specified behaviors and the time, place, and circumstances of their occurrence. Self-observation, sometimes referred to as *self-monitoring*, can be fairly reliable when the patient is carefully trained.

Interviews

Next to observation, interviewing is the oldest and most popular of all personality assessment methods. Even when personality tests and other psychometric devices are used, a personal interview is almost always conducted to confirm and expand the findings. Intake, diagnostic, and exit interviews in clinical situations have both structured and unstructured features and must be conducted by a person who is well-trained in interviewing techniques. The interviewer should be friendly but neutral, interested but not prying in reacting to the interviewee. Recognizing that the purpose of the interview is to understand the patient, the characteristics and causes of his or her problems, and what might be done about them, in most instances interviewers try to minimize the threat of the interview and the stress placed on the interviewee. An exception to this practice occurs in the case of a *stress interview,* in which the interviewer attempts to break down the interviewee's resistance or defensiveness by asking direct, pointed questions.

The particular approach and the questions asked vary with the purposes of the interview and the characteristics of the interviewee. Survey and polling interviews conducted in person or over the telephone are typically highly structured. On the other hand, obtaining in-depth information on personality and behavior for research or clinical purposes requires a more open-ended approach and a face-to-face format. Among the various kinds of clinical interviews are intake, diagnostic, therapeutic, and exit. *Intake interviews* of patients and their relatives are essential for obtaining case histories for medical and/or psychological diagnoses. *Diagnostic interviews* are designed to determine the causes and correlates of a person's problems. *Therapeutic interviews* (counseling, psychotherapy) constitute part of the psychological treatment process. *Exit interviews* are designed to determine whether a patient (or inmate) is ready for release.

A diagnostic or therapeutic interview can provide a great deal of information about a person, including:

- The nature, duration, and severity of the patient's problems, and how the problems are manifested,
- What past influences are related to the patient's current difficulties,
- The resources and limitations of the patient for coping with the problems,
- The kinds of psychological assistance the patient has had in the past, and
- What kinds of assistance the patient expects and might be of help now.

A checklist or rating scale may be used to obtain some of this information, but a personal interview is necessary for eliciting comprehensive, in-depth answers and details.

In certain instances, diagnostic interviewing can be made less difficult by using a standard form such as the Psychiatric Diagnostic Interview—Revised (PDI-R) (E. Othmer et al., Western Psychological Services) or the Structured Clinical Interview for DSM-III-R (Spitzer, Williams, Gibbon, & First, 1992). The last instrument consists of 170 items on which the interviewer checks 1 (Yes) or 2 (No) according to the observed behavior or answers of the interviewee. On some structured interview forms, the patient checks his or her symptoms or problems and rates their severity.

A special type of diagnostic interview known as a *mental status interview* is used to determine the mental competence of a person for legal and psychiatric purposes. A mental status interview is designed to yield in-depth information concerning the person's emotional state, intellectual and perceptual functioning, style and content of thought processes and speech, level of insight into mental status and personality problems, psychomotor activity, general appearance, attitude, and insight into his or her condition. The process of obtaining this information is facilitated by an interview and observation schedule such as the Schedule for Affective Disorders and Schizophrenia (Endicott & Spitzer, 1978). Each of the three forms of SADS—regular, lifetime version, and a version for measuring change—is composed of a structured interview guide and a rating form. Each form has two parts. Part 1 consists of a series of open-ended questions and rating scales pertaining to the occurrence and severity (on a scale of 0 to 6) of certain symptoms during the preceding week. Part 2, which consists of a series of checklists to be answered Yes, No, or No information, focuses mainly on information about the patient's history of psychiatric disturbances. SADS has been used in numerous psychiatric research investigations, and it provides diagnostic information consistent with the categories of the *Diagnostic and Statistical Manual* (DSM-III and DSM-III-R).

A mental status interview or other type of diagnostic interview can also be automated by storing a set of questions and instructions in a computer. The computer asks a question, receives an answer, and "decides" (conditionally branches) what question to ask next. Examples of computer software packages available for psychodiagnostic interviewing are the Diagnostic Interview for Children and Adolescents (from Multi-Health Systems), the Giannetti On-Line Psychosocial History (Giannetti, 1987; from National Computer Systems), and the Quickview Social History (from National Computer Systems). Computer interviewing is objective, efficient, and reliable, but it has limited utility in crisis cases and with children or adults of low mentality.

Furthermore, because only structured interviews can be conducted, computer-based interviewing is not as flexible as a typical unstructured clinical interview.

STANDARDIZED CHECKLISTS FOR PERSONALITY RESEARCH AND CLINICAL DIAGNOSIS

The findings of a lengthy observational session or a comprehensive, in-depth interview can be simplified and summarized to some extent by a properly constructed checklist or rating scale. Many standardized interview and observation instruments involve checking or rating observed characteristics, behaviors, or symptoms and hence consist in part of checklists and rating scales.

The major advantage of checklists and rating scales over interviews and observations are efficiency, objectivity, and comprehensiveness. These instruments can be administered to the individual himself (herself), as well as parents, teachers, and other interested persons to obtain multiple viewpoints. And because of their efficiency, many more questions or items, covering a wide range of problems and characteristics, can be presented.

Despite the ease with which they can be constructed, checklists for personality characteristics and clinical symptoms are usually fairly reliable. Many checklists are neither standardized nor commercially available, having been designed for specific investigations or other uses. An example is the Social Readjustment Scale, which was devised to test the theory that the stress of change, which requires behavioral and physiological readjustment, increases a person's susceptibility to disease (Holmes & Rahe, 1967). The magnitude of the increased susceptibility varies with the extent of the readjustment necessitated by the change. The events on the scale are scaled from 0 to 100, depending on the degree of readjustment required. According to the theory, the greater the degree of readjustment required in a given year, the greater the person's chances of developing a stress-related illness. Program I-7 on the diskette of computer programs accompanying this book presents and scores the Social Readjustment Scale.

Many standardized checklists are also designed for a specific purpose or to assess a specific characteristic, symptom, or group of people. In Chapter 6, we described several checklists for assessing adaptive behavior, school difficulties, learning disabilities, and other problems in children. Other standardized checklists have been constructed to

TABLE 7.1.   Representative Checklists for Personality and
Clinical Evaluations

Adjective Checklists

Adjective Check List (H. G. Gough & A. B. Heilbrun; CPP)

Multiple Affect Adjective Check List—Revised (M. Zuckerman & B. Lubin, EdITS)

Personality Adjective Checklist (21st Century Assessment)

Clinical Symptoms

Checklist for Child Abuse Evaluation (J. Petty, PAR)

Derogatis Symptom Checklist Series (L. R. Derogatis; NCS Assessments)

Hare Psychopathy Checklist-Revised (Multi-Health Systems)

Mental Status Checklist Series—Adolescent & Adult (J. A. Schinka, PAR)

Missouri Children's Behavior Checklist (Sines, Pauker, Sines, & Owen, 1969)

Symptom Checklist-90-Revised (SCL-90-R) (L. R. Derogatis; NCS Assessments)

Marital Evaluation

Marital Evaluation Checklist (L. Navran; PAR)

Personal History

Personal History Checklists—Adolescent and Adult (J. A. Schinka; PAR)

Problem Checklists

Child Behavior Checklist (T. M. Achenbach & C. Edelbrock; Thomas M. Achenbach)

Kohn Problem Checklist (J. Kohn; Psychological Corporation)

Mooney Problem Check Lists (R. L. Mooney & L. V. Gordon; Psychological Corporation)

Personal Problems Checklists—Children's, Adolescent, Adult (J. A. Schinka; PAR, Jastak)

Portland Problem Behavior Checklist—Revised (S. A. Waksman; PAR)

Problem Experiences Checklist (L. Silverton, WPS)

Revised Behavior Problem Checklist (H. C. Quay & D. R. Peterson; PAR)

evaluate marital or interpersonal relations, neuropsychological disorders, sexual desires and activities, depression, anxiety, hostility, and other behaviors, characteristics, or symptoms. The titles of a representative sample of these instruments are listed in Table 7.1.

Adjective Checklists

Several widely administered checklists for research on personality and the determination of personality adjustment difficulties consist of a list of adjectives. Two popular instruments of this type are the Adjective Check List and the Multiple Affect Adjective Check List. Both are omnibus or broad-band checklists, in that they can be scored on a number of variables rather than being restricted to a single variable such as anxiety, depression, or hostility.

The Adjective Check List (ACL)

The Adjective Check List (H. G. Gough & A. B. Heilbrun, Consulting Psychologists Press) consists of 300 adjectives, arranged alphabetically from *absentminded* to *zany*. It takes 15 to 20 minutes to mark those adjectives which respondents view as self-descriptive. Their responses can then be scored on 37 scales: 4 modus operandi scales, 15 need scales, 9 topical scales, 5 transactional analysis scales, and 4 origence-intellectence (creativity and intelligence) scales. Scores on the modus operandi scales (total number of adjectives checked, number of favorable adjectives checked, number of unfavorable adjectives checked, communality) pertain to the manner in which the respondent has dealt with the checklist. The need scales (scales 5–19) are based on Edwards's (1954) descriptions of 15 needs in Murray's (1938) need-press theory of personality. Each of the topical scales (scales 20–28) assesses a different topic or component of interpersonal behavior (counseling readiness, personal adjustment, creative personality, masculine attributes, etc.). The transactional analysis scales (scales 29–33) are measures of the five ego functions in Berne's (1966) transactional analysis theory. The origence-intellectence scales (scales 34–37) are measures of Welsh's origence-intellectence (creativity and intelligence) dimensions of personality.

The tendency for some people to check more items than other people, no matter whom or what they are evaluating—the so-called *frequency response set*—must be handled in some way on an adjective checklist. In scoring the Adjective Check List this is taken into account by separate norms tables for groups endorsing different numbers of items. Raw scores on the ACL scales may be converted to standard T scores for purposes of interpretation and counseling. To illustrate, the 37 T scores and the associated profile of the case described in Box 7.1 are given in Table 7.2. The T scores are interpreted with reference to norms, based on 5,238 males and 4,144 females. Profiles and associated interpretations for six sample cases, one of which is summarized in Box 7.1, are also provided. As listed in the 1983 manual, the test-retest reliability coefficients of the separate scales range from .34 for the

TABLE 7.2.   Scales and Sample T Scores on the Adjective Check List

Scale Name and Designation	T Scores for Case in Box 7.1
Modus Operandi	
1 Total number of adjectives checked (No Ckd)	37
2 Number of favorable adjectives checked	62
3 Number of unfavorable adjectives checked (Unfav)	59
4 Communality (Com)	68
Need Scales	
5 Achievement (Ach)	57
6 Dominance (Dom)	50
7 Endurance (End)	53
8 Order (Ord)	57
9 Intraception (Int)	57
10 Nurturance (Nur)	44
11 Affiliation (Aff)	53
12 Heterosexuality (Het)	46
13 Exhibition (Exh)	44
14 Autonomy (Aut)	49
15 Aggression (Agg)	58
16 Change (Cha)	58
17 Succorance (Suc)	41
18 Abasement (Aba)	56
19 Deference (Def)	49
Topical Scales	
20 Counseling Readiness (Crs)	55
21 Self-control (S-Cn)	48
22 Self-Confidence (S-Cfd)	59
23 Personal Adjustment (P-Adj)	53
24 Ideal Self (Iss)	64
25 Creative Personality (Cps)	63
26 Military Leadership (Mls)	52
27 Masculine Attributes (Mas)	54
28 Feminine Attributes (Fem)	69
Transactional Analysis	
29 Critical Parent (CP)	62
30 Nurturing Parent (NP)	48
31 Adult (A)	56
32 Free Child (FC)	46
33 Adapted Child (AC)	41
Origence-Intellectence	
34 High Origence, Low Intellectence (A-1)	47
35 High Origence, High Intellectence (A-2)	64
36 Low Origence, Low Intellectence (A-3)	44
37 Low Origence, High Intellectence (A-4)	63

Box 7.1
Case Description Accompanying Adjective Check List
Scores in Table 7.2

This 19-year-old undergraduate student majoring in biology maintained an A- grade average and planned to go to graduate school. She was brought up in a close-knit, large family, and had warm feelings about her parents and her childhood. Before college, she had always lived in small towns or semirural areas. Coming to an urban college required quite an adjustment, but she liked the excitement and stimulation of city life. She retained her religious beliefs and regularly attended church. She viewed herself as a political and economic conservative. Her life-history interviewer described her in the following way:

> She is an intelligent, vivacious, attractive young woman, enthusiastic about her life at the university. Although she views herself as introverted, her behavior is more extroverted; she was talkative, outgoing, candid, and not hesitant to assume a leadership role. Her parents were strict, expected the children to assume responsibilities, and placed a high value on academic achievement. She described her mother as a demanding, extremely shy woman who participated in social activities from a sense of duty. She said her father was somewhat intimidating, but affectionate; she feels closer to him now than she did when she was growing up. Being at school—away from home and the relative isolation of that environment—is very exciting.

Scores on her ACL profile are in agreement with the case history data and staff evaluations. Moderate elevations occur on the scales for Achievement, Self-confidence, and Personal Adjustment, and scores of 60 or greater on the scales for Ideal Self, Creative Personality, and A-2 (high origence, high intellectence). The ACL profile also revealed scores of 60 or greater on the scales for Favorable, Communality, Femininity, Critical Parent, and A-4 (low origence, high intellectence. Although the staff rating of 54 on Femininity was above average for the sample of 80 students included in this project, it is not as high as the score of 69 on her self-descriptive ACL. Because she had scores greater than 50 on both Masculinity and Femininity, she is in the androgynous cell in the interaction diagram between the two scales. The profile also reveals elevated scores on *both* Favorable and Unfavorable, which suggests she is more complex, internally differentiated, and less repressive than her peers.

High-Origence/Low-Intellectence scale to .77 for the Aggression scale (median of .65). The internal consistency reliability coefficients of the majority of the 37 scales are reasonably high. The ACL scales are significantly intercorrelated, and therefore should not be interpreted as independent factors. A factor analysis conducted by the author on the 15 need scales (scales 5–19) revealed three factors: Self-Confidence or Ego Strength, Goal Orientation, and Social Interactivity or Friendliness.

Despite the seeming simplicity of the instrument and the low to modest reliabilities of the scales, reviews of the Adjective Check List have been fairly positive (Teeter, 1985; Zarske, 1985). The instrument is well-developed and has been particularly useful in studies of self-concept. It has been used principally with normal people, but its validity in psychodiagnosis and treatment planning has not been determined.

Multiple Affect Adjective Check List-Revised (MAACL-R)

The MAACL-R (M. Zuckerman & B. Lubin, EdITS) consists of 132 adjectives descriptive of personal feelings; respondents check those adjectives that indicate how they generally feel (on the trait form) or how they feel today or at present (on the state form). Standard T scores on both the trait and state forms are obtained on five basic scales: Anxiety (A), Depression (D), Hostility (H), Positive Affect (PA), and Sensation Seeking (SS). Two summary standard scores—Dysphoria (Dys = A + D + H) and Positive Affect and Sensation Seeking (PASS = PA + SS) are also computed. Norms for the trait form of the MAACL-R are based on a representative national sample of 18-year-olds ($n = 1,491$); norms for the state form are based on a (nonrepresentative) sample of students ($n = 538$) enrolled in a midwestern college. With the exception of the Sensation Seeking scale, the internal-consistency reliability coefficients for both the trait and state scales are adequate. The test-retest reliabilities are satisfactory for the trait scales but, as expected, low for the state scales. The results of validity studies on various populations, including normal adolescents and adults, counseling clients, and patients from clinics and state hospitals, are reported in the MAACL-R manual (Zuckerman & Lubin, 1985). Scores on the MAACL-R correlate in the expected direction with other measures of personality (e.g., the Minnesota Multiphasic Personality Inventory, the Profile of Mood States, peer ratings, self-ratings, and psychiatric diagnoses).

Reviewing the MAACL-R, Templer (1985) concluded that it is definitely superior to its predecessor, the MAACL. He listed a number of advantages of the instrument: brevity and ease of administration, provision of both state and trait measures, assessment of five affect dimensions, sensitivity to changes over time, good reliability, relatively independent of response sets, commendable construct validity, and a wide range of research applications with normal and abnormal populations, especially in assessing temporal changes.

Problem Checklists

Perhaps the most widely administered of all types of checklists are problem checklists. The use of these instruments in the schools was discussed in Chapter 6. The informant need not be a teacher. Parents and other individuals who have spent a substantial amount of time with a child may know him or her behavior even better than a teacher.

Mooney Problem Check Lists

One of the oldest of all checklists is the Mooney Problem Check Lists. Designed for individuals from junior-high to adulthood, the four forms of the Mooney consist of 210 to 330 problems concerned with health and physical development, home and family, boy and girl relations, morals and religion, courtship and marriage, economic security, school or occupation, and social and recreational matters. Examinees begin by underlining problems of some concern to them, and then circle those problems of greatest concern. Finally, they write a summary of their problems. The Mooney is scored on the number of problems in each area, but responses are interpreted impressionistically rather than by comparing them with norms. The reliabilities of the area scores are satisfactory, and the case for the validity of the Mooney is made on the basis of content.

In contrast to *narrow-band instruments* designed for an in-depth examination of specific disorders or problem areas, the Mooney Problem Check Lists are *broad-band instruments:* they provide a fairly comprehensive overview of social, behavioral, and emotional functioning. Other examples of broad-band checklists are the Child Behavior Checklist and the Revised Behavior Problem Checklist. Unlike the Mooney, which is a *self-report instrument*, the last two checklists are *informant instruments* completed by a parent or teacher. Strictly speaking they are rating scales rather than checklists, in that responses are made on multiple categories.

Child Behavior Checklist (CBCL)

The CBCL (Achenbach & Edelbrock, 1983) is a broad-band instrument consisting of items related to academic and social competency. The Teacher's Report Form version of the CBCL is described in Chapter 6. The parent version consists of 118 Behavior Problem items to be rated on a scale of 0 (behavior "not true" of child), 1 (behavior "sometimes or somewhat true" of child), and 2 (behavior "very true or often true" of child). Scores on the social competency items are summed as Activities, Social, and School subscores.

The CBCL was standardized in 1981 on 1300 students in the Washington, D.C. area. Separate norms by gender and three age levels (4–5, 6–11, 12–16 years) on 8-9 factors are provided in the manual. The norms yield six different Child Behavior Profiles on 8 to 9 factors; they are grouped into Externalizing, Internalizing, and Mixed Syndromes. Test-retest reliability coefficients on the behavior problems and social competence variables are moderate to high; indexes of parental agreement are mixed. A substantial amount of validity data indicates that the CBCL measures what it is supposed to. Correlations with similar instruments, such as the Conners Parent Rating Scale and the Revised Behavior Problem Checklist are significant (Conners, 1973; Quay & Peterson, 1983).

Symptom checklists, such as the Mental Status Checklist Series (Adult and Adolescent) and the Derogatis Symptom Checklist Series, are useful in clinical diagnosis. The Mental Status Checklists consist of 120 items pertaining to matters typically included in comprehensive mental-status examinations of adults (presenting problem, referral data, demographics, mental status, personality function and symptoms, diagnosis, disposition).

Revised Behavior Problem Checklist (RBPC)

Based in part on research with its predecessor—the Behavior Problem Checklist, the RBPC is composed of 89 items to be answered by parents, teachers, or other informants on children in grades K-12. The child's behavior is checked on each item on a scale of 0 ("not at all"), 1 ("mild problem"), or 2 ("severe problem"). Responses can be made in approximately 10 minutes and scored in about 5 minutes on six factors: Conduct Problems, Personality Problems, Inadequate-Immature, Socialized Delinquency, Psychotic Behavior, and Motor Excess. The interrater and internal consistency reliability coefficients for the six factors are moderate to high; the test-retest coefficients are somewhat lower. Analysis of the construct validity of the RBPC indicate that it represents a consensus of what is known about maladaptive child behavior. Correlations between scores on the RBPC and criteria of behavior problems in children are impressive.

STANDARDIZED RATING SCALES FOR PERSONALITY RESEARCH AND CLINICAL DIAGNOSIS

As with checklists, many rating scales that are used in personality research and clinical diagnosis are neither standardized nor commercially available. They were designed for specific research investigations to test specific hypotheses and perhaps were published in a research paper or monograph or are available from the author(s). Other scales have been standardized, or partially standardized, on samples of patients or other groups of people. Certain rating scales and checklists are oriented toward behavioral assessment and modification, others stemmed from a trait-factor orientation, and still others were developed in a psychodynamic, psychopathological context. Some scales are used to record observations in non-interview situations, while other scales form a part of a structured interview.

Numerous published and unpublished scales for personality analysis and clinical diagnosis are described in the compendium by Bech (1993), the anthology by Butcher (1995), and in other sources (e.g., Goodwin & Jamison, 1990; Piacentini, 1993; Witt, Heffer, & Pfeiffer, 1990). Scales to measure aggression anxiety, depression, and mania are among the most popular of all unpublished instruments. Illustrative of instruments for measuring aggression is the Overt Aggression Scale (OAS) (Yudofsky, Silver, Jackson, & Endicott, 1986). Designed for inpatient settings, the OAS measures four categories of aggressive behavior over extended periods of time: verbal aggression, physical aggression against objects, physical aggression against self, and physical aggression against other people. For example, increasingly more severe levels of physical aggression against people include: (1) making threatening gestures, swinging at people, and grabbing at their clothes; (2) shaking, kicking, pushing, or pulling others' hair; (3) attacking others and causing mild to moderate physical injury; and (4) attacking others and causing severe physical injury. Suggested procedures for dealing with aggressive incidents are also noted. The OAS is scored by a computer program that can produce graphic representations of the results over extended time periods.

The Hamilton Anxiety Scale and the Hamilton Depression Scale are representative of unpublished narrow-band clinical scales; the latter has become a standard for identifying clinically depressed patients. Items on the Hamilton Scale are rated for severity on integer scales ranging from 0 to 2 or from 0 to 4. The reliability of this instrument can be increased by use of the Structured Interview Guide for the Hamilton Depression Scale (SIGH-D), which was designed to standardize its administration. A Revised Hamilton Rating Scale for Depression has recently been published by Western Psychological Services.

Other self-rating and observer-rating scales for depression and manic states are described by Goodwin and Jamison (1990). One of these, the Manic-State Rating Scale (Beigel, Murphy, & Bunney, 1971; Murphy, Beigel, Weingartner, & Bunney, 1974), is unique in that it requires rating the patient on a scale of 0 to 5 on *both* the frequency ("How much of the time?") and the intensity ("How intense is it?"—of each of 26 behaviors. As demonstrated by the author some years ago (Aiken, 1962), these two response modes (frequency and intensity) are not always closely related and provide different kinds of information.

Another popular rating scale designed to assist in psychiatric diagnosis, and one with a broader bandwidth than the Hamilton, is the Brief Psychiatric Rating Scale (Liberman, 1988; Overall & Gorham, 1962). Ratings of symptoms (somatic concern, anxiety, emotional withdrawal, guilt feelings, hostility, suspiciousness, unusual thought patterns, etc.) on the 18 scales of this instrument can be made by a clinician following an interview with the patient and then compared with ratings made on other diagnostic groups.

A number of interesting techniques have been devised to obtain ratings on psychological and somatic symptoms in therapeutic and research contexts. One type of rating scale, the *visual analogue scale,* has been used to measure subjective experiences such as pain, anxiety, and cravings for certain substances. Several scales of this type are shown in Figure 7.2 (Wewers & Lowe, 1990). The patient or research subject points to or marks the point on the line corresponding to the intensity of his or her experience (of pain or anxiety). Effective use of a visual analogue scale requires the respondent to represent his or her perception of an abstract concept such as anxiety or pain as a linear unit. Because some patients are unable to understand the method, its utility is limited.

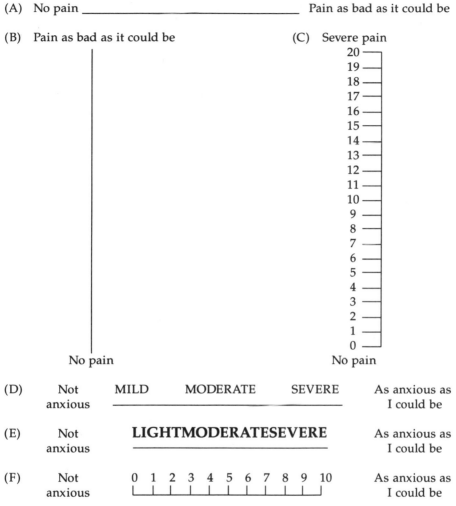

Figure 7.2. Various forms of visual analogue scales. Scales A, B, and C are for measuring intensity of pain; scales D, E, and F are for measuring intensity of anxiety.

A continuing problem in clinical medicine, and pediatric medicine in particular, is accurate communication of symptomatology from patient to physician. Not only are symptoms frequently "referred" and therefore not accurately localized by the patient, but communicating the intensity of the symptom (e.g., pain) to the doctor or nurse is not simple for many patients. The visual analogue procedure, Likert scales, and other rating procedures are sometimes but not invariably successful. In a study conducted by Zeltzer, Richie, LeBaron, and Reed (1988), a group of healthy children and a group of children with cancer were asked to rate "nausea," "vomiting," and "bother" on a scale of 0 to 10 in a series of vignettes with gradations of symptoms. Six faces of children showing increasing amounts of distress were placed as signposts along the "Bother" scale. The findings indicated that children as young as 5 years of age can understand and use rating scales to quantify descriptions of somatic symptoms, and that there is no difference between healthy children and children with cancer in this regard. However, the ratings given by older children and adolescents were closer than those of younger children to the ratings made by a sample of adults. Thus, the younger children had more difficulty than the older children in communicating the frequency and intensity of somatic symptoms by the procedures used in this investigation.

Illustrative Commercially Available Rating Scales

Several of the checklists described in this chapter and the preceding one consist not of single instruments but rather "families" or "systems" of instruments. (See Table 7.3 for a representative sample of these instruments.) This is true of the Mooney Problem Check Lists, which have different forms for different age groups, the Child Behavior Checklist (CBCL), and the Conners' Rating Scales. The Teacher's Report Form of the CBCL and the Conners' Teacher Rating Scales were described in Chapter 6. Like its companion instrument, the Conners' Parent Rating Scales are one of the most widely used of all behavioral instruments.

Conners' Parent Rating Scales (CPRS)

The CPRS was designed originally as a narrow-band instrument for identifying hyperactivity in children, but subsequently it was also found useful in diagnosing other behavior problems. There are two forms of the CPRS—a long (93-item) form and a short (48-item) form. On both forms, a parent or "significant other" rates each item on a scale of 0 ("not at all") to 3 ("very much") as it pertains to the child. The long form (CPRS-93) was standardized in 1970 on a sample of 6 14-year-olds, and is scored on eight factor scales: Conduct Disorder, Fearful-Anxious, Restless-Disorganized, Learning Problem-Immature, Psychosomatic, Obsessional, Antisocial, and Hyperactive-Immature. The short form (CPRS-48) was standardized in 1978 on a sample of

TABLE 7.3. Representative Commercially Distributed Rating Scales for Clinical Identification and Diagnosis

Beck Anxiety Inventory (A. T. Beck; Psychological Corporation)

Beck Depression Inventory (A. T. Beck; Psychological Corpora tion)

Beck Hopelessness Scale (A. T. Beck; Psychological Corporation)

Beck Scale for Suicide Ideation (A. T. Beck; Psychological Corporation)

Behavior Rating Instrument for Autistic & Other Atypical Children, 2nd ed. (B. A. Ruttenberg, C. Wenar, & E. G. Wolf; Stoelting)

Behavior Rating Profile-2 (L. Brown & D. D. Hammill; Pro.Ed)

Brief Derogatis Psychiatric Rating Scale (L. R. Derogatis; NCS)

Burks' Behavior Rating Scales (H. F. Burks; WPS)

Child Behavior Rating Scale (R. N. Cannell; WPS)

Childhood Autism Rating Scale (E. Schopler, R. J. Reichler, & B. R. Renner; WPS)

Cognitive Behavior Rating Scales (J. M. Williams; PAR)

Conners' Rating Scales (C. K. Conners; Jastak, Pro.Ed, Psychological Corporation)

Dementia Rating Scale (S. Mattis; PAR)

Derogatis Psychiatric Rating Scale (L. R. Derogatis; NCS Assessments)

Overt Aggression Scale (Yudofsky, Silver, Jackson et al., 1986)

Revised Hamilton Rating Scale for Depression (W. L. Warren; WPS)

SCL-90 Analogue (L. R. Derogatis; NCS Assessments)

children aged 3 to 17 years of age. Separate gender norms are available on five scales: Conduct Problem, Learning Problem, Psychosomatic, Impulsive-Hyperactive, and Anxiety. Because of its greater comprehensiveness and more extensive validation, CPRS-93 has been recommended over CPRS-48 (Conners & Barkley, 1985). However, greater brevity, combined with its more recent and more extensive standardization, would favor use of the CPRS-48 when the reduced number of variables is not a problem.

The Conners' Rating Scales are designed to identify behavior problems and other signs of adjustment disorders in children. Illustrative of groups of rating scales designed for adults are the Beck Scales and the Derogatis Symptom Checklist Series.

The Beck Scales

The four instruments in this group—the Beck Depression Inventory, the Beck Hopelessness Scale, the Beck Anxiety Scale, and the Beck Scale for Suicide Ideation—are all clinically based. One of the most widely used instruments for detecting and determining the intensity of depression in both normal and psychiatric populations of adults is the Beck Depression Inventory (BDI). The BDI consists of 21 sets of statements to be answered on a scale of 0 ("no complaint") to 3 ("severe complaint"), depending on the severity of the respondent's depression. The items were derived theoretically or judgmentally rather than empirically. Scores on two subscales (cognitive-affective and somatic-performance), as well as total score on the BDI, may be determined. Total scores of 0 to 9 are labeled "normal," scores of 10 to 18 are indicative of "mild-moderate depression, scores of 19 to 29 indicate "moderate-severe depression" and scores of 30 and above point to "extremely severe depression." Norms from various groups (major depressives, dysthymics, alcoholics, heroin addicts, and a mixed diagnostic group) are reported in the 1987 manual. The internal consistency reliabilities of the BDI scores are high; the test-retest reliabilities are moderate in psychiatric patient and nonpatient groups. Good evidence of the validity of the BDI, including high correlations with clinical ratings of depression, are given in the manual. Sundberg (1992) concluded that the BDI "has made an important contribution to clinical and research work on depression" (p. 80).

Similar in format to the BDI is the 20-item Beck Hopelessness Scale (BHS), which consists of 20 true-false item scale designed to measure negative beliefs concerning the future. Like the BDI, the BHS can be administered in 5 to 10 minutes. Scores on the BHS are moderately correlated with those on the BDI, but the former instrument is a better predictor of suicidal intention and behavior than the latter. The internal consistency reliabilities reported in the 1988 BHS manual are reasonably high (.82 to .93 in seven norm groups). The test-retest reliability coefficients are, however, quite modest (69 after 1 week and .66 after 6 weeks). Reviewing the BHS, Dowd (1992) concluded that it is "a well-constructed and validated instrument, with adequate reliability" (p. 82). Owen's (1992) review of the scale was also positive, but less enthusiastic than Dowd's.

Two other Beck scales similar in format to the BDI and BHS, and also available from The Psychological Corporation are the Beck Anxiety Inventory (BAI) and the Beck Scale for Suicide Ideation (BSI). Like their predecessors, these newer scales were designed for adults from 17 to 80 years; the 21 items can be answered in 5 to 10 minutes. Both instruments are available in English and Spanish. The BAI was designed to measure the severity of anxiety in adolescents and adults, and has been found to discriminate between anxious and nonanxious diagnostic groups. The anxious groups included patients with agoraphobia, panic disorder, social phobia, obsessive-compulsive disorder, and generalized anxiety. The BSI was designed to evaluate suicidal thinking and attitudes and thereby to identify individuals at risk for suicide. The internal consistency reliabilities of the BAI and the BSI are high, but the test-retest reliabilities are more modest. Studies of the clinical validity of the two instruments are reported in the BAI (1990) and BSI (1991) manuals.

Derogatis Symptom Checklist Series

Designed to identify symptoms of psychopathology in adults, the five instruments in this series are the Symptom Checklist-90-Revised, the Brief Symptom Inventory, the Derogatis Psychiatric Rating Scale, the Brief Derogatis Psychiatric Rating Scale, and the SCL-90 Analogue. The first two instruments are self-report inventories for screening patients for psychological disorders on intake, to record patient progress, and to serve as measures of treatment effectiveness. The last three instruments are observer-report instruments for measuring the same variables as the first two.

The 90 items on the SCL-90-R are rated by the patient on a scale of 0 ("not at all") to 5 ("extremely") in 12 to 15 minutes. Scores are obtained on nine primary symptom dimensions: Somatization, Obsessive Compulsive, Interpersonal Sensitivity, Depression, Anxiety, Hostility, Phobic Anxiety, Paranoid Ideation, and Psychoticism. In addition, three indices of stress measure the current level or depth of a disorder, the intensity of the symptoms, and the number of patient-reported symptoms. Normative data on groups of nonpatient adults, nonpatient adolescents, psychiatric outpatients, and psychiatric inpatients has been collected. Hundreds of studies concerned with the reliability, validity, and utility of the SCL-90-R have been conducted.

The 53 items on the BSI are, like those on the SCL-90-R, written at a sixth-grade level and rated by adults on a five-point scale. Designed to reflect psychological symptom patterns in psychiatric and medical patients, the BSI measures the same nine primary symptom dimensions as the SCL-90-R. Norms for nonpatient adults, nonpatient adolescents (13–17 years old), psychiatric outpatients, and psychiatric inpatients are available. Though not as widely researched and somewhat less reliable than the SCL-90-R, the BSI has adequate reliability and validity.

On the Derogatis Psychiatric Rating Scale (DPRS) and a shorter form—the Brief Derogatis Psychiatric Rating Scale (B-DPRS), the clinician rates his or her observations of the adult patient on the same nine dimensions as those measured by the SCL-90-R and the BSI. The DPRS can be filled out in 2 to 5 minutes and yields scores on 17 scales (9 primary dimensions plus eight additional dimensions) and a global index. The B-DPRS can be completed in 1 to 2 minutes and yields scores on the 9 primary dimensions plus a global index. Like the DPRS and the B-DPRS, the SCL-90 Analogue is completed by an observer of an adolescent or adult patient. Unlike the first four inventories in the Derogatis series, it can be used by health professionals who lack in-depth training or knowledge of psychopathology for the initial evaluation of patients and measurement of their progress during and after treatment. Taking only 1 to 3 minutes to complete, the SCL-90 Analogue is scored on the same nine primary dimensions as the other Derogatis inventories, plus a global psychopathology scale.

SUMMARY

The formal history of personality assessment begins with the researches and instrument developments of psychologists and psychiatrists during the late nineteenth and early twentieth centuries. Most objective and projective measures of personality during the first half of this century were designed originally to identify and diagnose adjustment problems and behavior disorders. Illustrative of these measures are the Kent-Rosanoff word association test, the Woodworth Personal Data Sheet, the Rorschach Inkblot Test, and the Thematic Apperception Test. Many other assessment instruments, including hundreds of checklists and scales, have been constructed since those instruments made their debuts.

Although this chapter deals primarily with two types of personality assessment instruments—rating scales and checklists, brief descriptions of observational and interview techniques are also given. Rating scales and checklists are often used to make more objective records of the findings of controlled or uncontrolled observations and structured or semi-structured interviews, whether conducted for research or clinical purposes. In addition, many of the observational and interviewing questionnaire-based schedules employed to make the results more objective contain checklists and rating scales of various kinds.

Theories of personality, including psychoanalysis, phenonmenological (self) theory, type theories, and trait/factor theories, have served as a foundation for the development of many personality assessment instruments and procedures. The largest number of these instruments have been constructed from a trait/factor framework. In addition, some of them, such as the Minnesota Multiphasic Personality Inventory, were developed on the basis of clinical experience without relying formal theory of personality. Among these empirically based instruments are numerous rating scales and checklists. Although some of these instruments have been standardized and are commercially available, even more were developed on an ad hoc basis for a particular investigation and have not been standardized or published. Good examples of such unpublished, unstandardized checklists and scales are those that were constructed to record responses in behavior modification programs.

The standardized checklists designed for personality research and clinical diagnoses described in this chapter include well-known instruments such as the Adjective Check List and the Multiple Affective Adjective Check List—Revised as well as problem checklists such as the Mooney Problem Check Lists, the Child Behavior Checklist, and the Revised Behavior Problem Checklist.

Among the standardized rating scales for personality research and clinical diagnosis are three families of instruments: the Conners' Parent Rating Scales, The Beck Scales (for depression, hopelessness, anxiety, and suicide ideation), and the Derogatis Symptom Checklist Series (the SCL-90-R, the Derogatis Psychiatric Rating Scale, the Brief Derogatis Psychiatric Rating Scale, and the SCL-90 Analogue). All of these instruments are widely used, fairly reliable, generally valid for the uses for which they were constructed, and objectively scored and analyzed by computer.

QUESTIONS AND ACTIVITIES

1. Define each of the following terms used in this chapter. Consult Appendix A and/or a dictionary if you need help.

adjective checklist	conditions of worth
agreeableness	conscientiousness
behavior modification	content analysis
body type theory	diagnostic interview
broad-band instrument	exit interview
cardinal traits	extraversion
central traits	five-factor model
cerebrotonic	frequency response set
conditional positive regard	informant instrument

intake interview
mental status interview
narrow-band instrument
need
neuroticism
openness
participant observation
phenomenal world
press
problem checklist
psychoanalysis
secondary traits
self
self theory

self-actualization
self-concept
self-monitoring
self-observation
self-report instrument
situational testing
somatotonic
somatotype
stress interview
therapeutic interview
trait theory
type theory
viscerontonic

2. One problem with the research literature on Type A behavior is that different assessment methods—for example, interview and questionnaire—do not yield the same results. Although questionnaires such as the Jenkins Activity Survey are more efficient than interviews, Rosenman (1986) and others have rejected such self-report measures because Type A personalities presumably have little insight into their own behavior. One way of testing this hypothesis is to compare self-ratings of behavior with ratings of behavior made by unbiased observers. With this in mind, select a few individuals who seem to fit the following description of the Type A personality:

A personality pattern characterized by a combination of behaviors, including aggressivity, competitiveness, hostility, quick actions, and constant striving.

Administer the following checklist to each person, and then ask someone who knows the person well to fill out the same checklist to describe that person. Use an appropriate statistical procedure to compare the self-ratings and the other-ratings. The checklist can also be completed by running program I-1 on the computer program diskette accompanying the book.

Checklist

Directions: Check each of the following terms or phrases that is descriptive of you.

_____ 1. achievement-oriented

_____ 2. aggressive

_____ 3. ambitious

_____ 4. competitive

_____ 5. constant worker

_____ 6. dislikes wasting time

_____ 7. easily angered

_____ 8. easily aroused to action

_____ 9. easily frustrated

_____ 10. efficient

_____ 11. emotionally explosive

_____ 12. fast worker

_____ 13. hard worker

_____ 14. highly motivated

_____ 15. impatient

_____ 16. likes challenges

_____ 17. likes to lead

_____ 18. likes responsibility

_____ 19. restless

_____ 20. tries hard to succeed

3. Construct a ten-item checklist of symptoms of depression and a second checklist of symptoms of anxiety. Administer your two checklists to a dozen people and determine the correlation between the number of items that they check on each list. Interpret the correlation.

4. Make a copy of the Behavioral Checklist for Performance Anxiety (Figure 7.1) and use it to record your observations of a person over eight time periods of 10 minutes each. Put a check mark after the behavior in the appropriate time period column if it occurred during that time. Make multiple check marks if the same behavior was observed more than once during the time period. How consistent was each of the behaviors across the eight time periods, and how many times did each behavior occur? Would you characterize the person whom you observed as "anxious?" Do you believe that all of the 20 behaviors listed in Figure 7.1 are indicative of "anxiety?" Why or why not?

5. Consult a dictionary or thesaurus, and select 50 adjectives referring to traits or characteristics of personality. Try to choose a
mixture of positive and negative adjectives that are not syn-
onyms or antonyms of each other. Make multiple copies of the
alphabetized list of adjectives. Leave a short blank line after
each adjective, and administer the list to a sample of people. Ask
the respondents to check each adjective that they feel is generally descriptive of themselves. Summarize the results, comparing them with what you already know about the individuals
from other reports and observations.

6. What are the pros and cons of psychodiagnosis, that is, classifying and assigning labels to people having specific psychological problems?

7. Administer the following checklist concerning psychotherapy anonymously to ten psychology majors (five men and
five women) and ten nonpsychology majors (five men and
five women). For each item, compare the number of men who
checked the statement with the number of women who
checked it. Also compare the number of psychology majors
who checked the item with the number of non-psychology
majors who checked it. What conclusions can you draw from
these comparisons?

Opinions of Psychotherapy

Directions: Check each of the following states with which you
agree.

_____ 1. Good psychotherapists are born, not made by a lot
of fancy education and training.

_____ 2. Effective psychotherapy is more of an art than a
science.

_____ 3. Psychotherapy is useful in treating both major and
minor mental health problems, ranging from mild
stress reactions all the way to psychoses.

_____ 4. Prolonged psychotherapy is usually unnecessary;
one or two sessions are typically enough for most
problems.

_____ 5. All that one needs to be an effective psychotherapist is the ability to listen carefully and nonjudg-
mentally.

_____   6. In many cases psychotherapy actually does more harm than good.

_____   7. Most people are better off after having received psychotherapeutic help.

_____   8. When psychotherapy works, it usually does so because of a placebo effect: the patient thinks he or she must be getting better because a prestigious person is trying to help.

_____   9. One reason why psychotherapy works is because the patient is paying so much money for it.

_____   10. In general, drugs such as Prozac are more effective than psychotherapy in treating serious mental disorders.

_____   11. In psychotherapy, as in many other things in life, "it takes one to know one." That is, a person who has had mental problems and worked through them is better able to help people with personal problems.

_____   12. A person needs little or no training to be an effective psychotherapist: it's mostly a matter of interpersonal warmth, understanding, common sense, and a genuine interest in helping people.

_____   13. Most people could benefit from psychotherapy at some time during their lives.

8. Complete the following Five-Factor Rating Scale, score it, and determine your percentile rank on each of the five factor variables.

Five-Factor Rating Scale

Directions: Check the number on each of the following bipolar scales that is most descriptive of your standing on that characteristic.

1. affectionate   1 2 3 4 5 6 7   reserved
2. calm   1 2 3 4 5 6 7   worrying
3. careful   1 2 3 4 5 6 7   careless
4. conforming   1 2 3 4 5 6 7   independent
5. disorganized   1 2 3 4 5 6 7   well-organized
6. down-to-earth   1 2 3 4 5 6 7   imaginative
7. fun-loving   1 2 3 4 5 6 7   sober
8. helpful   1 2 3 4 5 6 7   uncooperative

9. insecure   1 2 3 4 5 6 7   secure

10. prefer routine   1 2 3 4 5 6 7   prefer variety

11. retiring   1 2 3 4 5 6 7   sociable

12. ruthless   1 2 3 4 5 6 7   soft-hearted

13. self-disciplined   1 2 3 4 5 6 7   weak-willed

14. self-pitying   1 2 3 4 5 6 7   self-satisfied

15. suspicious   1 2 3 4 5 6 7   trusting

Scoring formulas for the five factors:

Agreeableness = 5 + Item 12 + Item 15 − Item 8

Conscientiousness = 13 − Item 3 + Item 5 − Item 13

Extroversion = 13 − Item 1 − Item 7 + Item 11

Neuroticism = 13 + Item 2 − Item 9 − Item 14

Openness = Item 4 + Item 6 + Item 10 − 3

Use the following norms table, based on the scores of a representative sample of college students, to determine your percentile ranks on the five variables. To interpret these percentile ranks, refer to the three items (see above scoring formulas) from which your score on each factor was determined. Recall that the percentile rank corresponding to a score is the percentage of people in the norm group who made lower scores than yours.

Percentile Rank for Factor Variable

Score	Agreeableness	Conscientiousness	Extroversion	Neuroticism	Openness
1				1	
2				3	
3		1		13	
4		3		30	2
5		6		47	7
6		8		57	10
7		13	1	64	15
8	2	19	5	72	26
9	2	19	14	79	38
10	7	26	24	87	51
11	19	34	31	87	70
12	33	41	42	87	85
13	41	48	58	94	85
14	55	57	69	96	90
15	74	74	76	99	92
16	88	87	87		94
17	95	92	95		99
18	99	98	99		99

8

Assessment of Attitudes and Values

The measurement of attitudes and values is truly cross-disciplinary or cross-situational, in that it has been of interest to every social or behavioral science, to administrators in industrial/organizational and educational contexts, to officials in government and the military, and even to the roving reporter and the man-in-the-street. Whether we realize it or not, many decisions concerning the products and services available to us, the people, commodities, and situations with which we interact, and our hopes and dreams for the future are affected by the results of surveys of our attitudes, opinions, and values. Every politician, every marketer, every newsperson, in fact everyone who wants to influence our purchases, our choices of entertainment and information, and in general how we behave, how we feel, and what we believe in has an interest in our attitudes, opinions, and values. Thus, the measurement of attitudes, opinions, and values is one of the most pragmatic and pervasive of all social/psychological assessments in our society.

ATTITUDE MEASUREMENT

The term *attitude* has never been very precisely defined and has varied in its meaning from one researcher to the next. Perhaps the most general definition was offered by Louis Guttman (Stouffer et al., 1950, p. 51), who characterized an attitude as "a delimited totality of behavior with respect to something." A definition that recognizes that attitudes cannot be observed directly but are inferred from behavior was offered by Gagné and Briggs (1974, p. 62), who described an attitude as "an internal state which affects an individual's choice of action toward some object, person, or event." Underscoring the relationship between attitudes and beliefs is Milton Rokeach's (1968, p. 112) definition of an attitude as "a relatively enduring organization of beliefs around an object or situation predisposing one to respond in some preferential manner."

By combining the common elements of several definitions, we may conceptualize an attitude as a learned predisposition to respond positively or negatively to certain objects, situations, institutions, concepts, or persons. As implied by this definition, attitudes possess cognitive (beliefs, knowledge, and expectations), affective (motivational and emotional), and performance (behavior or action) components. Though *attitude* is not distinct from psychological concepts such as interest, opinion, belief, and value, there are differences in the manner in which these concepts are employed.

Opinions and Beliefs

The meaning of *opinion* is similar to that of attitude, but opinions are perceived as being more specific, more changeable, and more factually based. People are always aware of their opinions, but they may not be fully conscious of their attitudes. Not only are attitudes less conscious; they are also more basic than opinions in that they combine with facts to determine opinions. The combination of attitudes and facts to produce opinions is, however, not necessarily additive: attitudes serve not only to organize facts into opinions according to some frame of reference but also affect the facts that will be selected for interpretation.

It is even more difficult to distinguish opinions from *beliefs:* both are judgments or acceptances of propositions as facts, but opinions are not held so tenaciously as beliefs and the factual support for opinions is usually weaker than for beliefs. In terms of the extent to which they are based on factual information, attitudes are in lowest place, opinions next, and beliefs at the top. However, attitudes are more pervasive or generalized and more resistant to change than either opinions or beliefs.

Methods of Measuring Attitudes

The scientific study of attitudes, which cuts across various disciplines, began in the 1920s with the work of E. S. Bogardus (1925, 1928), L. L. Thurstone (Thurstone & Chave, 1929), and other social psychologists and psychometricians. Research and theories concerning attitudes are still centered in social psychology, but important contributions, especially to attitude measurement, have been made by educational and industrial/organizational psychologists.

Like research on other psychological constructs, research on attitudes is only as effective as the method by which they are measured. Perhaps the most objective way of assessing attitudes toward specific ideas, persons, objects, or situations is to observe how people behave in relation to those things. What a person says or does in a situation where the attitude object or event is present may be viewed as an indicator of his or her attitude toward it. Examples of behavioral measures of attitudes are willingness to do a favor, sign a petition, or make a donation to some cause. Because it is not unusual for people to play roles, manipulate, or practice deception, even the direct observation of behavior is not always a valid indicator of attitude in a given situation or at a particular time. A representative sampling of behavior across time and situations would eliminate this objection, but such a procedure is likely to be time-consuming and expensive. Notwithstanding its inefficiency, it may be necessary to employ direct observations to assess the attitudes of certain groups, such as young children, or when other methods are considered obtrusive.

Inferring attitudes from direct observations of behavior often yields different results from other methods. One alternative to behavior observations is a projective technique, such as asking people to tell a story about each of several ambiguous pictures. Because the pictures can be interpreted in various ways, the stories should reveal something about the respondents' attitudes toward the characters, scenes, or situations in the pictures. Moyer's (1977) *Unobtrusive Survey of Environmental Attitudes* refers to two other projective techniques—word associations and sentence completions. There is, however, no good evidence that such procedures are any less obtrusive or possess greater validity than more direct measures of attitudes.

More popular than either behavioral observation or projective techniques is to ask specific questions in an interview or on a self-report inventory and to infer attitudes from the answers. An assumption of this method is that the respondent knows what his or her attitudes are and is willing to reveal them to the questioner. Because self-deception is fairly common, this is not always a reasonable assumption. A second implicit assumption of research employing attitude scales or inventories is that these methods are unobtrusive. That is, it is assumed that the very process of asking people what their attitudes are does not affect the attitudes under investigation. Again, this may or may not be true: People are not robots who respond only to specific questions or commands. They are dynamic, interactive, intelligent beings who constantly attempt to determine what other people really mean by what they say or do and what response might best serve their own personal interests.

Attitude Scales

An attitude scale consists of a series of statements expressing positive and negative feelings about a given institution, a group of people, or a concept. A person's score on an attitude scale is determined by the items with which he or she agrees or disagrees, the exact scoring procedure depending on the type of scale. Many techniques are available for constructing attitude scales, including Bogardus's cumulative scaling, Thurstone's pair comparisons and equal-appearing intervals, Likert's summated ratings, and Guttman's scalogram analysis.

The Bogardus Social Distance Scale (Bogardus, 1925), which was the first formally designed attitude scale, is a cumulative scale. Examinees are asked to indicate, by ranking them, the extent to which they would accept various social or religious groups in various capacities. The items are arranged in a hierarchy such that a positive response to a given item implies a positive response to all preceding items on the scale. The Bogardus scale proved useful in research on regional differences and other variables associated with racial prejudice, but it was somewhat crude by today's standards. Further development of cumulative scaling did not occur until Louis Guttman's work on scalogram analysis.

The Bogardus Social Distance Scale is basically a rank-ordering instrument. For this reason, it permits the measurement of attitudes only on an ordinal level. By applying the methods of paired comparisons and equal-appearing intervals, Thurstone hoped to improve upon Bogardus's approach and measure attitudes on an interval level. In constructing an attitude scale by the method of paired comparisons, a group of "experts" is asked to compare a large number of statements expressing a range of positive and negative attitudes toward a given topic and to make a judgment about which member in each pair expresses a more positive attitude. Because the method of pair comparisons is cumbersome and time consuming, it has not been used extensively in attitude measurement.[1]

Equal-Appearing Intervals

The first step in constructing an attitude scale by the method of *equal-appearing intervals* is to collect 200 or so statements expressing a wide range of positive and negative attitudes toward a given topic. Next, a large sample of people (50 to 300 so-called "judges") are directed to sort the statements into eleven response categories, varying from least favorable (category 1) to most favorable (category 11). The judges are told to think of the eleven categories as lying at equal intervals along a continuum. After all judges have completed the sorting process, for every statement a frequency distribution of the number of judges who placed the statement in each category is constructed. Then from each of the frequency distributions, the median score (scale value) and semi-interquartile range (ambiguity index) of the corresponding statement is computed. Statements having large ambiguity indexes are discarded. The final attitude scale consists of approximately twenty statements selected so their scale values are approximately equal numerical distances apart, the scale values range from one extreme to the other, and the ambiguity indexes of the statements are fairly low. The score on an attitude scale constructed in this way, such as the one of which the 12 statements in Figure 8.1 are representative, is the median of the scale values of the statements which the respondent endorses. Note that the scale values of the statements on this Scale of Attitudes Toward Capital Punishment range from .1 (highly negative toward capital punishment) to 11.0 (highly positive toward capital punishment). These 12 attitude statements can also be administered by program J-7 on the computer diskette accompanying this book.

Thurstone and his co-workers constructed some 30 attitude scales by the method of equal-appearing intervals. The procedure was generalized by Remmers (1960) in the Master Attitude Scales. These nine scales measure attitudes toward: any school subject, any vocation, any institution, any defined group, any proposed social action, any practice, any homemaking activity, individual and group morale, and the high school. As with Thurstone scales, the reliabilities of most of the Master Attitude Scales are in the .80s.

This is a study of attitude toward capital punishment. Below you will find a number of statements expressing different attitudes toward capital punishment.

√   Put a checkmark if you agree with the statement.

X   Put a cross if you disagree with the statement.

Try to indicate either agreement or disagreement for each statement. If you simply cannot decide about a statement you may mark it with a question mark.

This is not an examination. There are no right or wrong answers to these statements. This is simply a study of people's attitudes toward capital punishment. Please indicate your own convictions by a checkmark when you agree and by a cross when you disagree.

Scale Value	Item Number	
(0.1)	12	I do not believe in capital punishment under any circumstances.
(0.9)	16	Execution of criminals is a disgrace to civilized society.
(2.0)	21	The state cannot teach the sacredness of human life by destroying it.
(2.7)	8	Capital punishment has never been effective in preventing crime.
(3.4)	9	I don't believe in capital punishment but I'm not sure it isn't necessary.
(3.9)	11	I think the return of the whipping post would be more effective than capital punishment.
(5.8)	18	I do not believe in capital punishment but it is not practically advisable to abolish it.
(6.2)	6	Capital punishment is wrong but it is necessary in our imperfect civilization.
(7.9)	23	Capital punishment is justified only for premeditated murder.
(9.4)	20	Capital punishment gives the criminal what he deserves.
(9.6)	17	Capital punishment is just and necessary.
(11.0)	7	Every criminal should be executed.

Figure 8.1. Twelve of the 24 items on a scale of attitudes toward capital punishment. The items are arranged in order of their scale values, and the scale values are listed, neither of which is the case on the actual scale. From *Motion Pictures and the Social Attitudes of Children* by R. C. Peterson and L. L. Thurstone, 1933. New York: Macmillan. Reprinted by permission.

A number of objections have been raised to Thurstone-type attitude scales. One objection, which is not so serious in the light of new timesaving techniques, is the great amount of work required by the method. A second, more serious, shortcoming is the fact that a person's score on a Thurstone-type scale—the median of the scale values of checked items—is not unique. That is, the same score can be obtained by checking different combinations of items, such as two neutral items or one positive and one negative item. A third objection is that the scale values of the items may be influenced by the attitudes of the judges. As Thurstone seems to have recognized by requiring "expert judges" to sort the attitude items into 11 categories, not everyone is capable of playing the role of a neutral judge. Still, when the judges are carefully instructed, bias in rating attitude statements does not seem to seriously distort the equal-interval properties of Thurstone attitude scales (Bruvold, 1975; Goodstadt & Magid, 1977).

Summated Ratings

Although Thurstone-type scales represent an effort at interval-level measurement, they are actually somewhere between an interval and an ordinal measurement scale. Rensis Likert (1932) would probably not have quibbled with the allegation that scores on attitude scales constructed by his *method of summated ratings* are only ordinal-level measures. This method, which has proved more popular than the Thurstone procedures, also begins with the collection of a large number of statements expressing a variety of positive and negative attitudes toward a given topic. Edwards (1957) provided the following guidelines for selecting statements to be included in a Likert attitude scale:

- Avoid statements that refer to the past rather than to the present.
- Avoid statements that are factual or capable of being interpreted as factual.
- Avoid statements that may be interpreted in more than one way.
- Avoid statements that are irrelevant to the psychological object under consideration.
- Avoid statements that are likely to be endorsed by almost everyone or by almost no one.
- Select statements that are believed to cover the entire range of the affective scale of interest.
- Keep the language of the statements simple, clear, and direct.

- Statements should be short, rarely exceeding 20 words.
- Each statement should contain only one complete thought.
- Statements containing universals such as *all, always, none,* and *never* often introduce ambiguity and should be avoided.
- Words such as *only, just, merely,* and others of a similar nature, should be used with care and moderation in writing statements.
- Whenever possible, statements should be written in simple sentences rather than compound or complex sentences.
- Avoid the use of words that may not be understood by those who are to be given the completed scale.
- Avoid the use of double negatives. (p. 14)

After the statements are constructed, a group of 100 to 200 people—not necessarily unbiased or expert "judges"—indicate on a four- to seven-point scale the extent of their agreement or disagreement, approval or disapproval, with each statement. On a typical five-point scale, responses to positively worded items are scored 0 for *strongly disagree,* 1 for *disagree,* 2 for *undecided,* 3 for *agree,* and 4 for *strongly agree.* Responses to negatively worded items are scored 0 for *strongly agree,* 1 for *agree,* 2 for *undecided,* 3 for *disagree,* and 4 for *strongly disagree.*

The total score on the initial set of Likert-type items is the sum of the numerical weights of the response categories checked by the respondent. After all responses are scored, item analysis procedures (t-tests or item discrimination indexes) are applied to find the ten or so positively worded statements and an equal number of negatively worded statements that most closely distinguish respondents falling in the upper quartile from those falling in the lowest quartile on the total-score distribution. The total score in the final scale is the sum of the numerical weights of the responses checked by the person. An attitude scale developed by this procedure is shown in Figure 8.2.

Not all published attitude scales referred to as Likert-type scales were constructed by using item-analysis procedures. In many cases, a set of declarative statements, each with five agree/disagree response categories, is simply put together with no discernable underlying theoretical construct(s) and referred to as a Likert attitude scale. Consequently, one cannot be certain that an attitude inventory having the appearance of a Likert scale has actually been constructed by the Likert scaling procedures.

Despite misuses of the procedure, Likert scales have several advantages over Thurstone-type scales. Unlike a Thurstone scale, a

Directions: Write your name in the upper right corner. Each of the statements on this opinionnaire expresses a feeling or attitude toward mathematics. You are to indicate, on a five-point scale, the extent of agreement between the attitude expressed in each statement and your own personal feeling. The five points are: Strongly Disagree (SD), Disagree (D), Undecided (U), Agree (A), Strongly Agree (SA). Check the letter(s) which best indicate(s) how closely you agree or disagree with the attitude expressed in each statement as it concerns you.

1. I am always under a terrible strain in a math class.	SD	D	U	A	SA
2. I do not like mathematics, and it scares me to have to take it.	SD	D	U	A	SA
3. Mathematics is very interesting to me, and I enjoy math classes.	SD	D	U	A	SA
4. Mathematics is fascinating and fun.	SD	D	U	A	SA
5. Mathematics makes me feel secure, and at the same time it is stimulating.	SD	D	U	A	SA
6. My mind goes blank, and I am unable to think clearly when working math problems.	SD	D	U	A	SA
7. I feel a sense of insecurity when attempting mathematics.	SD	D	U	A	SA
8. Mathematics makes me feel uncomfortable, restless, irritable, and impatient.	SD	D	U	A	SA
9. The feeling that I have toward mathematics is a good feeling.	SD	D	U	A	SA
10. Mathematics makes me feel as though I'm lost in a jungle of numbers and can't find my way out.	SD	D	U	A	SA
11. Mathematics is something I enjoy a great deal.	SD	D	U	A	SA
12. When I hear the word *math*, I have a feeling of dislike.	SD	D	U	A	SA
13. I approach mathematics with a feeling of hesitation—resulting from a fear of not being able to do math.	SD	D	U	A	SA
14. I really like mathematics.	SD	D	U	A	SA
15. Mathematics is a school subject that I have always enjoyed studying.	SD	D	U	A	SA
16. I makes me nervous to even think about having to do a math problem.	SD	D	U	A	SA
17. I have never liked math, and it is my most dreaded subject.	SD	D	U	A	SA
18. I am happier in a mathematics class than in any other class.	SD	D	U	A	SA
19. I feel at ease in mathematics, and I like it very much.	SD	D	U	A	SA
20. I have a definite positive reaction to mathematics; it's enjoyable.	SD	D	U	A	SA

Figure 8.2.   Mathematics attitude scale. (See exercise 4 of Questions and Activities for explanation of scoring.)

Likert Scale allows items that are not clearly related to the attitude of concern to be included if they have significant correlations with total scores. Likert scales are also easier to construct, and are probably more reliable than Thurstone scales having the same number of items. In addition, many different patterns of response can yield the same score. This makes it difficult to assign a uniform meaning to a given attitude scale, and creates a problem with respect to the validity of the scale.

In the half-century since publication of Likert's original paper (1932), the method of summated ratings has undoubtedly been applied more than any other attitude-scaling technique. A sizable sample of attitude scales constructed by Likert's procedure may be found in various compendia (Shaw & Wright, 1967; Robinson, Athanasiou, & Head, 1974; Robinson, Rush, & Head, 1973; Robinson, Shaver, & Wrightsman, 1991). These scales range from those devised specifically for research designed to test a theoretical proposition to those constructed with more practical applications in clinical, educational, and industrial/organizational contexts in mind. Readers who wish to design their own attitude instruments will find procedures for facilitating the task of items analysis and scoring of summated ratings in the computer programs accompanying this book.

Spector (1976) suggested that the level of measurement represented by scores on Likert scales might be improved by replacing arbitrary response categories with categories scaled to have equal interval properties. Response category weights would be determined, in the manner of Thurstone, from ratings of the categories by representative judges (Spector, 1976). Andrich (1978a, 1978c) provided an even more complex unification of the procedures of Thurstone and Likert by a generalization of Rasch's binomial logistic model. As Andrich pointed out, Thurstone's equal-appearing intervals procedure provides for statement scaling but not for true measurement of an individual's attitude, whereas the reverse is true of Likert's method of summated ratings. Combining the Thurstone and Likert procedures with Rasch's (1972) model yields an attitude questionnaire constructed, in the Likert manner, with a category system of responses, but the statements are scaled and the overall attitudes of persons are measured on an interval scale.

Scalogram Analysis

The main purpose of Louis Guttman's (1944) *scalogram analysis* procedure is to determine whether the responses to the items designed to

measure a given attitude fall on a single dimension. The scale construction procedure begins with the selection of a large number of statements that apply to the attitude domain of interest. These statements
are then administered to a large representative sample of people, and
statements with which there is 80% or more agreement or disagreement
are discarded. Statements that fail to discriminate between respondents
having the largest number of favorable responses and those having the
smallest number of favorable responses are also discarded. Next, a response matrix, in which the statements are ordered on the columns
from the most favorable to the fewest favorable responses and the respondents are ordered on the rows from most favorable to fewest favorable responses, is constructed (see Table 8.1). If the statements selected
by this method constitute a true, unidimensional Guttman scale, then a
respondent who endorses a given statement will also endorse all statements that are endorsed by other respondents who endorse that particular statement.

As with the Bogardus approach, scalogram analysis aims to
produce a cumulative, ordinal scale. The conditions for a true cumulative scale can occasionally be found in the cognitive domain but
only rarely for items that measure attitudes or other affective variables. Guttman recognized this fact but he felt that the conditions
for a true scale could be approximated in many cases. The degree of

**TABLE 8.1   Response Matrix for Computing the
Reproducibility Coefficient**

Respondent	Statement							Score
	5	7	1	2	3	4	6	
I	yes	yes	yes	yes	yes	yes	yes	7
B	yes	yes	yes	yes	yes	no	yes	6
A	yes	yes	yes	yes	no	no	no	4
E	yes	yes	yes	yes	no	no	no	4
H	yes	yes	yes	no	no	yes	no	4
J	yes	yes	yes	yes	no	no	no	4
D	yes	yes	yes	no	no	no	no	3
C	yes	yes	no	no	no	no	no	2
F	no	no	no	no	yes	no	no	1
G	yes	no	no	no	no	no	no	1
Errors	1	0	0	1	1	1	0	

approximation to a true scale obtained with a set of attitude statements is indicated by a *reproducibility coefficient*. This coefficient, an acceptable value of which is .90, is the proportion of actual responses falling in the perfect pattern of a true Guttman scale. The reproducibility coefficient for a set of data is computed by (1) determining the number of errors (responses that deviate from the pattern) and (2) calculating

$$R = 1 - \text{number of errors/number of responses} \qquad (8.1)$$

In the example given in Table 8.1, there are 4 errors, or deviations from the pattern; so $R = 1 - 4/70 = .94$.

Other Attitude Scaling Procedures

Although the procedures devised by Thurstone, Likert, and Guttman have been the most popular techniques for scaling attitudes, other methods have been devised. Among these are the scale discrimination technique, the semantic differential technique, Q sort, multiple rank orders, and multidimensional procedures such as facet analysis and latent structure or latent class models. The *scale discrimination technique*, which purportedly produces a unidimensional interval scale, combines aspects of the Thurstone, Likert, and Guttman attitude-scaling procedures (Edwards & Kilpatrick, 1974). The semantic differential technique is described in Chapter 3, and the multiple rank orders and constant sum methods have not been used much. Q sort and multidimensional scaling are described next.

Q Sort. Another procedure that has been used to assess individual attitudes toward objects, persons, and situations is the Q sort. In this method, pioneered by William Stephenson (1953), the respondent sorts large numbers of cards containing statements pertaining to a given attitude object into nine to eleven piles. The procedure is similar to the first stage of the equal-appearing intervals method, but the examinee is directed to sort the statements in such a way that the number placed in each pile approximates a normal frequency distribution. Although Stephenson felt that factor analysis was essential in analyzing Q-sort data, there has been some disagreement concerning the appropriate data analysis procedure. Kerlinger's (1972) study of liberals and conservatives illustrates the use of factor analysis with Q-sort data and is recommended reading for anyone who plans to assess political attitudes by means of the Q-sort technique.

Multidimensional Scaling. One criticism of scalogram analysis, which applies to the method of equal-appearing intervals as well, is that attitudes are complex, multidimensional states that can rarely be represented by a single score. For example, two people may both have moderately positive attitudes toward, say, the church, but one person's attitude stems from the spiritual needs satisfied by the church while the other person is drawn to the opportunity for social interaction provided by church attendance. Although some attitudes appear to be fairly unidimensional, more complex attitudes toward institutions, products, political candidates, and the like are clearly multidimensional. In addition, the dimensionality of an attitude may vary with the particular sample of respondents.

The psychometrics of multidimensional scaling consists of analyzing the psychological or social "distance" between people, objects, or events as if it were physical distance (Euclidean difference) and then constructing a kind of "map" of how a person structures the attitude domain of interest. On such a map, short distances between statements or people represent high agreement and long distances represent high disagreement (see Schiffman, Reynolds, & Young, 1981).

Among the several multidimensional or multivariate procedures that have been applied to the construction of attitude scales are facet analysis, latent class, latent structure, and latent partition analysis, and the repertory grid technique (Abelson, 1967; Langeheine, 1988; Lazarsfeld & Henry, 1968; McCutcheon, 1987). *Facet analysis* is a complex, à priori, multidimensional paradigm for item construction and analysis that can be applied to any attitude, object, or situation (Castro & Jordan, 1977). This procedure has been used to construct cross-cultural attitude-behavior scales on a number of psychosocial conditions and situations, including mental retardation (Jordan, 1971) and racial-ethnic interaction (Hamersma, Paige, & Jordon, 1973). The basic postulate of *latent structure* and *latent class* models is that the observed relationships among a set of attitude statements (or other psychometric items) can be accounted for by a set of latent (unobserved) variables. Factor analysis and other multivariate statistical procedures are applied to the observed data to reveal the relationships among the latent class variables.

Psychometric Characteristics of Attitude Measures

As with any kind of measuring instrument, the practical value of attitude measures depends on their reliability, validity, and adequacy of standardization. In view of the careless way in which many attitude instruments have been constructed, it is not surprising that adequate information on many published and unpublished attitude instruments is unavailable.

Reliability

Although the reliability coefficients of attitude instruments are usually lower than those of cognitive measures, it is not unusual to find test-retest and internal consistency coefficients at levels of .80 and .90 for Thurstone- and Likert-type scales. One reason for these relatively high reliability coefficients is the influence of a strong general factor in what these scales are measuring. If a scale is fairly homogeneous with respect to item type, a split-half or alpha coefficient as well as coefficients of stability (test-retest) and equivalence (alternate forms) may be computed.

In addition to actual changes in attitudes produced by some manipulated condition, a number of situational and procedural variables can affect the reliability of an attitude instrument. Among such variables are testing conditions, number of response categories, and method of scoring.

Testing Conditions. Standardization of a psychometric instrument implies standard, uniform conditions of administration. Nevertheless, it is frequently impossible to hold testing conditions constant when attitude data are collected in many different situations. Because reliability implies consistency in differentiating among persons, it is lower when testing conditions affect the scores of respondents in different ways. For example, as on any psychological assessment procedure younger children are affected more than older children by variations in conditions of administering attitude scales. Consequently, the reliability of attitude scale scores increases with the age of the respondents.

Number of Response Categories. A possible reason why scores on Likert-type scales tend to be more reliable than those on Thurstone-type scales is that the larger number of response categories on instruments constructed by the former procedure increases the variance of the scores and hence their reliability. It may appear reasonable to assume that increasing the number of response categories beyond five would raise reliability even more, but this has not generally been found to be true. Increasing the number of response categories to 6, 9, or even 19 has little or no effect on the reliability of Likert scales. The reason appears to be that, when there is a large number of categories on a scale, respondents use only some of them. A possible exception to this typical behavior occurs when the range of attitudes toward the content being measured is small; in this case, increasing the number of response categories to six or seven increases reliability to some degree (Masters, 1974).

Scoring Weights. It is possible that increasing the number of response categories will improve the overall reliability if responses are transformed to normal deviation (z) scores (Wolins & Dickinson, 1973). This technique is one of the many efforts to increase the reliability and validity of attitude measures by some kind of item- or component-weighting procedure. Unfortunately, none of the various differential weighting schemes has been found to be superior with respect to effort and accuracy, compared to more traditional scoring methods. This is particularly true when the number of items on the single-score instrument is large.

Neutral Response Category? On certain kinds of attitude items, including some Thurstone-type scales, there is a middle or neutral response category (?, Don't know, Uncertain, etc.) in addition to the bipolar Yes/No categories. Use of this neutral category by respondents varies with instructions, the situation, and the type of attitude object. As might be expected, on two-and three-category formats, inclusion of a neutral response category may improve reliability somewhat. For this reason, inclusion of a neutral response category is generally recommended on scales that otherwise would have only dichotomous item scoring.

Validity of Attitude Measures

The validity of any cognitive or affective assessment instrument depends on the extent to which it measures what it was designed to measure. Validity depends, of course, on reliability, in that an instrument cannot be valid without being reliable. Consequently, both the reliability and validity of an attitude scale may be reduced by conditions that produce errors of measurement. Examples of factors that can cause measurement errors on attitude inventories are response sets (acquiescence, social desirability, indecisiveness) and faking.

As with other psychometric instruments, evidence for the validity of attitude inventories and scales is of three kinds: content validity, criterion-related validity, and construct validity. The *content validity* of an attitude inventory is related to the representativeness of the sample of questions in the inventory. Evidence for content validity is obtained from careful inspection of the inventory by attitude "experts" and their judgments of its validity. Information concerning the *criterion-related validity* of an attitude inventory is obtained by correlating scores on the instrument with other measures of the same or another variable obtained at the same time (concurrent validity) or at a later date (predictive validity). Although correlations obtained in this way are usually not very high, when combined with scores on ability tests they frequently make a small but significant contribution to the prediction of performance on the criterion measure. In addition, higher correlations between attitudes and behavior are obtained when the statements on the attitude inventory are expressed in behavioral terms (Ajzen & Fishbein, 1977; Fishbein & Ajzen, 1975).

The first step in designing an attitude instrument—identification of the theoretical construct to be measured—is often neglected (Gardner, 1975). Only after the construct has been identified is the investigator ready to search for a measure of the attitude construct among available instruments or to design a new measure. The most general method of determining whether a given instrument actually measures the appropriate variable is to search for evidence of its construct validity. The *construct validity* of an attitude instrument, concerned as it is with the extent to which the instrument measures the construct it purports to measure, cannot be determined by means of a single procedure. Various kinds of evidence must be sought—expert opinion, correlations of scores with other measures of the same construct, and comparing the scores of people who obviously have a high amount of the construct with the scores of people who have a low amount.

Sources of Information on Attitude Scales and Inventories

Many different inventories and scales for assessing social attitudes (Robinson, Shaver, & Wrightsman, 1991), political attitudes (Robinson, Rush, & Head, 1973), and occupational attitudes (Robinson, Athanasiou, & Head, 1974) are described in a series of books published by the Institute for Social Research at the University of Michigan. Other sources include the *American Social Attitudes Data Sourcebook, 1947–78* (Converse, Dotson, Hoag, & McGee, 1980), *A Sourcebook of Harris National Surveys: Repeated Questions, 1963–76* (Martin & McDuffee, 1981), and *General Social Surveys, 1973–1994: Cumulative Codebook* (Davis & Smith, 1994). Dozens of attitude measures in a wide range of areas are also listed in *Tests in Microfiche* (Educational Testing Service) and in Volume 5 of the *ETS Test Collection Catalog* (1991). Examples of attitude areas that have been assessed and studied extensively are attitudes toward:

aged (old) people	gender role	race (ethnic group)
AIDS	gifted children	school
any school subject	handicapped people	science
computers	gays and lesbians	sex
Congress	mainstreaming	smoking
day care	mathematics	teachers
drinking	politicians	testing
education	premarital sex	women
the environment	the president	work

Several publishers and distributors of psychological assessment instruments market attitude questionnaires and scales, a representative list of which is given in Table 8.2. In addition, you are encouraged to take the seven attitude inventories in Category J (Sample Inventories of Attitudes and Values) on the computer program diskette accompanying this book.

Problems in Measuring Differences and Changes in Attitudes

It might seem that determination of the significance of differences or changes in attitudes would pose no problem. Presumably, all one would need to do is subtract initial scores from final scores and analyze the differences in whatever way is considered appropriate.

One difficulty with raw final-minus-initial scores is that they are extremely unreliable and particularly so when the reliability coefficients of the initial and final scores are modest. This is even more likely to occur with scores on attitude scales and other affective instruments than with cognitive test scores. Another difficulty encountered in dealing with raw scores is regression toward the mean—the tendency for individuals whose initial scores are either very high or very low to make final scores that cluster closer to the mean. The use of regressed difference scores as a measure of attitude change is often recommended as a way of dealing with regression toward the mean, but such a procedure is not always appropriate.

TABLE 8.2   Some Representative Commercially Available Attitude Inventories and Scales

Alienation Index Survey: from Psychological Surveys Corporation; assesses work-related attitudes of adult job applicants.

Arlin-Hills Attitude Surveys: M. Arlin & D. Hills; from Psychologists and Educators, Inc.; measures attitudes of students in grades K–12.

Attitude Survey Program for Business and Industry: from London House, Inc.; measures the attitudes of adult employees and provides an overview of company conditions.

Attitude Survey Program for Business and Industry: Managerial Survey; from London House, Inc.; measures attitudes of managers above first-line supervisors toward the company and provides an overview of company conditions.

Attitude Survey Program for Business and Industry: Organization Survey: from London House, Inc.; measures the attitudes of hourly employees and first-line supervisors toward the company and provides an overview of company conditions.

Attitude Survey Program for Business and Industry: Professional Survey; from London House, Inc; measures attitudes of professions in staff positions (attorneys, editors, accountants, engineers, etc.) toward the company.

Attitude Survey Program for Business and Industry: Sales Survey: from London House, Inc.; measures attitudes of outside field sales representatives toward the company.

Attitude Toward School Questionnaire: G. P. Strickland, R. Hoepfner, & S. P. Klein; from Monitor; measures attitudes toward school in students in grades K–3.

Attitude Towards Disabled Persons Scale: H. E. Yuker & J. R. Block; from Center for the Study of Attitudes Toward Persons with Disabilities, Hofstra University; measures attitudes of students and adults toward disabled persons.

Bloom Sentence Completion Attitude Survey: W. Bloom; from Stoelting; assesses attitudes relating to eight important factors in everyday living.

Canadian Comprehensive Assessment Program: School Attitude Measure: from Guidance Center; evaluates affective responses of students in grades 4-9 to their school experiences.

Career Attitudes and Strategies Inventory: J. L. Holland & G. D. Gottfredson; from Psychological Assessment Resources; assesses career attitudes and obstacles in employed and unemployed adults.

Employee Attitude Inventory: from London House, Inc.; measures six variables designed to help identify an organization's potential exposure to employee theft and counterproductive behavior.

Easy.Gen Employee Attitude Survey Generator: from Wonderlic Personnel Test, Inc; Computer software for designing attitude questions and selecting questions from a database of 515 questions covering 41 topics; also administers attitude questionnaires by computer or paper-and-pencil and produces graphs and reports of results.

TABLE 8.2 *(Continued)*

Marriage and Family Attitude Survey: D. V. Martin & M. Martin; from Psychologists and Educators, Inc.; assesses attitudes of adolescents and adults toward various aspects of marriage and family life (parenting, communication expectations and privacy rights, social needs, sexuality, sex roles, marriage and divorce, etc.)

Opinions Toward Adolescents: W. T. Martin; from Psychologists and Educators, Inc.; examines opinions and attitudes of adults toward adolescents on eight bipolar scales.

Sex-Role Egalitarianism Scale (SRES): L. A. King & D. W. King; from Sigma Assessment Systems; measures attitudes toward the equality of men and women and judgments about both men and women assuming nontraditional roles.

Study Attitudes and Methods Survey: W. B. Michael, J. J. Michael, & W. S. Zimmerman; from EdITS; developed to assess dimensions of a motivational, noncognitive nature that are related to school achievement and which contribute to student performance beyond what is measured by traditional ability tests.

Survey of Study Habits and Attitudes: W. F. Brown & W. H. Holtzman; from The Psychological Corporation; measures study methods, motivation for studying, and certain attitudes toward scholastic activities that are important in the classroom.

The Sales Attitude Checklist: E. K. Taylor; from London House; measures the attitudes and behaviors toward selling of sales applicants.

Because most research on attitudes is fundamentally correlational in nature, investigators should be familiar with a variety of correlational procedures for determining the significance of differences and changes. Among these procedures are part (semipartial) and partial correlation, two-way part correlation, cross-lagged panel correlation, and time-series analysis. For example, if a researcher is interested in the correlation between ability and changes in work-related attitudes associated with the introduction of a new procedure, an appropriate statistic is part correlation. Using this method, initial attitude scores are partialed out from final attitude scores and the resulting regressed difference scores are correlated with the measure of ability.

A traditional approach to determining the effects of experimental treatments on intergroup differences or intragroup changes in dependent variables involves analysis of variance designs. The mean attitude scores of two or more groups can be compared by using a randomized groups design, or the means of the same group or correlated groups can be compared in a repeated measures design. One difficulty with the first design is that the two groups may not be strictly comparable at the beginning of the experiment. Initial attitude scores can be used as a covariate to correct statistically for initial differences in attitudes, but the initial test may sensitize the subjects in such a way that final attitude scores are affected. The same criticism can be applied to the repeated measures design, where initial testing may sensitize the subjects and thereby affect scores on the final test. It is possible, of course, to employ a procedure such as the Solomon four-group design (Solomon & Lessac, 1968) to determine the effects of initial testing on final attitude scores. Another way of reducing the sensitizing effects of testing is to administer the initial attitude inventory several weeks before the study is conducted and disguise the purpose of the study by making the attitude inventory part of a longer questionnaire on a variety of topics (Mussen et al., 1979).

The practice of using analysis of covariance in studies that include such organismic variables as sex, grade level, and intelligence as independent variables also causes problems. Suppose, for example, that a scale of attitudes toward premarital sex is administered to a group of girls and a group of boys both before and after they listen to a lecture on AIDS. To determine the differential effects of the lecture on changes in attitudes toward premarital sex, the researcher uses an analysis of covariance design with initial attitude scores as the covariate, final attitude scores as the dependent variable, and sex as the independent variable. Because in this case the covariate is confounded with the independent variable, an important assumption underlying the analysis of covariance has been violated and the results cannot be interpreted clearly (Evans & Anastasio, 1968). What is required is a partial correlation analysis, not an analysis of covariance.

Another common situation calling for a partial correlation analysis rather than an analysis of covariance is as follows. An educational researcher wishes to determine whether increases in competence, resulting from instruction in a subject, are accompanied by improvements in attitude toward the subject. Method of instruction is the independent variable, initial scores on an appropriate achievement test and a measure of attitudes toward the subject are the covariates, and final scores on the last two variables are the dependent variables. Two analyses of covariance are conducted, one with achievement test scores and the other with attitude scores as the covariate and dependent variable. The results of the two analyses are compared to determine whether statistically significant changes in achievement are accompanied by significant changes in attitudes. Unfortunately, there is no way in which a univariate analysis of covariance can yield an unambiguous conclusion in this situation. The reason is that this approach takes into account the correlation between the dependent variable and the covariate *within* each analysis but not *across* the two analyses. A better, and perhaps simpler, procedure is to compute the correlations among the dependent variables and covariates and apply the following special semipartial correlation formula (Aiken, 1981):

$$r_{(1.2)(3.4)} = [r_{13} - r_{12}r_{23} - r_{34}(r_{14} - r_{12}r_{24})]/(\sqrt{1 - r_{12}^2}\sqrt{1 - r_{34}^2}) \qquad (8.2)$$

where 1 = posttest achievement score, 2 = pretest achievement score, 3 = posttest attitude score, and 4 = pretest attitude score. The value of $r_{(1.2)(3.4)}$ is the correlation between residual posttest achievement scores (after pretest achievement scores have been partialled out) and residual posttest attitude scores (after pretest attitude scores have been partialled out).

MEASURES OF VALUES

Related but not identical to attitudes are values, which are concerned with the utility, importance, or worth attached to particular activities or objects. Most questionnaires and inventories for measuring values are designed for a specific research purpose or application and are not commercially available; examples of such unpublished instruments are the author's Educational Values Inventory and Altruism Inventory (see programs J-5 and J-6 of *Computer Programs for Rating Scales and Checklists*). A number of values inventories are commercially-available, and the list in Table 8.3 is representative. In this section, we shall describe five of these instruments—the Rokeach Value Survey, the Study of Values, the Work Values Inventory, The Values Scale, and the Temperament and Values Inventory.

Among the pioneers in the study of values were Gordon Allport, L. L. Thurstone, and Milton Rokeach. Rokeach, in particular, conducted extensive international and cross-cultural research on the topic. He defined a value as "an enduring belief that a specific mode of conduct or end-state of existence is personally or socially preferable to an opposite or converse mode of conduct or end-state of existence" (Rokeach, 1973, p. 5). This definition considers two kinds of values—those pertaining to modes of conduct (*instrumental values*) and those concerned with end-states (*terminal values*). Vocational psychologists have in large

TABLE 8.3.   Some Representative Commercially Available Values Inventories

Career Orientation Placement and Evaluation: L. F. Knapp & R. R. Knapp; from EdITS; designed to measure those personal values which have been observed to be related to the type of work one chooses and the satisfactions derived from the work one does.

Rokeach Value Survey: M. Rokeach; from Consulting Psychologists Press; assesses the relative important of 18 instrumental values and 18 terminal values to the respondent.

Study of Values: G. W. Allport; from Riverside Publishing Company; measures six values (Theoretical, Economic, Aesthetic, Social, Political, Religious), useful in vocational guidance, personnel work, personality research, and classroom demonstrations in psychology courses.

Survey of Interpersonal Values: L. V. Gordon; from SRA Product Group; measures six values (support, conformity, recognition, independence, benevolence, leadership) involving relationships with others that are important in many work situations.

Survey of Personal Values: L. V. Gordon; from SRA Product Group; measures six values (practical mindedness, achievement, variety, decisiveness, orderliness, goal orientation) that influence the manner in which people cope with problems and choices of everyday living; provides information about how people are likely to approach jobs or training programs.

Temperament and Values Inventory: C. B. Johannson & P. L. Webber; from NCS Assessments; measures personality factors that may affect contentment in work situations.

The Values Scale (2nd ed.): D. E. Super & D. D. Nevill; from Consulting Psychologists Press; measures extrinsic and intrinsic values related to career development and most personally satisfying career.

Work Values Inventory: D. E. Super; from Riverside Publishing Company; measures the relative importance of work values in grades 7-12; provides guidance counselors, teachers, and administrators with profiles of student values for counseling them in occupational choices and course selections.

measure limited their attention to terminal values, but Rokeach defined several subcategories of both instrumental and terminal values and designed an instrument to measure them.

Rokeach Value Survey

According to Milton Rokeach, there are two types of instrumental values—*moral values* and *competence values*. The former type pertains to interpersonal modes of conduct, which precipitate feelings of guilt when they are violated. The latter type, competence values, has to do with intrapersonal, self-actualizing modes of conduct; violation of these values leads to feelings of inadequacy. Terminal values are divided further into *personal values* and *social values*. Personal values, including such end-states as peace of mind and salvation, are self-centered; social values, including end-states such as equality and world peace, are society-centered.

The Rokeach Value Survey consists of 18 instrumental and 18 terminal value terms or phrases for assessing the relative importance of these values. The respondent is directed to rank order the 18 items in each list according to their importance to him or her. No other instrument attempts to measure as many values as the Rokeach Value Survey, a fact which, together with speed of administration and scoring and inexpensiveness, may account for its popularity. The reliability of the instrument for comparing different groups of people, a purpose for which it has been used in hundreds of investigations, is adequate. Individuals of different nationalities and in different living circumstances rank the items on the survey differently. Rokeach (1973) reported, for example, that Israeli students gave the highest ranking to the terminal values of "a world at peace" and "national security." American students, in contrast, ranked the terminal value of "a comfortable life" and the instrumental value of "ambitious" highest.

Study of Values

Social and vocational psychologists have designed many different instruments to measure values. The most popular of these, the Study of Values (G. W. Allport, P. E. Vernon, & G. Lindzey), has been used in numerous research investigations concerned with education and learning, perception, personality, perception, social psychology, and vocational guidance. It has also been found useful in vocational guidance, personnel work, and for classroom demonstrations in psychology courses.

The design and scoring of the Study of Values is based on Eduard Spranger's (1928) classification of people into six types: theoretical, economic, aesthetic, social, political, and religious. The Study of Values can be completed in approximately 20 minutes by high school or college students and adults. On Part I, respondents indicate a relative preference for each of 30 pairs of activities by dividing three points among them, or by dividing the three points between affirmative and negative responses. On Part II, respondents rank the four choices on each of 15 items in order of preference. Scores on the six values areas are plotted as a profile showing the relative strength of the respondent's values. Because the scores are ipsative (correlated), if a person scores high on some areas he or she will score low on others. Mean scores on each of the six areas measured by the Study of Values based on a sample of over 8,000 college students of both sexes and various occupational groups are listed in the manual. The most recent norms, based on a nationwide sample of 6,000 high school students, were obtained in 1968. The test-retest reliabilities of scores on the separate values areas are reported as in the .80s over an interval of two months.

Rabinowitz (1984) and others have criticized the theoretical formulation, the ipsative nature of the scoring system, and the fair amount of education required to understand the items on the Study of Values. In addition to having outdated norms, some of the content appears old-fashioned for the 1990s. Be that as it may, the Study of Values continues to be used for instructional and research purposes.

Vocational Values

The Rokeach Value Survey and the Study of Values can be administered in vocational counseling situations, but these inventories were not designed specifically for this purpose. Instruments such as the Work Values Inventory, The Values Scale, and the Temperament and Values Inventory are more closely related to occupational choice and satisfaction. These *vocational values* vary with the person and the situation. Super (1973) found, for example, that people in upper-level occupations were more motivated by the need for self-actualization, an intrinsic goal, whereas extrinsic values were more likely to be subscribed to by those in lower-level occupations.

Work Values Inventory

This inventory (D. E. Super), which can be completed in about 15 minutes by individuals from grade 7 on up, consists of 45 Likert-type items designed to assess 15 values considered important in vocational success and satisfaction. Each of the 15 values (e.g., achievement, supervisory relations, independence, aesthetics, creativity) is measured by only three items. Examinees rate each statement on a five-point scale, depending on the degree of importance attached to the value represented by the statement. The combined ratings for the three statements on a particular scale determine the strength of that value. Percentile norms by grade (7-12) are based on data collected in 1968 on a representative national sample of approximately 9,000 high school students. Reliability coefficients (test-retest), obtained from retesting 99 tenth graders after two weeks, range from .74 to .88 for the 15 scales. Statistics and other information concerning the content, concurrent, and construct validity of the Work Values Inventory is described in the manual.

Bolton (1985) praised the Work Values Inventory for its excellent psychometric foundations and its continuing research uses, but it has been criticized on a number of points. A revised, up-to-date manual that incorporates the findings of research conducted since 1970, in particular occupational validity studies based on the current form of the inventory, is needed. Also needed are reliability data based on college students and adults, not just tenth graders, and new, representative norms.

The Values Scale

This instrument, which was developed by the Work Importance Study, an international consortium of vocational psychologists from America, Asia, and Europe, has characteristics of both the Work Values Inventory and the Rokeach Value Survey. The goal of both the consortium and The Values Scale was to obtain a better understanding of the values that people seek or hope to find in various life roles and to assess the relative importance of the work role as a means of value realization in the context of other life roles. The scale consists of 106 items and takes 30 to 45 minutes to complete. It is scored for the following 21 values, with five items per value:

Ability Utilization	Creativity	Social Interaction
Achievement	Economic Rewards	Social Relations
Advancement	Life Style	Variety
Esthetics	Personal Development	Working Conditions
Altruism	Physical Activity	Cultural Identity
Authority	Prestige	Physical Prowess
Autonomy	Risk	Economic Security

Reliabilities of the scores on these 21 values are satisfactory for individual assessment at the adult level, the reliabilities of the scores on ten scales are high enough for individual assessment at the college level, and the reliabilities of eight scales are adequate for the high school level. The manual provides means and standard deviations for three samples (high school, college, and adult), as well as information on the construct validity of The Values Scale. The instrument appears to have good potential for research on vocational counseling and selection, and particularly for cross-cultural or cross-national comparisons.

Temperament and Values Inventory (TVI)

This inventory is the result of careful construction by the authors, C. B. Johansson and P. L. Webber, to provide a measure of temperament and values that would complement information obtained from ability tests and vocational interest inventories. Designed primarily for high school students and adults, it takes approximately 30 minutes to complete. There are 230 items, divided into two sections: 133 true-false items scored on seven Temperament Scales (Personal Characteristics) and 97 Likert-type items scored on seven Values Scales (Reward Values). The seven bipolar Temperament Scales on which the TVI is scored are Routine-Flexible, Quiet-Active, Attentive-Distractible, Serious-Cheerful, Consistent-Changeable, Reserved-Social, and Reticent-Persuasive. It is also scored on seven Values Scales, including Social Recognition, Managerial-Sales Benefits, Leadership, Social Services, Task Specificity, Philosophical Curiosity, and Work Independence. Scoring and score interpretation are both done by computer.

An initial sample of 802 males and females was used to develop the 14 TVI scales, which were verified on a separate sample of 456 high school students. Standard T-score norms for the scales are based on three age groups (15–19, 20–25, and 26–53 years) of males and females. The test-retest reliabilities, which were obtained on small samples retested over 1 to 2 weeks, are fairly satisfactory (.79–.93). Comparisons between the TVI and other related inventories substantiate the construct validity of the inventory. Data on the ability of the TVI to differentiate between relatively small samples of individuals in a rather narrow range of occupations is reported as evidence for concurrent validity.

Fairly positive evaluations (Wheeler, 1985; Zuckerman, 1985) have been given to the TVI, especially for its careful construction and well-designed manual. Among its psychometric shortcomings are a lack of long-term reliability data, a lack of convergent and discriminant validity studies, and norms that are based on fairly small and nonrepresentative samples.

SUMMARY

Attitudes are defined as learned predispositions to respond positively or negatively to some object, situation, or person. They are more pervasive than opinions, but more superficial than beliefs and values. Various methods—direct observation, interview, projective techniques, questionnaires—can be used to in assess attitudes, but the most efficient and popular procedure is to administer an attitude scale. The methods devised by Thurstone (equal-appearing intervals), Likert (summated ratings), and Guttman (scalogram analysis) for scaling attitudes have been applied extensively to the construction of attitude scales. Other attitude-scaling procedures include the semantic-differential technique, Q sorts, and facet analysis. Factor analysis, multidimensional scaling, latent-structure analysis, latent-partition analysis, the repertory grid technique and other multivariate statistical procedures have also been applied in scaling attitudes.

An individual can have an attitude toward almost anything—any school subject, any vocation, any defined group, any institution, any proposed social action, any practice. Most of the hundreds of attitude scales and questionnaires listed in various reference sources are unstandardized instruments designed for a particular research investigation or application. But a number of standardized instruments for assessing attitudes, especially attitudes toward school and school subjects, work and work supervisors, are available from publishers of psychological and educational tests.

On a Q sort the respondent sorts a set of a 100 or so cards containing descriptive statements pertaining to attitudes, opinions, values, or some other psychological construct into nine piles to form a normal distribution of statements across piles. This forced-distribution procedure has been used in studies concerned with the effectiveness of psychological counseling and in other research and applied contexts.

The concept of value refers to the usefulness, importance, or worth attached to particular activities or objects. Rokeach distinguished between two kinds of values: instrumental and terminal. He devised a checklist, the Rokeach Value Survey, to measure two kinds of instrumental values (moral and competence) and two kinds of terminal values (personal and social). The most time-honored measure of values is the Study of Values. This ipsatively scored inventory measures a person's values in six areas: theoretical, economic, aesthetic, social, political, and religious. Studies of work-related values have led to the development of instruments such as the Work Values Inventory, and the Values Scale. Relationships between values and personality are seen in data obtained by administering the Temperament and Values Inventory, which is scored on seven bipolar Temperament Scales and seven Values Scales.

QUESTIONS AND ACTIVITIES

1. Define each of the following terms:

    attitude   pair comparisons
    attitude scale   personal values
    belief   reproducibility coefficient
    competence values   scalogram analysis
    equal-appearing intervals   social values
    facet analysis   summated ratings
    instrumental values   terminal values
    interest   value
    moral values   vocational values
    opinion

2. To construct an attitude scale by Thurstone's method of equal appearing intervals, suppose that each of 50 judges sorts 200 attitude statements into 11 piles. The numbers of judges who place statements X, Y, and Z into each of the 11 categories are given in the three frequency distributions listed below. Compute the scale value (median) and ambiguity index (semi-interquartile range) of each statement (see Chapter 2). Use the pile number (1, 2, . . . , 11) plus .5 as the upper exact limit of the interval.

Pile Number	Statement X	Statement Y	Statement Z
1	3		
2	4		
3	6	8	
4	8	10	
5	13	12	6
6	10	9	9
7	6	8	10
8		3	18
9			7
10			
11			

3. Make multiple copies of the attitude scale in Figure 8.1 ("Attitudes Toward Capital Punishment") for administration to several people. Before administering the scale, the statements in Figure 8.1 will have to be retyped in order of their item numbers, omitting the scale values enclosed in parentheses. The respondent's total score on the scale of attitudes toward capital punishment is determined by adding the scale values of the statements that are checked and dividing the sum by the total number of statements (12). Ask the examinees to explain the reasons for their attitudes toward capital punishment, and summarize the results. What personality variables do you believe are related to attitudes toward capital punishment? (Note: This scale can also be administered and scored by program J-7.)

4. Make multiple copies of the Mathematics Attitude Scale in Figure 8.2 and administer the scale to several men and the same number of women. Compute their scores on the scale as follows: For items 1, 2, 6, 7, 8, 10, 12, 13, 16, and 17: SD = 4, D = 3, U = 2, A = 1, SA = 0. For the remaining items, SD = 0, A = 1, U = 2, A = 3, SA = 4. Total score, the sum of the scores on all 20 items, ranges from 0 to 80. The higher the score, the more positive the respondent's attitude toward mathematics. Compare the mean scores of men and women be using a t test or other appropriate statistic. (Note: This scale can also be administered and scored by program J-1.)

5. Run all of the programs in Category J ("Sample Inventories of Attitudes, Opinions, and Values") of the computer program diskette accompanying this book.

6. Differentiate among attitudes, beliefs, interests, opinions, and values. Which of these constructs is easiest to measure? Which is more useful, i.e., practical, to measure?

Appendix A
Glossary

Acquiescence response set (style).   Tendency of a person to answer affirmatively (yes or true) of personality test items and in other alternative response situations.

Adaptive behavior.   The extent to which a person is able to interact effectively and appropriately with the environment.

Affective assessment.   Measurement of noncognitive (nonintellective) variables or characteristics. Affective variables include temperament, emotional, interests, attitudes, personal style, and other behaviors, traits or processes typical of an individual. See **Cognitive assessment.**

Alternate-forms reliability.   An index of reliability determined by correlating the scores of individuals on one form of a test with their scores on another form.

Analytic scoring.   Scoring performance in terms of set of individual elements rather than by an overall impression of the product as a whole. See **Holistic scoring.**

Anchoring.   Setting the points on a rating scale, including the ends and various intermediate categories between them.

Aptitude.   Capability of learning to perform a particular task or skill. Traditionally, aptitude was thought to depend more on inborn potential than on actual practice.

Aptitude test.   A measure of the ability to profit from additional training or experience, that is, become proficient in a skill or other ability.

Arithmetic mean.   A measure of the average or central tendency of a group of scores. The arithmetic mean is computed by dividing the sum of the scores by the number of scores.

Assessment.   Appraising the presence or magnitude of one or more personal characteristics. Assessing human behavior and mental processes includes such procedures as observations, interviews, rating scales, checklists, inventories, projectives techniques, and tests.

Attitude.   Tendency to react positively or negatively to some object, person, or situation.

Attitude scale.   A paper-and-pencil instrument, consisting of a series of statements concerning an institution, situation, person, event, and so on. The examinee responds to each statement by endorsing it or indicating his degree of agreement or disagreement with it.

Attribution error. Tendency of supervisors to rate high performers higher and low performers lower when they attribute the causes of a given level of job performance to internal rather than external factors.

Aunt Fanny error. See **Barnum effect.**

Automated assessment. Use of test-scoring machines, computers, and other electronic or electromechanical devices to administer, score, and interpret psychological assessments.

Average. Measure of central tendency of a group of scores; the most representative score.

Barnum effect. Acceptance as accurate a personality description phrased in generalities, truisms, and other statements that sound specific to a given person but are actually applicable to almost anyone. Same as **Aunt Fanny error.**

Base rate. Proportion of individuals having a specified condition who are identified or selected without the use of new selection procedures.

Behavior analysis. Procedures that focus on objectively describing a particular behavior and identifying the antecedents and consequences of that behavior. Behavior analysis may be conducted for research purposes or to obtain information in planning a behavior modification program.

Behavior expectation scale (BES). Technique of evaluating employee performance in which evaluators rate, in terms of their expectations, employee behaviors that are considered critical.

Behavioral observation scale (BOS). Technique of evaluating employee performance in which evaluators rate the frequency employee behaviors that are considered critical.

Behaviorally anchored rating scale (BARS). Technique of performance evaluation in which evaluators rate critical employee behaviors.

Belief. Confidence in the truth or existence of something not immediately susceptible to rigorous proof. See **Attitude** and **Opinion.**

Bias. Any one of a number of factors that cause scores on psychometric instruments to be consistently higher or lower than they should be if measurement were accurate. An example of bias in rating is the *leniency error*—the tendency to rate a person consistently higher than he or she should be rated.

Bimodal distribution. A frequency distribution having two modes (maximum points). See **Frequency distribution; Mode.**

Bipolar scale. A rating scale with antonyms (good-bad, fast-slow, weak-strong, etc.) at opposite ends of the scale.

Central tendency. Average, or central, score in a group of scores; the most representative score (e.g., arithmetic mean, median, mode).

Central tendency error. The tendency to rate in the middle category to a greater extent than justified.

Checklist. List of words, phrases, or statements descriptive of personal characteristics; respondents endorse (check) those items that are characteristic of themselves (self-ratings) or other people (other-ratings).

Classification. The use of test scores to assign a person to one category rather than another.

Cluster sampling. Sampling procedure in which the target population is divided into sections or clusters, and the number of units selected at random from a given cluster is proportional to the total number of units in the cluster.

Coefficient alpha. An internal-consistency reliability coefficient, appropriate for tests comprised of dichotomous or multipoint items; the expected correlation of one test with a parallel form.

Coefficient of equivalence. A reliability coefficient (correlation) obtained by administering a test to the same group of examinees on two different occasions. See **Test-retest reliability.**

Coefficient of internal consistency. Reliability coefficient based on estimates of the internal consistency of a test (for example, split-half coefficient and alpha coefficient).

Coefficient of stability. A reliability coefficient (correlation) obtained by administering a test to the same group of examinees on two different occasions. See **Test-retest reliability.**

Coefficient of stability and equivalence. A reliability coefficient obtained by administering two forms of a test to a group of examinees on two different occasions.

Cognition. Having to do with the processes of intellect; remembering, thinking, problem solving, and the like.

Cognitive assessment. Measurement of intellective processes, such as perception, memory, thinking, judgment, and reasoning. See **Affective assessment.**

Communality. Proportion of variance in a measured variable accounted for by variance that the variable has in common with other variables.

Composite score. The direct or weighted sum of the scores on two or more tests or sections of a test.

Concurrent validity. The extent to which scores obtained by a group of people on a particular psychometric instrument are related to their simultaneously determined scores on another measure (criterion) of the same characteristic that the instrument is supposed to measure.

Constant errors. Errors in rating, such as being too lenient, too severe, or rating in the middle category, that tend to bias the ratings.

Construct validity. The extent to which scores on a psychometric instrument designed to measure a certain characteristic are related to measures of behavior in situations in which the characteristic is supposed to be an important determinant of behavior.

Content analysis. Method of studying and analyzing written (or oral) communications in a systematic, objective, and quantitative manner to assess certain psychological variables.

Content validity. The extent to which a group of people who are experts in the material with which a test deals agree that the test or other psychometric instrument measures what it was designed to measure.

Contrast error. In interviewing or rating, the tendency to evaluate a person more positively if an immediately preceding individual was assigned a highly negative evaluation or to evaluate a person more negatively if an immediately preceding individual was given a highly positive evaluation.

Convergent validity. Situation in which an assessment instrument has high correlations with other measures (or methods of measuring) the same construct. See **Discriminant validity.**

Correction for attenuation. Formula used to estimate what the validity coefficient of a test would be if both the test and the criterion were perfectly reliable.

Correlation. Degree of relationship or association between two variables, such as a test and a criterion measure.

Correlation coefficient. A numerical index of the degree of relationship between two variables. Correlation coefficients usually range from −1.00 (perfect negative relationship), through .00 (total absence of a relationship) to +1.00 (perfect positive relationship). Two common types of correlation coefficient are the product-moment coefficient and the point-biserial coefficient.

Criterion. A standard or variable with which scores on a psychometric instrument are compared or against which they are evaluated. The validity of a test or other psychometric procedure used in selecting or classifying people is determined by its ability to predict a specified criterion of behavior in the situation for which people are being selected or classified.

Criterion contamination. The effect of any factor on a criterion such that the criterion is not a valid measure of an individual's accomplishment. Intelligence test scores are frequently used to predict grades in school, but when teachers use intelligence test scores in deciding what grades to assign, the grades are not a valid criterion for validating the intelligence test; the criterion has become contaminated.

Criterion-related validity. The extent to which a test or other assessment instrument measures what it was designed to measure, as indicated by the correlation of test scores with some criterion measure of behavior.

Critical incident. A measure of performance, used primarily in industrial-organizational contexts, in which an individual's overall criterion score is determined by the extent to which behavior thought to be critical for effective performance in a given situation is manifested.

Cross-validation. Re-administering an assessment instrument that has been found to be a valid predictor of a criterion for one group of persons to a second group of persons to determine whether the instrument is also valid for that group. There is almost always some shrinkage of the validity coefficient on cross-validation, since chance factors spuriously inflate the validity coefficient obtained with the first group of examinees.

Cumulative scale. Rating scale, such as Bogardus's Social Distance Scale or Guttman's scales, on which items are arranged in a hierarchy so that endorsing (or answering correctly) a particular item correctly implies the endorsement of (or answering correctly) all items below it on the hierarchy.

Cutoff score (cutting score).   Score on a test or other selection measure, below which all applicants (candidates) are rejected and at or above which all applicants are accepted. The cut-off score depends on the validity of the test, the selection ration, and other factors.

Deferred rating system.   Procedure, as in most federal government positions at GS-9 and above, of waiting until specific vacancies become available before rating applicants for positions. Registers of applicants are not ranked or assigned numerical scores at the time of application. Only when openings in the positions occur are applicants on the register rated and the best-qualified applicants placed at the top of the list and referred to the agency for employment consideration.

Derived score.   A score obtained by performing some mathematical operation on a raw score, such as multiplying the raw score by a constant and/or adding a constant to the score. See **Standard scores; T-score; z-score.**

Developmental quotient (DQ).   An index, roughly equivalent to a mental age, for summarizing an infant's behavior as assessed by the Gesell Developmental Schedules.

Differential accuracy.   Tendency of supervisors in rating their subordinates to focus on, and therefore be more accurate in rating, effective rather than ineffective performance of the subordinates.

Discriminant validity.   Situation in which a psychometric instrument has low correlations with other measures of (or methods of measuring) different psychological constructs.

Ectomorph.   In Sheldon's somatotype system, a person with a tall, thin body build; related to the cerebrotonic (thinking, introversive) temperament type.

Efficiency rating.   Dated term for performance appraisal.

Empirical scoring.   A scoring system in which an examinee's responses are scored according to a key constructed from responses made by people in certain criterion groups, such as schizophrenics or physicians. This scoring procedure is employed with various personality and interest inventories.

Endomorph.   In Sheldon's somatotype system, a person having a rotund body shape (fat); related to the viscerotonic (relaxed, sociable) temperament.

Equal-appearing intervals (method of).   Method of attitude scaling devised by Thurstone, in which a large sample of "judges" sort attitude statements into 11 piles. The scale value of a statement is computed as the median, and the ambiguity index as the semi-interquartile range, of the judges' ratings.

Equipercentile method.   Traditional method of converting the score units of one test to the score units of a parallel test. The scores on each test are converted to percentile ranks, and a table of equivalent scores is produced by equating the score at the pth percentile on the first test to the score at the pth percentile on the second test.

Evaluation.   To judge the merit or value of an examinee's behavior from a composite of test scores, observations, and reports.

Exceptional (special) child.   A child who deviates significantly from the average in mental, physical, or emotional characteristics.

Experiment. Research investigation in which certain factors (independent variables) are varied, others (control or extraneous variables) are held constant, and the effects on the dependent variable(s) on randomly assigned subjects are measured.

Face validity. The extent to which the appearance or content of the materials (items and the like) on a test or other psychometric instrument is such that the instrument appears to be a good measure of what it is supposed to measure.

Factor. A dimension, trait, or characteristic of personality revealed by factor analyzing the matrix of correlations computed from the scores of a large number of people in several different tests or items.

Factor analysis. A mathematical procedure for analyzing a matrix of correlations among measurements to determine what factors (constructs) are sufficient to explain the correlations.

Factor loadings. In factor analysis, the resulting correlations (weights) between tests (or other variables) and the extracted factors.

Factor rotation. A mathematical procedure applied to a factor matrix for the purpose of simplifying the matrix for interpretation purposes by increasing the number of high and low factor loadings in the matrix. Factor rotation may be either *orthogonal,* in which case the resulting factors are at right angles (uncorrelated) to each other, or *oblique,* in which the resulting factor axes form acute or obtuse angles with each other and hence are correlated.

False negative. Selection error or diagnostic decision error in which an assessment procedure incorrectly predicts a maladaptive outcome (for example, low achievement, poor performance, or psychopathology).

False positive. Selection error or diagnostic decision error in which an assessment procedure incorrectly predicts an adaptive outcome (for example, high achievement, good performance, or absence of psychopathology).

Forced-choice item. Item on a personality or interest inventory, arranged as a dyad (two options), a triad (three options), or a tetrad (four options) of terms or phrases. The respondent is required to select the option viewed as most descriptive of the personality, interests, or behavior of the person being evaluated and perhaps another option perceived to be least descriptive of the personality, interests, or behavior of the person being evaluated. Forced-choice items are found on certain personality inventories (for example, the Edwards Personal Preference Schedule, interest inventories (Kuder General Interest Survey), and rating forms to control for response sets.

Forced-distribution technique. Technique in which raters are told to assign ratings to each of several categories on rating scales according to fixed percentages, so that a specified number of ratings will fall in each category.

Frequency distribution. A table of score intervals and the number of cases (scores) falling within each interval.

Generalizability theory. A theory of test scores and the associated statistical formulation that conceptualizes a test score as a sample from a universe of scores. Analysis of variance procedures are used to determine the generalizability from score to universe value, as a function of examinees, test items, and situational contexts. A generalizability coefficient may be computed as a measure of the degree of generalizability from sample to population.

Graphic rating scale.   A rating scale containing a series of items, each consisting of a line on which the rater places a check mark to indicate the degree of a characteristic that the ratee is perceived as possessing. Typically, at the left extremity of the line is a brief verbal description indicating the lowest degree of the characteristic, and at the right end is a description of the highest degree of the characteristic. Brief descriptions of intermediate degrees of the characteristic may also be located at equidistant points along the line.

Guess-who technique.   Procedure for analyzing group interaction and the social stimulus value of group members, in which children are asked to "guess who" in a classroom or other group situation possesses certain characteristics or does certain things.

Halo effect.   Rating a person high on one characteristic merely because he or she rates high on other characteristics.

Heritability index (h^2).   Ratio of the test score variance attributable to heredity to the variance attributable to both heredity and environment.

Holistic scoring.   Scoring based on an overall impression of the product rather than a consideration of individual elements.

Idiographic approach.   Approach to personality assessment and research in which the individual is viewed as a lawful, integrated system in his or her own right.

In-basket technique.   A procedure for evaluating supervisors or executives in which the candidate is required to indicate what action should be taken on a series of memos and other materials of the kind typically found in a supervisor's or executive's in-basket.

Incident (event) sampling.   In contrast to *time sampling*, an observational procedure in which certain types of incidents or events, such as those indicative of aggressive behavior, are selected for observation and recording.

Informed consent.   A formal agreement made by an individual, or the individual's guardian or legal representative, with an agency or another person to permit use of the individual's name and/or personal information (test scores and the like) for a specified purpose.

Interest.   Attentiveness, concern, or curiosity about something. See **Attitude, Belief, Opinion,** and **Value.**

Interest inventory.   A test or checklist, such as the Strong Interest Inventory or the Kuder General Interest Survey, designed to assess an individual's preferences for certain activities and topics.

Internal consistency.   The extent to which all items on a test measure the same variable or construct. The reliability of a test computed by the Spearman-Brown, Kuder-Richardson, or Cronbach-alpha formulas is a measure of the test's internal consistency.

Interpersonal affect.   The personal relationship (feelings or emotions) between rater and ratee, which can affect the ratings given.

Interrater (interscorer) reliability. Two scorers assign a numerical rating or score to a sample of people. Then the correlation between the two sets of numbers is computed.

Interval scale. A measurement scale on which equality of numerical differences implies equality of differences in the attribute or characteristic being measured. The scale of temperature (Celsius, Fahrenheit) and, presumably, standard score scales z, T), are examples of interval scales.

Interview. A systematic procedure for obtaining information by asking questions and, in general, verbally interacting with a person (the interviewee).

Inventory. A set of questions or statements to which the individual responds (for example, by indicating agreement or disagreement), designed to provide a measure of personality interest, attitude, or behavior.

Ipsative measurement. Test item format (e.g., forced-choice) in which the variables being measured are compared with each other, so that a person's score on one variable is affected by his or her scores on other variables measured by the instrument.

Item. One of the units, questions, or tasks of which a psychometric instrument is composed.

Item analysis. A general term for procedures designed to assess the utility or validity of a set of test items.

Item characteristic curve. A graph, used in item analysis, that depicts the proportion of examinees passing a specified item against the total test score.

Item-response (characteristic) curve. Graph showing the proportion of examinees who get a test item right, plotted against an internal (total test score) or external criterion of performance.

Item sampling. Procedure for selecting subsets of items from a total item pool; different samples of items are administered to different groups of examinees.

Job analysis. A general term for procedures used to determine the factors or tasks making up a job. A job analysis is usually considered a prerequisite to the construction of a test for predicting performance on a job.

Kuder-Richardson formulas. Formulas used to compute a measure of internal-consistency reliability from a single administration of a test having 0–1 scoring.

Latent trait theory. Any one of several theories (for example, item characteristic curve theory, Rasch model) and associated statistical procedures that relate a person's test performance to his or her estimated standing on some hypothetical latent ability trait or continuum; used in item analysis and test standardization.

Leaderless group discussion (LGD). Six or so individuals (e.g., candidates for an executive position) are observed while discussing an assigned problem to determine their effectiveness in working with the group and reaching a solution.

Leniency error. Tendency to rate an individual higher on a positive characteristic and less severely on a negative characteristic than he or she actually should be rated.

Likert scale. Attitude scale in which respondents indicate their degree of agreement or disagreement with a particular proposition concerning some object, person, or situation.

Linear regression analysis. Procedure for determining the algebraic equation of the best-fitting line for predicting scores on a dependent variable from one or more independent variables.

Linear transformation. Converting a score to a new scale by multiplying the score by a constant and/or adding another constant.

Man-to-man (person-to-person) scale. Procedure in which ratings on a specific trait (e.g., leadership) are made by comparing each person to be rated with several other people whose standings on the trait have already been determined.

Measurement. Procedures for determining (or indexing) the amount or quantity of some construct or entity; assignment of numbers to objects or events.

Median. Score point in a distribution of scores below and above which 50% of the scores fall.

Mentally retarded. A person who is significantly above average in intellectual functioning, variously defined as an IQ of 130 or 140 and above.

Merit ratings. Appraising employees by assigning ratings to them on one or more variables indicative of their performance on the job.

Mesomorph. W. H. Sheldon's term for a person having an athletic physique; correlated with a somatotonic temperament (active, aggressive, energetic).

Mode. The most frequently occurring score in a group of scores.

Most-recent-performance error. In evaluating employee performance, the rater evaluates the most recent behavior of the employee rather than the employee's behavior during the entire period since the last performance evaluation.

Multiple correlation coefficient (R). A measure of the overall degree of relationship, varying between -1.00 and $+1.00$, of several variables with a single criterion variable. For example, the multiple correlation of a group of scholastic aptitude tests with school grades is typically around .60 to .70, a moderate degree of correlation.

Multiple-regression analysis. Statistical method for analyzing the contributions of two or more independent variables in predicting a dependent variable.

Multivariate statistics. A set of statistical procedures (factor analysis, discriminant analysis, multivariate analysis of variance, canonical correlation, etc.) that analyze multiple variables and take the relationships among them into account.

Nielsen rating. Estimate of the audience share of a network television program captured at a given period. Recognized as the index to success or failure in television program, Nielsen ratings are accomplished by means of boxes (Audimeters) connected to selected television sets to record which channels are being watched and when.

Nominal scale. The lowest type of measurement, in which numbers are used merely as descriptors or names of things, rather than designating order or amount.

Nomination technique.   Technique of studying social structure and personality in which students, workers, or other groups of individuals are asked to indicate the persons with whom they would like to do a certain thing or the person(s) whom they feel possesses certain characteristics.

Norm group.   Sample of people on whom a test is standardized.

Normal distribution.   A smooth, bell-shaped frequency distribution of scores, symmetrical about the mean and described by an exact mathematical function. The test scores of a large group of examinees are frequently distributed in an approximately normal manner.

Normalized scores.   Scores obtained by transforming raw scores in such a way that the transformed scores are normally distributed with a mean of 0 and a standard deviation of 1 (or some linear function of these numbers).

Norms.   A list of scores and the corresponding percentile ranks, standard scores, or other transformed scores of a group of examinees on whom a test has been standardized.

Numerical scale.   A rating scale on which the categories or points are numerals.

Objective test.   A test scored by comparing the examinee's responses to a list of correct answers (a key) prepared beforehand, in contrast to a subjectively scored test. Examples of objective test items and multiple-choice and true-false.

Oblique rotation.   In a factor analysis, a rotation in which the factor axes are allowed to form acute or obtuse angles with each other. Consequently, the factors are correlated.

Odd-even reliability.   The correlation between total scores on the odd-numbered and total score on the even-numbered items of a test, corrected by the Spearman-Brown reliability formula. See **Spearman-Brown formula.**

Opinion.   Judgment of a person or thing with respect to character, merit, etc. See **Attitude** and **Belief.**

Ordinal scale.   Type of measurement scale on which the numbers refer merely to the ranks of objects or events arranged in order of merit (e.g., numbers referring to order of finishing in a contest).

Orthogonal rotation.   In factor analysis, a rotation that maintains the independence of factors, that is, the angles between factors are kept at 90 degrees and hence the factors are uncorrelated.

Pair(ed) comparisons (method of).   Method by which every individual is compared with every other individual in a group on some characteristic. There are $n(n-1)/2$ such comparisons in a group of n people.

Parallel forms.   Two tests that are equivalent in the sense that they contain the same kinds of items of equal difficulty and are highly correlated. The scores made by examinees on one form of the test are very close to those made by them on the other form.

Parallel forms reliability.   An index of reliability determined by correlating the scores of individuals on parallel forms of a test.

Percentile.   The pth percentile is the test score at or below which p percent of the examinees' test scores fall.

Percentile band.   A range of percentile ranks within which there is a specified probability that an examinee's true score on a test will fall.

Percentile norms.   A list of raw scores and the corresponding percentages of the test standardization group whose scores fall below the given percentile.

Percentile rank.   The percentage of scores falling below a given score in a frequency distribution or group of scores; the percentage corresponding to the given score.

Performance appraisal (evaluation).   Periodic, formal evaluation of on-the-job performance of employees.

Personality.   Sum total of the qualities, traits, and behaviors characterizing a person and by which, together with his or her physical attributes, the person is recognized as a unique individual.

Personnel psychology.   Branch of industrial/organizational psychology that deals with selection, placement, training, performance evaluation, and other psychological matters pertaining to employees.

Point-biserial coefficient.   Correlation coefficient computed between scores on a dichotomous variable and a continuous variable; derived from the product-moment correlation coefficient.

Predictive validity.   Extent to which scores on a test are predictive of performance on some criterion measure assessed at a later time; usually expressed as a correlation between the test (predictor variable) and the criterion variable.

Primacy effect.   Tendency of raters to assign more weight to initial behaviors or performances than to subsequent behaviors of ratees.

Product scale.   Consists of a series of sample products representing various degrees of quality, e.g., scales for evaluating handwriting or works of art.

Q sort.   Assessment procedure that centers on sorting cards or other materials containing self-descriptive statements into categories on some continuum and correlating the responses of different individuals or the same individuals at different times.

Quartile.   A score in a frequency distribution below which either 25% (first quartile), 50% (second quartile), 75% (third quartile), or 100% (fourth quartile) of the total number of scores fall.

r.   A symbol for the Pearson product-moment correlation coefficient.

Random sample.   A sample of observations (e.g., test scores) drawn from a population in such a way that every member of the target population has an equal chance of being selected in the sample.

Range.   A crude measure of the spread or variability of a group of scores computed by subtracting the lowest score from the highest score.

Rank performance rating.   Rank-ordering employees according to their merit.

Ranking.   Placing a group of individuals in order according to their judged standing on some characteristic; placing a list of characteristics of an individual in order according to their salience or significance.

Rapport.   A warm, friendly relationship between examiner and examinee.

Rasch model.   One-parameter (item difficulty) model for scaling test items for purposes of item analysis and test standardization. The model is based on the assumption that indexes of guessing and item discrimination are negligible parameters. As with other latent trait models, the Rasch model relates examinees' performances on test items (percentage passing) to their estimated standings on a hypothetical latent ability trait or continuum.

Rating scale.   A list of words or statements concerning traits or characteristics, sometimes in the form of a continuous line divided into sections corresponding to degrees of the characteristics, on which the rater indicates judgments of either his or her own behavior or characteristics or the behavior or characteristics of another person (ratee). The rater indicates how or to what degree the behavior or characteristic is possessed by the ratee.

Ratio scale.   A scale of measurement, having a true zero, on which equal numerical ratios imply equal ratios of the attribute being measured. Psychological variables are typically not measured on ratio scales, but height, weight, energy, and many other physical variables are.

Raw score.   An examinee's unconverted score on a test, computed as the number of items answered correctly or the number of correct answers minus a certain portion of the incorrect answers.

Regression equation.   A linear equation for forecasting criterion scores from scores on one or more predictor variables; a procedure often used in selection programs or actuarial prediction and diagnosis.

Reliability.   The extent to which a psychological assessment device measures anything consistently. A reliable instrument is relatively free from errors of measurement, so the scores obtained on the instrument are close in numerical value to the true scores of examinees.

Reliability coefficient.   A numerical index, between .00 and 1.00, of the reliability of an assessment instrument. Methods for determining reliability include test-retest, parallel-forms, and internal consistency.

Representative sample.   A group of individuals whose characteristics are similar to those of the population of individuals for whom a test is intended.

Response sets (styles).   Responding in relatively fixed or stereotyped ways in situations in which there are two or more response choices, such as on a personality inventory. Examples of response sets are the tendency to guess, to answer true (acquiescence), and to give socially desirable responses.

Sampling from lists.   From a list of telephone subscribers, home owners, or any other relevant list, selecting every mth person on the list for a sample. The starting place on the list is chosen at random, and from that point on every $N/n = m$th person (where N is the size of the population and n the size of the sample) is selected.

Scalogram analysis.   Method of attitude-scaling pioneered by Louis Guttman. The attitude statements are arranged in a hierarchy in such a way that endorsing an item at any point in the hierarchy implies endorsement of all items below it. The extent to which this occurs is indicated by a reproducibility coefficient.

Scatter diagram.   A cluster of points plotted from a set of X-Y values, in which X is the independent variable and Y the dependent variable.

Screening.   A general term for any selection process, usually not very precise, by which some applicants are accept and other applicants are rejected.

Selection.   The use of tests and other devices to select those applicants for an occupation or educational program who are most likely to succeed in that situation. Applicants who fall at or above the cutoff score on the test are selected (accepted); those who fall below cutoff are rejected.

Selection ratio.   The proportion of applicants who are selected for a job or training (educational) program.

Self-ratings.   Performance appraisal technique in which individuals evaluate their own abilities and performance.

Semantic differential.   Rating scale technique for evaluating the connotative meanings that selected concepts have for a person. Each concept is rated on a 7-point, bipolar adjectival scale.

Semi-interquartile range (Q).   A measure of the variability of a group of ordinal-scale scores, computed as half the difference between the first and third quartiles.

Severity error.   The tendency to be severe in rating, i.e., to assign lower ratings than justified.

Skewness.   Degree of asymmetry in a frequency distribution. In a positively skewed distribution, there are more scores to the left of the mode (low scores), as in a test that is too difficult for the examinees. In a negatively skewed distribution, there are more scores to the right of the mode (high scores), as in a test that is too easy for the examinees.

Social desirability response set.   Response set or style affecting scores on personality inventories. Refers to the tendency on the part of a person to respond to the assessment materials in what he or she judges to be a more socially desirable direction, rather than responding in a manner that is truly characteristic or descriptive of the person.

Sociogram.   A diagram consisting of circles representing persons in a group, with lines drawn indicating which people chose (accepted) each other and which ones did not choose (rejected) each other. Terms used in referred to particular elements of a sociogram include *star, clique, isolate,* and *mutual admiration society.*

Sociometric technique.   Technique for determining and describing the pattern of acceptances and rejections among a group of people. See **Sociogram.**

Spearman-Brown formula.   An estimate of reliability determined by applying the Spearman-Brown formula for $m = 2$ to the correlation between two halves of the same test, such as the odd-numbered items and the even-numbered items.

Specificity.   The proportion of the total variance of a test that is due to factors specific to the test itself.

Split-half coefficient.   See **Spearman-Brown formula.**

Standard deviation.   The square root of the variance; used as a measure of the dispersion or spread of a group of scores.

Standard error of estimate.   The standard deviation of obtained criterion scores around the predicted criterion score; used to estimate a range of actual scores on a criterion variable for an individual whose score on the predictor variable is equal to a specified value.

Standard error of measurement.   An estimate of the standard deviation of the normal distribution of test scores that an examinee would theoretically obtain by taking a test an infinite number of times. If an examinee's obtained test score is X, then the chances are two out of three that he or she is one of a group of people whose true scores on the test fall within one standard error of measurement of X.

Standard rating scale.   Scale on which there is a set of standards with which the persons being rated are to be compared. See **Man-to-man scale.**

Standard scores.   A group of scores, such as z-scores, T-scores, or stanine scores, having a desired mean and standard deviation. Standard scores are computed by transforming raw scores to z-scores, multiplying the z-scores by the desired standard deviation, and then adding the desired mean to the product.

Standardization.   Administering a carefully constructed test to a large, representative sample of people under standard conditions for the purpose of determining norms.

Standardization sample.   The subset of a target population on which a test is standardized.

Stanine.   A standard score scale consisting of the scores 1 through 9, having a mean of 5 and a standard deviation of approximately 2.

Statistic.   A number used to describe some characteristic of a sample of test scores, such as the arithmetic mean or standard deviation.

Stratified random sampling.   A sampling procedure in which the population is divided into strata (e.g., men and women; blacks and whites, lower class, middle class, upper class), and samples are selected at random from the strata; sample sizes are proportional to strata sizes.

Summated ratings (method of).   Technique of attitude-scale construction devised by R. Likert. Raters check the numerical values on a continuum with 3–7 (usually 5) categories corresponding to the degree of positivity or negativity of each of a large number of attitude statements concerned with the topic in question. Twenty or so statements are selected by certain statistical criteria to comprise the final attitude scale.

T-scores.   Converted, normalized standard scores having a mean of 50 and a standard deviation of 10. Z-scores are also standard scores with a mean of 50 and a standard deviation of 10, but in contrast to T-scores they are not normalized.

Target population.   The population of interest in standardizing a test or other assessment instrument; the norm group (sample) must be representative of the target population if valid interpretations of (norm-referenced) scores are to be made.

Taylor-Russell tables.   Tables for evaluating the validity of a test as a function of the information contributed by the test beyond the information contributed by chance.

Test.   Any device used to evaluate the behavior or performance of a person. Psychological tests are of many kinds—cognitive, affective, and psychomotor.

Test-retest reliability.   A method of assessing the reliability of a test by administering it to the same group of examinees on two different occasions and computing the correlations between their scores on the two occasions.

Time sampling.   Observational sampling procedure in which observations lasting only a few minutes are made over a period of a day or so.

True score.   The hypothetical score that is a measure of the examinee's true knowledge of the test material. In test theory, an examinee's true score on a test is the mean of the distribution of scores that would result if he or she took the test an infinite number of times.

Validity.   The extent to which an assessment instrument measures what it was designed to measure. Validity can be assessed in several ways: by analysis of the instrument's content *(content validity)*, by relating scores on the test to a criterion *(predictive* and *concurrent validity)*, and by a more thorough study of the extent to which the test is a measure of a certain psychological construct *(construct validity)*.

Validity generalization.   The application of validity evidence to situations other than those in which the evidence was obtained.

Value.   The worth, merit, or importance attached to something.

Variability.   The degree of spread or deviation of a group of scores around their average value.

Variable.   In contrast to a *constant*, any quantity that can assume more than one state or numerical value.

Variance.   A measure of variability of test scores, computed as the sum of the squares of the deviations of raw scores from the arithmetic mean, divided by one less than the number of scores; the square of the standard deviation.

z-score.   Any one of a group of derived scores varying from $-\infty$ to $+\infty$, computed from the formula $z = $ (raw score $-$ mean)/standard deviation, for each raw score. In a normal distribution, over 99% of the cases lie between $z = -3.00$ and $z = +3.00$.

Appendix B

Computer Programs for Rating Scales, Checklists, and Other Psychometric Instruments

To use the accompanying diskette, insert it into the A drive. Switch to the A drive, and then run the programs by typing "menu" or "prog" at the A prompt (A:\>). The command "menu" will get you into the menu, from which you can make a choice of programs to run. The command "prog" is followed by the query "Category and number of program?" You specify the category (A through I) and the number of the program you wish to run. The programs will run faster if they are stored in a directory on your hard disk. You can also run the programs when you are in Windows: Use the File Menu's "Run" command, type a:menu or a:prog in the dialog box, and select the "OK" button. Or, if you have stored the programs in a directory, named "ratings" for example, on your hard disk, then type c:\ratings\menu in the dialog box. You can escape from a running program by pressing function key 1 (F1).

The output for some of the programs is printed on the screen and/or in a disk output file named "results." On many programs you will be queried as to whether you wish to print the results on a line printer. Follow the directions for each program carefully and you should have few problems. All the programs are in color, but they will work with a black-and-white monitor as well. Keep in mind that the rating scales, checklists, and other instruments administered by some of the programs are meant to be illustrative exercises or demonstrations rather than serious efforts at assessment. Very few of the instruments have norms, and for those that do the norms are tentative. Consequently, you should view the results as suggestive rather than definitive and advise others to do likewise.

Brief descriptions of the programs follow.

CATEGORY A. CONSTRUCTING AND SCORING RATING SCALES AND CHECKLISTS

1. "Constructing a Custom-Designed Rating Scale or Checklist." This program assists in constructing a checklist or rating scale having any desired number of rating categories and items. The scale constructor enters the name of the rating scale or checklist, the directions, the number of rating categories, the label and definition for each category, the number of items to be rated, and then types each item. Items are limited to 50 characters per line. The completed scale is stored in output file "results" and can be printed at run time or later.

2. "Constructing and Scoring Several Types of Rating Scales and Checklists." This program consists of a set of 11 menu-driven procedures for constructing several types of rating scales, attitude scales, and checklists, as well as for scoring responses to the constructed instruments. The program can facilitate the construction and scoring of bipolar, forced-choice, graphic, numerical, semantic differential, and standard rating scales, as well as Likert attitude scales, questionnaires for comparing and ranking persons, and checklists of behaviors and characteristics.

3. "Scoring a Rating Scale or Checklist." This program scores a specified number of rating scale or checklist questionnaires. The user enters the number of questionnaires to be scored, the number of response categories per item, the label for each category, the numerical value corresponding to each category of every item, and the response to each item on each questionnaire. In addition to each respondent's raw score, a frequency distribution of responses made by the respondent to all items is obtained.

4. "Constructing a Questionnaire for Intragroup Ratings." This program generates and prints an intragroup ratings questionnaire from the names of the members of any kind of group. Group members fill out the printed questionnaires by rating each name on a scale of 1 to 7 according to how much they would like or dislike to engage in some activity with the person, how important the person is to the group, how close the respondent feels toward the person, likes to cooperate with him or her, considers the person important to the successful functioning of the group, or any other interpersonal perception or attitude. The questionnaire can be administered at the beginning and again at the end of a course or other regularly meeting group to determine changes in intragroup perceptions and attitudes.

5. "Scoring and Interpreting an Intragroup Ratings Questionnaire." This program scores the ratings obtained from the questionnaires generated by the program A-4 and computes several indices of intragroup perceptions or attitudes. The measures include (1) a coefficient for each rater indicating how he or she feels toward the other members of the group, (2) a coefficient for each ratee revealing how the rest of the group feels toward him or her, and (3) a coefficient reflecting how the entire group feels about the group as a whole.

6. "Scoring Ratings on Bipolar Scales and Large-Sample Probabilities." This program computes a B (bidirectional) coefficient, ranging in value from −1

to +1 and thereby providing information on both the magnitude and direction of a set of ratings. B and its statistical significance are determined on large samples of items or raters. The statistical significance of a mean of B values, computed across items or raters, can also be assessed by applying a normal approximation test.

7. "Probabilities of Bipolar (B) Coefficients Based on Small Samples." This program computes the right-tail probabilities for B coefficients determined on sets of ratings on bipolar scales. The distribution of ratings in the population may be assumed to be either normal or uniform.

8. "Scoring Ranking Items." This program scores ranking or rearrangement items two procedures (absolute values of difference scores and squares of difference scores) devised by the author. The user specifies the number of categories, lists the correct (keyed) ranks by category, and the examinee's rankings by category. Scores may be printed (1) in decimal form or (2) rounded to the nearest whole number.

9. "Assigning Grades by the Modified Cajori Procedure." Using a modification of the Cajori procedure, this program determines a frequency distribution of grades and grade ranges. The user must specify the number of scores, the maximum possible score, the minimum possible score, and the median ability level of the group on a scale of 1 to 100 (see Aiken, 1983b).

CATEGORY B. ANALYZING ERRORS IN RATINGS

1. "Eight Rating Error Coefficients." This program can be used to compare either items across raters or raters across items on eight coefficients: (1) leniency, (2) severity, (3) leniency/severity, (4) central tendency, (5) homogeneity (halo), (6) proximity, (7) uniformity, and (8) contrast. All coefficients except number 3, which ranges from -1 to 1, range from 0 to 1. Large sample probability values are conducted on coefficients 1, 2, 3, 4, 5, and 8.

2. "Probabilities for Rating Error Coefficients in Program B-1." This program computes and prints out the probability distribution for the eight coefficients (leniency, severity, leniency/severity, central tendency, homogeneity (halo), proximity, uniformity, contrast) computed on small samples of ratings by program B-1.

3. "Evaluating Constant Rating Errors by Analysis of Variance." Based on Guilford's (1954) analysis, this program computes a raters $\times$ ratees $\times$ traits analysis of variance to determine the significance of various constant rating errors (leniency, halo, contrast) by examination of the raters $\times$ ratees, raters $\times$ traits, and ratees $\times$ traits interactions as well as the main effects for raters, ratees, and traits.

4. "Coefficients of Response Homogeneity and Congruence." This program computes and evaluates the statistical significance of two coefficients (H and C) for determining the homogeneity or congruence of a set of n ratings or scores. Tests for determining the statistical significance of the coefficients in

both small and large samples are provided. These procedures may be used to evaluate the consistency of measurements made on n persons or in situations on one characteristic or on one person or in one situation on n characteristics.

CATEGORY C. ITEM ANALYSIS AND MEASURES OF RELATIONSHIP

1. "Eight Simple Item Analysis Statistics and Significance Tests." This program computes eight indexes for item analyses of small samples of test scores. These indexes include measures of: (1) item difficulty (proportion or respondents selecting the keyed response), (2) performance of examinees on the instrument as a whole, (3) similarity between an examinee's response to an item and his or her responses to other items, (4) similarity between an examinee's response to an item and the responses of other examinees to that item, (5) uniformity of responses to non-keyed item options, (6) relationship between item and total scores (item discrimination index) (7) differences among item total scores, and (8) differences among examinees' total scores. Each index and a corresponding statistical significance test is defined. The program will compute all indexes or any subset of them for a given data matrix and determine the right-tail probability of obtained values for indexes 1–4. The program also computes chi square and the associated right-tail probability for indexes 5–8.

2. "Plotting Item Characteristic and Item Response Curves." This program plots item characteristic curves from raw data or from a specified item response model. The user indicates whether he (she) wishes to compute an item characteristic curve from (1) raw data or (2) an item-response model, then enters the total number of scores, the number of intervals, and, for each interval, the midpoint of the interval, the number of scores on the interval, and the number of examinees on the interval who passed the item. If an item-response model is selected, the user must indicate whether a one-parameter (Rasch), a two-parameter, or a three-parameter model is desired. The output, which is printed on the screen, is a graphical plot of the item characteristic curve.

3. "Measures of Association for Nominal and Ordinal Data." Three measures of association or relationship between data on a nominal measurement scale (lambda, Cramer's V, phi coefficient) and four measures of association on an interval measurement scale (gamma, Spearman's rho, Somer's d, Kendall's tau-b) may be computed with this program. The z value for a test of significance of gamma in large samples and the t value for a test of significance of Spearman's rho are also computed.

4. "Point-Biserial and Rank-Biserial Correlation Coefficients." This program computes the point-biserial and rank-biserial correlation coefficients. The user enters the total number of examinees, the mean criterion score, the standard deviation of the criterion scores, and the total number of items. For each item, the user indicates the number of examinees who passed the item and the mean criterion score of examinees who passed the item. The resulting

coefficients are stored, by item number, in disk file "results" and can be printed on the screen or a line printer.

5. "Pearson Correlation and Regression Equation." This program computes the product-moment correlation coefficient between two variables (X and Y), the linear regression equation for predicting Y from X, and the means and standard deviations of X and Y for 3-100 pairs of values. The number of false positive and false negative errors, hits, and correct rejections for a specified criterion cutoff score (minimum acceptable performance) can also be determined.

6. "Multiple Regression and Multiple Correlation." This program computes the standardized and unstandardized regression weights, the multiple correlation coefficient (R), the standard errors of the regression weights, and t tests for the significance of the regression weights for a linear regression analysis with one, two, or three independent variables. The last variable is the dependent variable. Input data are the means, standard deviations, and intercorrelations of the variables.

CATEGORY D. SCORE TRANSFORMATIONS AND NORMS

1. "Normal Deviates and Areas Under the Normal Curve." This program may be used to compute either (1) the normal probability for a given z value or (2) the z value corresponding to a given cumulative normal probability.

2. "Transforming Proportions to Arc Sines." This program makes an arc sine transformation of proportion scores (Y = 2 arc sin X), thereby stabilizing the variances preparatory to analysis of variance computations.

3. "Transforming Scores on One Rating Scale to a Scale Having a Different Origin and a Different Number of Categories." This program transforms scores and statistics on a rating scale having any number of categories to a scale having a specified origin and number of categories. The origins of the two scales may be any negative or positive integers; the scales may increase in the same or opposite directions and have any category widths. The transformation formulas provide not only a procedure for equating scores on different scales but also a method of investigating a variety of research questions involving ratings.

4. "Converting Raw Scores to Simple Ranks." This program converts sets of n raw scores on each of m variables to ranks, with the highest score receiving the lowest rank (1). A table of raw scores and the corresponding ranks for each variable are printed on the computer screen and recorded in a disk file "results."

5. "Converting Raw Scores to Percentile Ranks, Deciles, and Quartiles." This program converts sets of raw scores on multiple variables, entered from the keyboard or a file, into percentile ranks, deciles, and quartiles. The conversions are done separately for each variable, and the results printed as a table on the screen and in disk file "results."

6. "Converting Raw Scores to Non-Normalized Standard Scores." This program converts sets of raw scores on multiple variables, entered from the keyboard or a file, into non-normalized standard z-scores and T-scores. The conversions are done separately for each variable, and the results printed as a table on the screen and in disk file "results."

7. "Converting Raw Scores to Normalized Standard Scores." This program converts sets of raw scores on multiple variables, entered from the keyboard or a file, into normalized standard z scores and T scores. The conversions are done separately for each variable, and the results printed as a table on the screen and in disk file "results."

8. "Converting Rating Categories to Standard Score Scales." From a frequency distribution of responses to unipolar or bipolar rating scales, this program transforms the numerical values of the rating categories to three standard scales: (1) TA scores based on a standard z transformation with a mean equal to (high + low)/2 and a standard deviation equal to (high − low)/6, where "high" is the highest rating category and "low" the lowest rating category; (2) TN scores based on normalized standard z scores having a mean and standard deviation of (high + low)/2 and (high − low)/2; (3) TR scores based on the proportional deviation of the actual frequency distribution from a theoretical uniform distribution across rating categories. The user specifies the number of rating categories, the value of the highest category, and the frequency of each rating. A table listing the rating, the frequency, the corresponding mid-percentile rank, and the values of TA, TN, and TR for each rating is printed on the screen and in disk file "results."

CATEGORY E. RELIABILITY COEFFICIENTS

1. "Coefficient Alpha." This short program computes coefficient alpha, a measure of the internal consistency reliability of a test. The user enters the number of items and the number of examinees, and then enters the score for each examinee on each item. The numerical value of coefficient alpha is printed on the computer screen.

2. "Kuder-Richardson Reliability Coefficients." This program computes the internal consistency reliability of a test by using Kuder-Richardson formulas 20 and 21. The user enters the number of items, the arithmetic mean of total test scores, the variance of total test scores, and, for each item, the proportion of examinees answering the item correctly. Kuder-Richardson 20 and Kuder-Richardson 21 coefficients are printed on the computer screen.

3. "Kappa Coefficient." This program computes a weighted or unweighted value of coefficient kappa (kap) and the coefficient of agreement (p_o), maximum values of kap and p_o, 95% and 99% confidence limits and approximated right-tail normal curve probabilities of kap and p_o in large samples (n > 29), and exact right-tail hypergeometric probabilities of kap and p_o in small samples (n < 30). The number of rows or columns in the square matrix of observed frequencies may range from 2 to 5. For observed frequencies on the major diagonal, disagreement weights are set equal to 0. For unweighted kappa, disagreement

weights in off-diagonal frequencies are set equal to 1. For weighted kappa, the user specifies the values of weights for off-diagonal frequencies.

4. "Intraclass Coefficient." This program computes an intraclass (interrater) correlation coefficient among the ratings assigned by several raters to the same ratees, in addition to an intraclass correlation of a sum or average.

5. "Concordance Coefficient." This program determines the amount of agreement among the ranks assigned by several raters to the same ratees. In addition to the coefficient of concordance and the corresponding value of chi square, the program computes the average rank correlation and the expected correlation among the set of rankings with a comparable set.

6. "Absolute Difference Coefficients (V, R, and H)." This set of programs computes numerical coefficients (V, R, and H) for analyzing the validity and reliability of ratings. Each coefficient, which ranges in value from 0 to 1, is computed as the ratio of an obtained to a maximum sum of differences in ratings, or as 1 minus that ratio. Programs for calculating the coefficients, their associated individual and cumulative right-tail probabilities, and the population mean and standard deviation of each coefficient are included. Individual and right-tail probabilities for specified values of the three coefficients can be generated for any number of rating categories, raters, or items. When the number of items or raters is large ($n > 25$), the right-tail probability associated with any value of a V, R, or H may be estimated by a z-score procedure. The three coefficients are applicable not only to validity and reliability (test-retest and internal consistency) determinations but also to item analysis, agreement analysis, and cluster of factor analysis of rating-scale data.

CATEGORY F. SAMPLE SELECTION AND ASSIGNMENT

1. "Random Sampling and Random Permutations." This program randomly selects a sample of m numbers, with or without replacement, from a population of n numbers. When $m = n$, the numbers are selected without replacement and the result is a random permutation of the numbers.

2. "Random Assignment of Observational Elements to Conditions." This program randomly assigns n observational elements to g groups. If $q = n/g$ is an integer, then q elements are assigned to each group. If $n/g = q + f$, where q is an integer and f is a fraction, then $q + 1$ elements are assigned to some groups and q elements to the remaining groups in a random fashion to total n.

3. "Stratified Random Sampling—Selection and Assignment." A sample of n observational units is randomly selected from or assigned to b strata, levels, or blocks, each consisting of g groups. The number of elements selected from or assigned to each stratum is proportional to the total number of elements contained in the stratum in the population of interest. Within a given stratum, the sample elements are assigned to groups in the same manner as in program F-2.

4. "Multistage Cluster Sampling." In this program, a designated number of clusters is randomly selected at each stage from clusters randomly selected

at the preceding stage. Up to five sampling stages are possible. At the final stage, all observational elements, or a random sample selected by program F-1 may be examined.

5. "Required Sample Size for Tests on Population Proportions." This program computes the required sample size for z tests on population proportions. The user specifies the population size, the hypothesized population proportion, the desired confidence level, and the degree of accuracy expressed as a proportion. Procedures for both finite and infinite populations are provided.

6. "Power and Minimum Sample Sizes for Binomial or Sign Tests." This program estimates power and minimum sample size for binomial or sign tests. The binomial probability and power are computed by adaptation of a procedure described by Pagano (1994). The user enters the value of alpha, whether a one- or a two-tailed test is desired, and the proportion of positive signs under the alternative hypothesis. The program prints out the critical number of positive signs needed to reject the null hypothesis, the power of the test, and the probability of a Type II error.

7. "Sample Sizes for Conditions in Randomized Groups ANOVA." This program is based on the tables and approach described by Bratcher, Morgan, and Zimmer (1970). The user enters the power of the test (.7, .8, .9, or .95), the effect size (1.0, 1.25, 1.75, 2.0, 2.5, or 3.0), the alpha level (.20, .10, .05, or .01) and the number of treatment levels or blocks (1, 2, 3, 4, 5, 6, 7, 8, 9, 10, 11, 13, 16, 21, 25, or 31). Although the required sample sizes for the various numbers of levels or blocks are computed only for completely randomized designs, the resulting values are also very close to those for randomized blocks designs.

8. "Matching Groups on a Control Variable." This program matches two or more groups of people or other observational elements on a control variable. The data may be entered either from the keyboard or from a data file, and the results are recorded in output file "results." The user indicates the number of sample groups to match, the number of persons or other observational units per group, and the corresponding scores. The scores in each group are ranked and paired with the ranks of scores in the other groups. The output consists of a table indicating the sample or group, the observation or person number, the corresponding score, and the rank of the score.

9. "Matching and Assigning Observational Elements to Groups." This program matches people or other sampling elements and assigns the matched elements at random to a specified number of groups. The data may be entered either from the keyboard or from a designated data file. The user indicates the number of observations, the number of groups to which they are to be assigned, and the numerical values of the observations. The output is a table consisting of the group numbers, the person (unit) numbers, and the corresponding scores.

10. "Constructing Latin Squares for Counterbalanced Assignment of Subjects to Groups." This program constructs Latin square designed for counterbalanced assigned of subjects to groups, or conditions to treatment levels or other designated conditions. The program constructs squares up to 50 rows × 50 columns in size and may be easily extended to even larger dimensions

if desired. One square is constructed when the dimensions of the square are even, and two squares when the dimensions are odd.

CATEGORY G. NONPARAMETRIC STATISTICAL TESTS OF HYPOTHESES

1. "Binomial Test." This program computes the right-tail binomial probability for a one-sample statistical test on dichotomous data. The data are entered as 1's and 0's, where 1 is a "hit" (yes, agree, pass, etc.) and 0 a "miss." The program tests the null hypothesis that the probability of a hit is equal to a specified value between 0 and 1.

2. "Chi Square Tests of Goodness of Fit and Independence." This program performs a chi square test of goodness of fit (one basis of classification) or independence (two bases of classification). When there is only one degree of freedom, the user has the choice of whether or not to employ Yates' correction. For the goodness of fit test, the value of chi square, the degrees of freedom, and the expected frequency is printed. For the test of independence, in addition to the value of chi square and the degrees of freedom, the observed and expected frequencies in each cell are printed.

3. "Cochran Q Test & McNemar Test of Significance of Changes." The Cochran Q Test is a nominal-level test of equality of distributions of dichotomous responses of a group of individuals to two or more conditions. It is the nominal-level counterpart of the one-factor repeated measures analysis of variance and the Friedman analysis of variance by ranks. The McNemar test is appropriate for only two conditions, but the Cochran test can be applied to two or more conditions.

4. "Fisher Exact Probability Test." This test computes the exact probability of a particular combination of frequencies in two independent samples with a dichotomous criterion.

5. "Friedman Two-Way Analysis of Variance by Ranks." This program computes the sums of ranks for the k conditions, the value of chi square, and the degrees of freedom for a Friedman Two-Way Analysis of Variance by Ranks. This is a nonparametric procedure parallel to the one-way repeated measures design in the analysis of variance.

6. "Kruskal-Wallis H Test." This program conducts a Kruskal-Wallis H test for two or more independent samples. In addition to the value of H and the degrees of freedom for the equivalent chi square test, the raw data and ranked scores may be printed.

7. "Mann-Whitney U Test." This program conducts a Mann-Whitney U test for two independent samples. The values of U_1, U_2, and U, in addition to the large sample approximation for U, are printed. The user may also choose to have the raw data and the ranked scores printed.

8. "Sign Test." This program conducts a sign test on correlated (matched) samples. The user enters the number of scores and paired values of observations

in the two groups. The observations are entered as paired values separated by a comma. Printed results are the number of plus signs, the number of minus signs, and the right-tail binomial probabilities associated with the number of plus and minus signs.

9. "Wilcoxon Matched-Pairs Signed-Ranks Test." This program conducts a Wilcoxon matched-pairs signed-ranks test for two matched (dependent or correlated) samples. The user specifies the number of paired data values and enters each data pair separated by a comma. The raw data, their ranked values (when requested), and the values of R+, R−, and T, and (for large samples) the z value equivalent to T, are printed.

CATEGORY H: STATISTICAL SIGNIFICANCE TESTS BASED ON ABSOLUTE VALUES OF DIFFERENCES

1. "D Coefficients for Tests of Goodness of Fit and Independence." This program computes difference (D) coefficients from observed frequencies in $1 \times c$ (one basis of classification) or $r \times c$ (two bases of classification tables. D_1 is a goodness of fit statistic, and D_2 an independence statistic. Larger values of D_1 and D_2 indicate greater deviations of the observed frequencies from a specified theoretical frequency distribution. The values of D_1 and D_2 range from a maximum value of 1.00 to a minimum value of 0 or near 0. D_1' and D_2' are linear transformations of D_1 and D_2, respectively, having a range of .00 to 1.00.

2. "Determining Probabilities for D_1 Values Computed by Program H-1." This program computes discrete and right-tail probabilities of D_1 and D_1' coefficients determined by program H-1. The user specifies the number of categories (c), the number of observations (n), and the high and low limits for the right-tail probabilities (significance levels).

3. "Determining Probabilities for D_2 Values Computed by Program H-1." As in program H-2, the procedure on which this program is based makes use of a D statistic ranging from a minimum value equal to or close to 0 to a maximum value of 1. To test the independence of observations in r × c contingency tables, the program computes discrete and right-tail probabilities of the D_2 and D_2' coefficients determined from the observed frequencies in the tables.

4. "Difference Tests for Distributions of Ratings." Three exact probability tests, counterparts of t tests for single samples, independent samples, and dependent samples, can be conducted by means of this program. The data may be obtained from ratings on m scales by a single rater or ratings on a single scale by n raters. The statistical tests, which involve computing a difference ratio (d), require fewer assumptions and restrictions than the t test or nonparametric procedures such as the Mann-Whitney and Wilcoxon tests. Exact probabilities associated with each difference ratio (d_1, d_2, d_3) are computed for small samples; one-tail normal probabilities associated with each different ratio and with the means of a sample of such ratios, are given

for large samples. Program "d1" computes the probability tables for one-sample difference ratio for rating scale data. Program "d_2" computes probability tables for independent samples difference ratio for rating scale data. Program "d_3" computes probability tables for dependent (paired) samples difference ratio for rating scale data. Program "comp" computes the values of d_1, d_2, and d_3 from data supplied by the user. A menu of options, from which programs "d_1," "d_2," "d_3," and "comp" may be run, is provided.

5. "Comparing Ratings in Several Samples." This program computes difference and similarity indexes based on several independent or dependent samples of ratings and determines their statistical significance. The procedures employed by the program are exact probability analogues of the randomized groups and repeated measures analyses of variance for small samples.

CATEGORY I. SAMPLE CHECKLISTS, RATING SCALES, AND RANKING QUESTIONNAIRES

1. "Checklist for Type A Behavior." This is a 20-item adjective checklist for the Type A behavior pattern. The respondent enters "y" (yes) if he (she) considers the term or phrase to be self-descriptive and "n" (no) if not self-descriptive. The score (number of adjectives responded to with "y") and the percentage of the total possible score are printed on the screen.

2. "Ranking Adjectives for Your Real and Ideal Selves." This program randomly presents a series of 20 adjectives twice. The examinee ranks them according to how descriptive they are of his (her) real and ideal selves. A percentage agreement between the real and ideal self rankings is computed.

3. "Checklist for Comparing Self With Others." This program administers and scores a checklist for determining the congruence between responses to self-descriptive and other-descriptive adjectives. The respondent is asked to indicate whether each of 25 adjectives is descriptive of him (her) personally and whether it is descriptive of people in general in the respondent's chronological age and sex group. The raw score (number of agreements between self and other responses) and the percentage of total possible agreements between self and other responses are printed on the screen.

4. "Five-Factor Personality Rating Scale." This program administers and scores a five-factor personality inventory consisting of 15 self-rating items. Scores on the five factors (Agreeableness, Conscientiousness, Extraversion, Neuroticism, Openness), which range from 0 to 18, are printed on the screen.

5. "Rating Personality of Instructor." This program presents a set of 12 adjectives on which the examinee is asked to rate any college or university professor. The adjectives are: considerate, courteous, creative, friendly, helpful, interesting, knowledgeable, motivating, organized, patient, prepared, punctual. The following directions are given: "On a scale of 0 to 4, where 0 = lowest amount of characteristic and 4 = highest amount of characteristic, rate your professor on each of the following descriptive characteristics."

Overall Rating, which ranges from 0 to 48, and Percentage Rating, which ranges from 0 to 100, are both printed on the screen.

6. "College Course and Instructor Evaluation Questionnaire." This program presents 14 items to be answered on a scale from 1 (not at all descriptive) to 5 (very descriptive) according to how descriptive of a particular course or instructor the respondent judges the statement to be. Eight of the statements are concerned with the characteristics of the course and six items with the instructor. Separate "Course" and "instructor" scores, in addition to a "Total" score, are provided. Although quite short, the form has fairly good internal consistency and test-retest reliabilities (high .70s to high .80s).

7. "Social Readjustment Scale." The respondent indicates ("y" or "n") whether he or she has experienced each of 43 events during the past year. Each event is weighted from 0 to 100, depending on the degree of readjustment required. The respondent's total score on the scale is the sum of the weights corresponding to the items he or she indicates having experienced. Total score and percent of possible score are printed on the screen.

CATEGORY J. SAMPLE INVENTORIES OF ATTITUDES, OPINIONS, AND VALUES

1. "Attitudes Toward Mathematics or Science." This is a Likert-type, "master attitude scale" consisting of 24 statements. Except for the subject (mathematics or science) referred to, the statements are the same when assessing attitudes toward either subject. Each statement expresses a feeling or attitude toward the subject. The examinee is instructed to indicate, on a five-point scale, the extent of agreement between the attitude expressed in the statement and his (her) own personal attitude: sd = "Strongly Disagree," d = "Disagree," u = "Undecided," a = "Agree," sa = "Strongly Agree." The 12 positively-worded and 12 negatively-worded statements on the inventory are presented in random order. The scale is scored on four variables consisting of six items each: Enjoyment of Mathematics (or Science), Motivation in Mathematics (or Science), Importance of Mathematics (or Science), Fear of Mathematics (or Science), plus a composite Total Attitude Toward Mathematics (or Science) score.

2. "Attitudes Toward Intelligence Testing." This program administers and scores a ten-item Likert-type inventory of attitudes and beliefs concerning intelligence testing. The items are concerned with a variety of assumptions and empirical findings pertaining to intelligence and intelligence testing. The examinee types "sa" (Strongly Agree), "a" (Agree), "u" (Undecided), "d" (Disagree), or "sd" (Strongly Disagree) in response to each statement.

3. "Attitudes Toward Personality Assessment." This program administers and scores a ten-item Likert-type inventory of attitudes and beliefs concerning personality assessment. The items consist of a set of statements pertaining to the theory, methods, and uses of personality assessment procedures. The

examinee enters "sa" ("Strongly Agree"), "a" ("Agree"), "u" ("Undecided"), "d" ("Disagree"), or "sd" ("Strongly Disagree") in responding to each statement.

4. "Attitudes Toward the Roles of Women." This program consists of two ten-item questionnaires to assess the respondent's opinion of (1) equal rights for women and (2) the treatment of women in advertising. Total scores on both questionnaires are computed and presented on the screen. A high score on the first questionnaire indicates a more feministic attitude. A high score on the second questionnaire indicates a strong belief that women are exploited by advertising in negative ways.

5. "Altruism Inventory." The inventory administered and scored by this program is designed to measure the personality characteristic of altruism. Eight items of the 15-item inventory are worded in the positive direction and the remaining seven items in the negative direction. The examinee types "sa" (strongly agree), "a" (agree), "u" (undecided), "d" (disagree), or "sd" (strongly disagree) in response to each of the randomly arranged statements. Total score ranges from 0 to 60. The Altruism Inventory has been used by the author in a variety of student research projects involving correlational methodology. The internal consistency reliabilities of the inventory are in the high .80's.

6. "Educational Values Questionnaire." This questionnaire consists of 24 items concerned with six educational values: Aesthetic, Leadership, Philosophical, Social, Scientific, and Vocational. Each item is answered on a five-point scale. The 12 items in Part I refer to possible goals or emphases of higher education; the respondent is instructed to type the appropriate letter when a statement is presented to indicate how important he or she believes the corresponding goal should be (u = "Unimportant," s = "Somewhat important," i = "Important," v = "Very important," e = "Extremely important"). On the six items of Part II the respondent enters the appropriate letter to indicate how valuable the particular kinds of college courses are to students in general n = "Not at all valuable," s = "Somewhat valuable," v = "Valuable," q = "Quite valuable," e = "Extremely valuable"). On the six items of Part III the respondent enters the appropriate letter to indicate how much attention he or she feels should be given to each kind of college course in the education of most students (n = "No attention at all," l = "Little attention," m = "Moderate amount of attention," a = "Above average amount of attention," or e = "Extensive amount of attention"). Responses are scored on a scale of 0 to 4, yielding scores ranging from 0 to 24 on each of the six scales. Various published and unpublished investigations have been conducted with this inventory, providing information on how educational values vary with sex, ethnic group, educational level, socioeconomic status, and decade.

7. "Attitude Toward Capital Punishment." This attitude scale, which was constructed by Thurstone's method of equal-appearing intervals, consists of 12 statements expressing favorable or unfavorable attitudes toward capital punishment. Each statement is presented individually, and the respondent indicates whether he (she) agrees (a) or disagrees (d) with it. The respondent's overall score, which is printed on the screen, is the median of the scale values of the statements endorsed by the respondent.

Appendix C

Commercial Suppliers of Rating Scales, Checklists, and Other Psychometric Instruments

American Guidance Service (AGS)
4201 Woodland Road
P.O. Box 99
Circle Pines, MN 55014-1796
(800) 328-2560

California Test Bureau (CTB)
20 Ryan Ranch Road
Monterey, CA 93940-5703
(800) 538-9547

Consulting Psychologists Press, Inc.
  (CPP)
3803 East Bayshore Road
P.O. Box 10096
Palo Alto, CA 94303
(800) 624-1765

CPPC
4 Conant Square
Brandon, VT 95733
(800) 433-8234

DLM
One DLM Park
Allen, TX 75002
(800) 527-4747

Educational and Industrial Testing Service
  (EdITS)
P.O. Box 7234
San Diego, CA 92167
(619) 226-1666

George Spivack and Marshall Swift
Department of Mental Health Sciences
Hahnemann Medical College
  and Hospital
Hahnemann University
Philadelphia, PA 19102
(215) 499-1211

Hawthorne Educational
  Services, Inc.
800 Gray Oak Drive
Columbia, MO 65201
(800) 542-1673

Institute for Personality and Ability
  Testing (IPAT)
P.O. Box 1188
Champaign, IL 61824-1188
(800) 225-4728

Jastak Associates
P.O. Box 3410
Wilmington, DE 19804-0250
(800) 221-WRAT

London House
9701 West Higgins Road
Rosemont, IL 60018
(800) 221-8378

MetriTech, Inc.
4106 Fieldstone Road
P.O. Box 6479
Champaign, IL 61826-6479
(217) 398-4868

Multi-Health Systems, Inc.
908 Niagara Falls Boulevard
North Tonawanda, NY 14120-2060
(800) 456-3003

NCS Assessments
5605 Green Circle Drive
P.O. Box 1416
Minneapolis, MN 55440
(800) 627-7271

Pro-Ed
8700 Shoal Creek Boulevard
Austin, TX 78757-6897
(512) 451-3246

Psychological and Educational
   Publications, Inc.
1477 Rollins Road
Burlingame, CA 94010-2316
(800) 523-5775

Psychological Assessment Resources, Inc.
   (PAR)
P.O. Box 998
Odessa, FL 33556
(800) 331-TEST

Psychological Corporation (The)
555 Academic Court
San Antonio, TX 78204-2498
(800) 228-0752

Psychological Publications, Inc.
290 Conejo Ridge Avenue
Suite 100
Thousand Oaks, CA 91361
(800) 345-TEST

Psychologists and Educators, Inc.
P.O. Box 513
Chesterfield, MO 63006

Riverside Publishing Co.
8420 Bryn Mawr Ave.
Chicago, IL 60631
(800) 767-TEST

Scholastic Testing Service, Inc. (STS)
480 Meyer Road
Bensenville, IL 60106-1617
(708) 766-7150

Sigma Assessment Systems, Inc.
P.O. Box 610984
Port Huron, MI 48061-0984
(800) 265-1285

Slosson Educational Publications, Inc.
P.O. Box 280
East Aurora, NY 14052-0280
(800) 828-4800

SRA Product Group
London House
9701 West Higgins Road
Rosemont, IL 60018
(800) 237-7685

SOI Systems
P.O. Box D
45755 Goodpasture Rd.
Vida, OR 97488
(503) 896-3936

Stoelting
Oakwood Center
620 Wheat Lane
Wood Dale, IL 60191
(708) 860-9700

Thomas M. Achenbach
Department of Psychiatry
University of Vermont
1 S. Prospect Street
Burlington, VT 05401-3444
(802) 656-4563

Western Psychological Services (WPS)
12031 Wilshire Boulevard
Los Angeles, CA 90025-1251
(800) 648-8857

Wonderlic Personnel Test, Inc.
1509 N. Milwaukee Ave.
Libertyville, IL 60048-1380
(800) 963-7542

Endnotes

CHAPTER 1

1. A set of computer programs for analyzing the results of elections is available from the author.

CHAPTER 2

1. Related to the forced-choice method is the *method of pair comparisons,* in which all the persons, objects, or events in the domain of interest are compared with each other in terms of preference or some specified characteristic or quality. Because the number of possible pairings of n objects, i.e. $n(n - 1)/2$, can become quite large as n increases, a balanced incomplete blocks procedure is an efficient alternative to complete pairing (Gulliksen & Tucker, 1961). In this procedure, subsets of the persons, objects, or events to be compared are ranked in such a way that the results of all possible pair comparisons can be inferred.
2. The formula $S = n\{1 - 3\Sigma d_i^2/[c(c^2 - 1)]\}$ may be used when disproportionately large weights are assigned to larger values of d_i.

CHAPTER 3

1. A procedure and a corresponding computer program for determining an optimum set of numerical weights for the parts of a composite in order to maximize the reliability of the composite is described in Aiken (1988).
2. The generalized Spearman-Brown formula for estimating reliability (r_{mm}) when test length is increased by a factor m is $r_{mm} = mr_{11}/[r_{11}(m - 1) + 1]$. Solving this formula for m yields $m = r_{mm}(1 - r_{11})/[r_{11}(1 - r_{mm})]$, the estimated factor by which the test must be lengthened in order to increase the reliability from r_{11} to r_{mm}.

CHAPTER 4

1. Generally, the name, age, and sex of the patient are also provided.
2. The same hypothesis can be tested with the D_1 statistic computed by program H-1 and the corresponding right-tail probability by program H-2. This test also yields a nonsignificant probability for the example.
3. Statistical tests based on absolute values of differences in one or two independent or dependent samples (program H-4) or as analogues to the randomized groups or repeated measures analysis of variance (program H-5) can be conducted with the programs in category H.

CHAPTER 5

1. Rather than writing a job description in paragraph form, in some cases a checklist of duties, tasks, and job specifications, such as in Control Data's

Occupational Analysis Questionnaire, may be used to summarize the components of a job.

2. Combining the traditional functions of job analysis and job evaluation into a single package is the Common-Metric Questionnaire: A Job Analysis System (CMQ). The CMQ, available from The Psychological Corporation, consists of a 32-page booklet to be filled out by employees, supervisors, or human resource administrators to describe, analyze, and evaluate any job.

3. Program C-5 will compute the numbers of false positive and false negative errors for specified cutoff scores and the regression equation determined from data entered by the user.

4. In general, labor unions have not been greatly supportive of performance appraisal programs, but have tended to view seniority as the only justifiable basis for advancement.

CHAPTER 6

1. Program I-6 on the computer diskette accompanying this book may be used to administer this "College Course and Instructor Evaluation Questionnaire."

2. Although subject to the leniency error, as revealed by the following poem, student ratings of faculty are not always positive:

> His lectures were so dull and elementary
> And his humor was not even supplementary,
> That his students learned no more
> Than they had known long before,
> Consequently rating him not complimentary.

3. An exception may occur when a teacher wants very much to have a difficult child removed from the classroom. In such cases, the teacher may bias the ratings negatively to make the child appear worse than he or she actually is.

CHAPTER 7

1. A short poem may facilitate remembering the distinctions among the three types of body build and the three temperament types:

> Mesmorphs are very tough,   Viscerotonics are quite gay,
> And ectomorphs are thin.   And cerebrotonics think.
> Endomorphs eat lots of stuff, Somatotonics love to play
> Except when dietin'.   When physically "in the pink."

CHAPTER 8

1. Shoemaker (1971) described an application of item-examinee sampling to scaling attitudes by the method of pair comparisons, a procedure that can result in substantial savings in time and effort while providing a good approximation to results obtained by the full pair comparisons procedure. Also see endnote 1 for Chapter 2.

References

Abelson, R. P. (1967). A technique and a model for multi-dimensional attitude scaling. In M. Fishbein (Ed.), *Readings in attitude theory and measurement* (pp. 147–156). New York: Wiley.

Achenbach, T. M., & Edelbrock, C. (1983). *Manual of the Child Behavior Checklist and Revised Child Behavior Profile*. Burlington, VT: University of Vermont, Department of Psychiatry.

Aiken, L. R. (1962). Frequency and intensity as psychometric response variables. *Psychological Reports, 11,* 535–538.

Aiken, L. R. (1966). Another look at weighting test items. *Journal of Educational Measurement, 3,* 183–185.

Aiken, L. R. (1975). A program for computing rank correlations from ordered contingency tables. *Educational and Psychological Measurement, 35,* 181–183.

Aiken, L. R. (1979). Relationships between item difficulty and discrimination indexes. *Educational and Psychological Measurement, 39,* 821–824.

Aiken, L. R. (1980). Content validity and reliability of single items or composites. *Educational and Psychological Measurement, 40,* 955–959.

Aiken, L. R. (1981). Analysis of covariance or partial correlation: What is the question? *Educational Research Quarterly, 6*(2), 13–16.

Aiken, L. R. (1983a). The case for oral achievement testing. *ERIC Reports ED, 222,* 578.

Aiken, L. R. (1983b). Determining grade boundaries on classroom tests. *Educational and Psychological Measurement, 43,* 759–762.

Aiken, L. R. (1985a). Evaluating ratings on bidirectional scales. *Educational and Psychological Measurement, 45,* 195–202.

Aiken, L. R. (1985b). Three coefficients for analyzing the reliability and validity of ratings. *Educational and Psychological Measurement, 45,* 131–142.

Aiken, L. R. (1988). A program for computing the reliability and maximum reliability of a weighted composite. *Educational and Psychological Measurement, 48,* 703–706.

Aiken, L. R. (1992). Some measures of interpersonal attraction and group cohesiveness. *Educational and Psychological Measurement, 52,* 63–67.

Aiken, L. R. (1994a). *Psychological testing and assessment* (8th ed.). Boston: Allyn & Bacon.

Aiken, L. R. (1994b). Some observations and recommendations concerning research methodology in the behavioral sciences. *Educational and Psychological Measurement, 54,* 848–860.

Aiken, L. R. (in press). Programs for alternative voting systems. *Educational and Psychological Measurement.*

Ajzen, I., & Fishbein, M. (1977). Attitude-behavior relations: A theoretical analysis and review of empirical research. *Psychological Bulletin, 84,* 888–918.

Aleamoni, L. (1978). Development and factorial validation of the Arizona counsel instructor evaluation questionnaire. *Educational and Psychological Measurement, 38,* 1063–1067.

American Psychological Association. (1992). Ethical principles of psychologists and code of conduct. *American Psychologist, 47,* 1597–1611.

Andrich, D. (1978a). A binomial latent trait model for the study of Likert-style attitude questionnaires. *British Journal of Mathematical and Statistical Psychology, 31*(1), 84–98.

Andrich, D. (1978b). A rating formulation for ordered response categories. *Psychometrika, 43*(4), 561–573.

Andrich, D. (1978c). Scaling attitude items constructed and scored in the Likert tradition. *Educational and Psychological Measurement, 38,* 665–680.

Andrich, D. (1994). Rating scale analysis. In T. Husén & T. N. Postlethwaite (Eds.), *The international encyclopedia of education* (2nd ed., pp. 4918–4923). New York: Elsevier Science.

Apgar, V. (1953). A proposal for a new method of evaluation in the newborn infant. *Current Research in Anesthesia and Analegesia, 32,* 260.

Bakan, D. (1966). The influence of phrenology on American psychology. *Journal of the History of the Behavioral Sciences, 2,* 200–220.

Bass, B. M., & Barrett, G. V. (1982). *People, work, and organizations.* Boston: Allyn & Bacon.

Beaty, J. J. (1994). *Observing development of the young child* (3rd ed.). New York: Merrill/Macmillan.

Bech, P. (1993). *Rating scales for psychopathology, health status and quality of life.* New York: Springer-Verlag.

Beigel, A., Murphy, D. L., & Bunney, W. E. (1971). The Manic-State Rating Scale: Scale construction, reliability, and validity. *Archives of General Psychiatry, 25,* 256–262.

Bernardin, H. J. (1986). Subordinate appraisal: A valuable source of information about managers. *Human Resource Management, 25,* 421–439.

Berne, E. (1966). *Principles of group treatment.* New York: Oxford University Press.

Bogardus, E. S. (1925). Measuring social distances. *Journal of Applied Sociology, 9,* 299–308.

Bogardus, E. S. (1928). *Immigration and race attitudes.* Boston: Heath.

Bolton, B. (1985). Work Values Inventory. In D. J. Keyser & R. C. Sweetland (Eds.), *Test critiques* (Vol. 2, pp. 835–843). Kansas City, MO: Test Corporation of America.

Bowmas, D. A., & Bernardin, J. J. (1991). Suppressing illusory halo with forced-choice items. *Journal of Applied Psychology, 76,* 592–594.

Brams, S. J., & Fishburn, P. C. (1991). Alternative voting systems. In L. S. Maisel (Ed.), *Political parties and elections in the United States: An encyclopedia* (Vol. 1, pp. 23–31). New York: Garland Publishing.

Bratcher, R. L., Morgan, M. A., & Zimmer, W. J. (1970). Tables of sample sizes in the analysis of variance. *Journal of Quality Technology, 2,* 156–164.

Bruvold, W. H. (1975). Judgmental bias in the rating of attitude statements. *Educational and Psychological Measurement, 35,* 605–611.

Burdock, E. L., Hardesty, A. S., Hakerem, G., Zubin, J., & Beck, Y. M. (1968). *Ward Behavior Inventory*. New York: Springer-Verlag.

Burisch, M. (1984a). Approaches to personality inventory construction. *American Psychologist, 39*, 214–227.

Burisch, M. (1984b). You don't always get what you pay for: Measuring depression with short and simple versus long and sophisticated scales. *Journal of Research in Personality, 18*, 81–98.

Buros, O. K. (Ed.). (1978). *The eighth measurements yearbook* (Vols. 1–2). Highland Park, NJ: Gryphon Press.

Butcher, J. N. (Ed.). (1995). *Clinical personality assessment.* New York: Oxford University Press.

Campbell, D. P., & Fiske, D. W. (1959). Convergent and discriminant validation by the multitrait-multimethod matrix. *Psychological Bulletin, 56*, 81–105.

Campbell, D. T., & Stanley, J. C. (1966). *Experimental and quasiexperimental designs for research.* Chicago: Rand McNally.

Carmody, D. (1987, December 2). Picking college guides: No easy task. *The New York Times, 137*, p. 19.

Cascio, W. F. (1991). *Applied psychology in personnel management* (4th ed.). Englewood Cliffs, NJ: Prentice-Hall.

Castro, J. G., & Jordan, J. E. (1977). Facet theory attitude research. *Educational Researcher, 6*, 7–11.

Champion, C. H., Green, S. B., & Sauser, W. I. (1988). Development and evaluation of shortcut-derived behaviorally anchored ratings scales. *Educational and Psychological Measurement, 48*, 29–41.

Chen, C., Lee, S., & Stevenson, H. W. (1995). Response style and cross-cultural comparisons of rating scales among East Asian and North American students. *Psychological Science, 6*, 170–175.

Chester, R. D., & Dulin, K. L. (1977). Three approaches to the measurement of secondary school students' attitudes toward books and reading. *Research in Teaching English, 11*, 193–200.

Chinn, P. C., Drew, C. J., & Logan, D. R. (1975). *Mental retardation: A life cycle approach.* St. Louis: Mosby.

Chun, K. T., Cobb, S., & French, J. R. P. (1976). *Measures for psychological assessment.* Ann Arbor, MI: University of Michigan, Institute for Social Research.

Ciminero, A. R., Calhoun, K. S., & Adams, H. E. (Eds.). (1986). *Handbook of behavioral assessment* (2nd ed.). New York: Wiley.

Cleveland, J. N., & Murphy, K. R. (1992). Analyzing performance appraisal as goal-directed behavior. In G. Ferris & K. Rowland (Eds.), *Research in personnel and human resources management* (Vol. 10, pp. 121–185). Greenwich, CT: JAI Press.

Cohen, J. (1988). *Statistical power analysis for the behavioral sciences* (2nd ed.). New York: Academic Press.

Comrey, A. L., Bacher, T. E., & Glaser, F. M. (1973). *A source book for mental health measures.* Los Angeles: Human Interaction Research Institute.

Conners, C. K. (1973). Rating scales for use in drug studies with children. *Psychopharmacology Bulletin, 24*–84.

Conners, C. K., & Barkley, R. A. (1985). Rating scales and checklists for child psychopharmacology. *Psychopharmacology Bulletin, 21*, 809–815.

Conoley, J. C., & Impara, J. C. (Eds.). (1995). *The twelfth mental measurements yearbook.* Lincoln: University of Nebraska and Buros Institute of Mental Measurements.

Conoley, J. C., & Kramer, J. J. (Eds.). (1989). *The tenth mental measurements yearbook.* Lincoln: University of Nebraska and Buros Institute of Mental Measurements.

Converse, P. E., Dotson, J. D., Hoag, W. J., & McGee, W. H., III. (1980). *American social attitudes data sourcebook, 1947–78.* Cambridge, MA: Harvard University Press.

Costa, P. T., Jr., & McCrae, R. R. (1986). Personality stability and its implications for clinical psychology. *Clinical Psychology Review, 6,* 407–423.

Cronbach, L. J., Gleser, G. C., Nanda, H., & Rajaratnam, N. (1972). *The dependability of behavioral measurements: Theory of generalizability for scores and profiles.* New York: Wiley.

Davis, J. A., & Smith, T. W. (1994). *General social surveys, 1972–1994: Cumulative codebook.* Chicago: National Opinion Research Center. (Distributed by Roper Center for Public Opinion Research, University of Connecticut, Storrs.)

Dowd, E. T. (1992). Review of the Beck Hopelessness Scale. In J. J. Kramer & J. C. Conoley (Eds.), *The eleventh mental measurements yearbook* (pp. 81–83). Lincoln: University of Nebraska and Buros Institute of Mental Measurements.

Driscoll, L. A., & Goodwin, W. L. (1979). The effects of varying information about use and disposition of results on university students' evaluation of faculty and courses. *American Educational Research Journal, 16,* 25–37.

DuBois, P. H. (1970). *The history of psychology testing.* Boston: Allyn & Bacon.

Duffy, K. E., & Webber, R. E. (1974). On "relative" rating systems. *Personnel Psychology, 27*(2), 307–311.

Edelbrock, C. (1988). Informant reports. In E. S. Shapiro & T. R. Kratchowill (Eds.), *Behavioral assessment in schools: Conceptual foundations and practical applications* (pp. 351–383). New York: Guilford.

Edelbrock, C., & Achenbach, T. M. (1984). The teacher version of the Child Behavior Profile 2: Boys aged 6–11. *Journal of Consulting and Clinical Psychology, 52,* 207–212.

Edwards, A. L. (1954). *Manual—Edwards Personal Preference Schedule.* New York: The Psychological Corporation.

Edwards, A. L. (1957). *Techniques of attitude scale construction.* New York: Appleton-Century-Crofts.

Edwards, A. L., & Kilpatrick, F. P. (1974). A technique for the construction of attitude scales. In G. M. Maranell (Ed.), *Scaling: A sourcebook for behavioral scientists.* Chicago: Aldine.

Endicott, J., & Spitzer, R. L. (1978). A diagnostic interview: The Schedule for Affective Disorders and Schizophrenia. *Archives of General Psychiatry, 35,* 837–844.

Equal Employment Opportunity Commission, Civil Service Commission, Department of Labor and Department of Justice. (1978). Adoption by four agencies of Uniform Guidelines on Employee Selection Procedures. *Federal Register, 43*(166), 38290–38315.

ETS test collection catalog (Vol. 5). (1991). Phoenix, AZ: Oryx Press.

Evans, S. H., & Anastasio, E. J. (1968). Misuse of analysis of covariance when treatment effect and covariate are confounded. *Psychological Bulletin, 69,* 225–239.

Farh, J. L., & Dobbins, G. H. (1989). Effects of comparative performance information on the accuracy of self-ratings and agreement between self- and supervisor ratings. *Journal of Applied Psychology, 74,* 606–610.

Feldt, L. S., & Brennan, R. L. (1989). Reliability. In R. L. Linn (Ed.), *Educational measurement* (3rd ed., pp. 105–146). New York: American Council on Education.

Fishbein, M., & Ajzen, I. (1975). *Belief, attitude, intention, and behavior: An introduction to theory and research.* Reading, MA: Addison-Wesley.

Flanagan, J. C. (1954). The critical incident technique. *Psychological Bulletin, 51,* 327–358.

Fox, S., & Dinur, Y. (1988). Validity of self-assessment: A field evaluation. *Personnel Psychology, 41,* 581–592.

Fraser, B. J., Anderson, G. J., & Walberg, H. J. (1982). *Learning Environment Inventory manual.* South Bentley, Western Australia: Western Australian Institute of Technology.

Gagné, R. M., & Briggs, L. J. (1974). *Principles of instructional design.* New York: Holt, Rinehart & Winston.

Gardner, P. L. (1975). Attitude measurement: A critique of some recent research. *Educational Research, 17,* 101–109.

Giannetti, R. A. (1987). The GOLPH psychosocial history: Response-contingent data acquisition and reporting. In J. N. Butcher (Ed.), *Computerized psychological assessment* (pp. 124–144). New York: Basic Books.

Gillmore, G. M., Kane, M. T., & Naccarato, R. W. (1978). The generalizability of student ratings of instruction. *Journal of Educational Measurement, 15,* 1–14.

Glass, G. V. (1966). None on rank-biserial correlation. *Educational and Psychological Measurement, 26,* 623–631.

Goldman, B. A., & Busch, J. C. (Eds.). (1978). *Directory of unpublished experimental mental measures* (Vol. 2). New York: Human Sciences Press.

Goldman, B. A., & Mitchell, D. F. (Eds.). (1990). *Directory of unpublished experimental mental measures* (Vol. 5). Dubuque, IA: William C. Brown.

Goldman, B. A., & Osborne, W. L. (Eds.). (1985). *Directory of unpublished experimental mental measures.* (Vol. 4). New York: Human Sciences Press.

Goldman, B. A., & Saunders, J. L. (Eds.). (1974). *Directory of unpublished experimental mental measures* (Vol. 1). New York: Human Sciences Press.

Goodstadt, M. S., & Magid, S. (1977). When Thurstone and Likert agree: A confounding of methodologies. *Educational and Psychological Measurement, 37,* 811–818.

Goodwin, F. K., & Jamison, K. R. (1990). *Manic-depressive illness* (pp. 318–331). New York: Oxford.

Grant, D. L. (1987). Personnel selection. In R. J. Corsini (Ed.), *Concise encyclopedia of psychology* (pp. 839–841). New York: Wiley.

Gresham, F. M. (1992). Review of the Teacher Evaluation Rating Scales. In J. J. Kramer & J. C. Conoley (Eds.), *The eleventh mental measurements yearbook* (pp. 915–916). Lincoln: University of Nebraska and Buros Institute of Mental Measurements.

Guilford, J. P. (1954). *Psychometric methods* (2nd ed.). New York: McGraw-Hill.

Gulliksen, H., & Tucker, L. R. (1961). A general procedure for obtaining paired comparisons from multiple rank orders. *Psychometrika, 26,* 173–184.

Guttman, L. (1944). A basis for scaling quantitative data. *American Sociological Review, 9,* 139–150.

Hamersma, R. J., Paige, J., & Jordan, J. E. (1973). Construction of a Guttman facet designed cross-cultural attitude-behavior scale toward racial ethnic interaction. *Educational and Psychological Measurement, 33,* 565–576.

Hammill, D. D., Brown, L., & Bryant, B. R. (1992). *A consumer's guide to tests in print* (2nd ed.). Austin, TX: Pro-Ed.

Harrington, R. G. (Ed.). (1986). *Testing adolescents.* Kansas City, MO: Test Corporation of America.

Harris, M. M., & Schaubroeck, J. (1988). A meta-analysis of self-supervisor, self-peer, and peer-supervisor ratings. *Personnel Psychology, 41,* 43–62.

Hattendorf, L. C. (Ed.). (1995). *Educational rankings annual.* New York: Gale Research, Inc.

Haynes, S. N. (1990). Behavioral assessment of adults. In G. Goldstein & M. Hersen (Eds.), *Handbook of psychological assessment* (2nd ed., pp. 423–463). New York: Pergamon.

Haynes, S. N., & Wilson, C. C. (1979). *Behavioral assessment.* San Francisco: Jossey-Bass.

Healey, J. F. (1993). *Statistics: A tool for social research* (3rd ed.). Belmont, CA: Wadsworth.

Hersen, M., & Bellack, A. S. (Eds.). (1982). *Behavioral assessment: A practical handbook* (2nd ed.). New York: Pergamon.

Holmes, T. H., & Rahe, R. H. (1967). The Social Readjustment Scale. *Journal of Psychosomatic Research, 11,* 213–218.

Honigfeld, G., & Klett, C. (1965). The Nurses' Observation Scale for Inpatient Evaluation (NOSIE): A new scale for measuring improvement in schizophrenia. *Journal of Clinical Psychology, 21,* 65–71.

Johnson, O. G. (1976). *Tests and measurements in child development: Handbook II.* San Francisco: Jossey-Bass.

Johnson, O. G., & Bommarito, J. W. (1971). *Tests and measurements in child development.* San Francisco: Jossey-Bass.

Jordan, J. E. (1971). Construction of a Guttman facet designed cross-cultural attitude-behavior scale toward mental retardation. *American Journal of Mental Deficiency, 76,* 201–219.

Kane, J. S., & Lawler, E. E., III. (1978). Methods of peer assessment. *Psychological Bulletin, 85,* 555–586.

Kane, J. S., & Lawler, E. E., III. (1980). In defense of peer assessment: A rebuttal to Brief's critique. *Psychological Bulletin, 88,* 80–81.

Kanungo, B. N. (1985). Review of Work Environment Scale. In J. V. Mitchell, Jr. (Ed.), *The ninth mental measurements yearbook* (pp. 1776–1777). Lincoln: University of Nebraska and Buros Institute of Mental Measures.

Kendall, M. G. (1970). *Rank correlation methods* (4th ed.). London: Charles Griffin.

Kendall, P. C., & Korgeski, G. P. (1979). Assessment and cognitive-behavioral interventions. *Cognitive Therapy and Research, 1,* 1–21.

Kerlinger, F. N. (1972). A Q validation of the structure of social attitudes. *Educational and Psychological Measurement, 32,* 987–995.

Keyser, D. J., & Sweetland, R. C. (Eds.). (1984–1994). *Test critiques* (Vols. 1–10). Austin, TX: Pro-Ed.

Kinicki, A. J., & Bannister, B. D. (1988). A test of the measurement assumptions underlying behaviorally anchored rating scales. *Educational and Psychological Measurement, 48*, 17–27.

Kleinmuntz, B. (1982). *Personality and psychological assessment.* New York: St. Martin's Press.

Kramer, J. J., & Conoley, J. (1992). *The eleventh mental measurements yearbook.* Lincoln: University of Nebraska and Buros Institute of Mental Measurements.

Krug, S. E. (1993). *Psychware sourcebook (4th ed.).* Champaign, IL: MetriTech.

Kubiszyn, T., & Borich, G. (1990). *Educational testing and measurement* (3rd ed.). Glenview, IL: Scott Foresman/Little, Brown.

Kulik, J. A., & McKeachie, W. J. (1975). The evaluation of teachers in higher education. In F. N. Kerlinger (Ed.), *Review of research in education* (pp. 210–240).

Lake, D. G., Miles, M. B., & Earle, R. B. (1973). *Measuring human behavior: Tools for the assessment of social functioning.* New York: Teachers College Press.

Landy, F. J., & Farr, J. I. (1983). *The measurement of work performance: Methods, theory, and applications.* New York: Academic Press.

Langeheine, R., & Rost, J. (Eds.). (1988). *Latent traits and latent class models.* New York: Plenum.

Lastovicka, J. L., Murray, J. P., Joachimsthaler, E. A., Bhalla, G., & Scheurich, J. (1987). A lifestyle topology to model young male drinking and driving. *Journal of Consumer Research, 14*, 257–263.

Lazarsfeld, P. F., & Henry, N. W. (1968). *Latent structure analysis.* Boston: Houghton Mifflin.

Levy, P., & Goldstein, H. (1984). *Tests in education: A book of critical reviews.* New York: Academic Press.

Liberman, R. P. (Ed.). (1988). *Psychiatric rehabilitation of chronic mental patients.* Washington, DC: American Psychiatric Press.

Likert, R. (1932). A technique for the measurement of attitudes. *Archives of Psychology, 22*(140).

Litwin, G. H., & Stringer, R. A., Jr. (1968). *Motivation and organizational climate.* Cambridge, MA: Harvard University, Graduate School of Business.

London, M., & Wohlers, A. J. (1991). Agreement between subordinate and self-ratings in upward feedback. *Personnel Psychology, 44*, 375–390.

Lyerly, S. B. (1978). *Handbook of psychiatric rating scales* (2nd ed.). Rockville, MC: National Institute of Mental Health.

Marsden, D. B., Meisels, S. J., Steel, D. M., & Jablon, J. R. (1993). *The work sampling system: The portfolio collection process for early childhood and early elementary classrooms.* Ann Arbor, MI: University of Michigan, Center for Human Growth and Development.

Marsh, H. W. (1977). The validity of students' evaluations: Classroom evaluations of instructors by graduating seniors. *American Educational Research Journal, 14*, 441–447.

Martin, E., & McDuffee, D. (1981). *A sourcebook of Harris national surveys: Repeated questions, 1963–76.* Chapel Hill: University of North Carolina, Institute for Research in Social Science.

Martin, R. P. (1988). Basic methods of objective test construction. In *Assessment of personality and behavior problems: Infancy through adolescence* (pp. 43–67). New York: Guilford.

Masters, J. R. (1974). Relationship between number of response categories and reliability of Likert-type questionnaires. *Journal of Educational Measurement, 11,* 49–53.

McCall, W. A. (1939). *Measurement.* New York: Macmillan.

McCutcheon, A. L. (1987). *Latent class analysis.* Newbury Park, CA: Sage.

McEvoy, G. M., & Buller, P. F. (1987). User acceptance of peer appraisals in an industrial setting. *Personnel Psychology, 40,* 785–797.

McReynolds, P. (1984). History of assessment in clinical and educational settings. In R. O. Nelson & S. C. Hayes (Eds.), *Conceptual foundations of behavioral assessment* (pp. 42–79). New York: Guilford.

Mislevy, R. J., & Bock, R. D. (1983). *BILOG: Marginal estimation of item parameters and subject ability under binary logistic models.* Chicago: International Educational Services.

Mitchell, J. V., Jr. (Ed.). (1985). *The ninth mental measurements yearbook.* Lincoln: University of Nebraska and Buros Institute of Mental Measurements.

Moos, R. H. (1986). *Work Environment Scale manual* (2nd ed.). Palo Alto, CA: Consulting Psychologists Press.

Moos, R. H. (1988). *University Residence Environment Scale manual* (2nd ed.). Palo Alto, CA: Consulting Psychologists Press.

Moos, R. H., & Billings, A. G. (1991). Understanding and improving work climates. In J. W. Jones, B. D. Steffy, & D. W. Bray (Eds.), *Applying psychology in business: The handbook for managers and human resource professionals* (pp. 552–562). Lexington, MA: Heath.

Moos, R., & Trickett, E. (1987). *The Classroom Environment Scale manual* (2nd ed.). Palo Alto, CA: Consulting Psychologists Press.

Morrow, J. R. (1977). Some statistics regarding the reliability and validity of student ratings of teachers. *The Research Quarterly, 48,* 372–375.

Moyer, R. H. (1977). Environmental attitude assessment: Another approach. *Science Education, 61,* 347–356.

Muchinsky, P. M. (1990). *Psychology applied to work: An introduction to industrial and organizational psychology* (3rd ed.). Chicago: Dorsey Press.

Murray, H. A. (1938). *Explorations in personality.* New York: Oxford University Press.

Murphy, D. L., Beigel, A., Weingartner, H., & Bunney, W. E. (1974). The quantification of manic behavior. *Modern Problems in Pharmacopsychiatry, 7,* 203–220.

Murphy, K. R., & Constans, J. I. (1987). Behavioral anchors as a source of bias in rating. *Journal of Applied Psychology, 72,* 573–577.

Murphy, K. R., & Davidshofer, C. O. (1994). *Psychological testing: Principles and applications.* Englewood Cliffs, NJ: Prentice-Hall.

Murphy, L. L., Conoley, J. C., & Impara, J. C. (Eds.). (1994). *Tests in print IV.* Lincoln: University of Nebraska and Buros Institute of Mental Measurements.

Mussen, P. (1979). *Psychology: An introduction.* Lexington, MA: Heath.

Ollendick, T. H., & Green, R. (1990). Behavioral assessment of children. In G. Goldstein & M. Hersen (Eds.), *Handbook of psychological assessment* (2nd ed., pp. 403–422). New York: Pergamon.

Oppler, S. H., Campbell, J. P., Pulakos, E. D., & Borman, W. C. (1992). Three approaches to the investigation of subgroup bias in performance measurement: Review, results, and conclusions. *Journal of Applied Psychology, 77,* 201–217.

Osgood, C. E., Suci, G. J., & Tannenbaum, P. H. (1957). *The measurement of meaning*. Urbana, IL: University of Illinois Press.

Overall, J. E., & Gorham, D. R. (1962). The Brief Psychiatric Rating Scale. *Psychological Reports, 10,* 799–812.

Owen, S. V. (1992). Review of the Beck Hopelessness Scale. In J. J. Kramer & J. C. Conoley (Eds.), *The eleventh mental measurements yearbook* (pp. 82–83). Lincoln: University of Nebraska and Buros Institute of Mental Measurements.

Pagano, R. R. (1994). *Understanding statistics in the behavioral sciences* (4th ed.). St. Paul, MN: West.

Peterson, R. C., & Thurstone, L. L. (1933). *Motion pictures and the social attitudes of children*. New York: Macmillan.

Piacentini, J. (1993). Checklists and rating scales. In T. H. Ollendick & M. Hersen (Eds.), *Handbook of child and adolescent assessment* (pp. 82–97). Boston: Allyn & Bacon.

Pulakos, E. D. (1991). Rater training for performance appraisal. In J. W. Jones, B. D. Steffy, & D. W. Bray (Eds.), *Applying psychology in business: The handbook for managers and human resource professionals* (pp. 326–332). Lexington, MA: Heath.

Quay, H. C., & Peterson, D. R. (1983). *Interim manual for the Behavior Problem Checklist*. Unpublished manuscript, University of Miami.

Rabinowitz, W. (1984). Study of Values. In D. J. Keyser & R. C. Sweetland (Eds.), *Test critiques* (Vol. 1, pp. 641–647). Kansas City, MO: Test Corporation of America.

Rasch, G. (1972). Objektivitet i Samfundsvidenskaberne et Metodeproblem. Paper presented at the University of Copenhagen.

Reckase, M. D. (1990). Scaling techniques. In G. Goldstein & M. Hersen (Eds.), *Handbook of psychological assessment* (2nd ed., pp. 41–56). New York: Pergamon.

Remmers, H. H. (1960). *Manual for the Purdue Master Attitude Scales*. Lafayette, IN: Purdue Research Foundation.

Robinson, J. P., Athanasiou, R., & Head, K. B. (1974). *Measurement of occupational attitudes and occupational characteristics*. Ann Arbor: University of Michigan, Institute for Social Research.

Robinson, J. P., Rush, J. G., & Head, K. B. (1973). *Measures of political attitudes*. Ann Arbor: University of Michigan, Institute for Social Research.

Robinson, J. P., Shaver, P. R., & Wrightsman, L. S. (1991). *Measures of personality and social psychological attitudes*. New York: Academic Press.

Roethlisberger, F. J., & Dickson, W. J. (1939). *Management and the worker: An account of a research program conducted by the Western Electric Company, Chicago*. Cambridge, MA: Harvard University Press.

Rogers, C. R., & Dymond, R. F. (Eds.). (1954). *Psychotherapy and personality change*. Chicago: University of Chicago Press.

Rokeach, M. (1968). *Beliefs, attitudes, and values: A theory of organization and change*. San Francisco: Jossey-Bass.

Rokeach, M. (1973). *The nature of human values*. New York: Free Press.

Rosenman, R. H. (1986). Current and past history of Type A behavior pattern. In T. H. Schmidt, T. M. Dembroski, & G. Blumchen (Eds.), *Biological and psychological factors in cardiovascular disease* (pp. 15–40). New York: Springer-Verlag.

Rossi, P. H., & Freeman, H. E. (1993). *Evaluation: A systematic approach* (5th ed.). Beverly Hills, CA: Sage Publications.

Rotem, A., & Glasman, N. S. (1979). On the effectiveness of students' evaluative feedback to university instructors. *Review of Educational Research, 49,* 497–511.

Rothkopf, A. J. (1995, July 14). Devising better ways to measure the quality of colleges and universities. *The Chronicle of Higher Education,* p. B3.

Schiffman, S. S., Reynolds, M. L., & Young, F. W. (1981). *Introduction to multidimensional scaling.* New York: Academic Press.

Schultz, D. P., & Schultz, S. E. (1994). *Psychology and work today: An introduction to industrial and organizational psychology* (6th ed.). New York: Macmillan.

Shaw, M. E., & Wright, J. M. (1967). *Scales for the measurement of attitudes.* New York: McGraw-Hill.

Sheldon, W. H., & Stevens, S. S. (1942). *The varieties of temperament.* New York: Harper & Row.

Sheldon, W. H., Stevens, S. S., & Tucker, W. B. (1940). *The varieties of human physique.* New York: Harper & Row.

Shoemaker, D. M. (1971). Application of item-examinee sampling to scaling attitudes. *Journal of Educational Measurement, 8,* 279–282.

Sines, J. O., Pauker, J. D., Sines, L. K., & Owen, D. R. (1969). Identification of clinically relevant dimensions of children's behavior. *Journal of Consulting and Clinical Psychology, 33,* 728–734.

Smith, P. C., Kendall, L. M., & Hulin, C. L. (1969). *The measurement of satisfaction in work and retirement.* Chicago: Rand McNally.

Smith, P. L. (1979). The generalizability of student ratings of courses: Asking the right questions. *Journal of Educational Measurement, 16,* 77–88.

Snider, J. G., & Osgood, C. E. (Eds.). (1969). *Semantic differential technique: A sourcebook.* Hawthorne, NY: Aldine.

Solomon, R. L., & Lessac, M. S. (1968). A control group design for experimental studies of developmental processes. *Psychological Bulletin, 70,* 145–150.

Spector, P. E. (1976). Choosing response categories for summated rating scales. *Journal of Applied Psychology, 61,* 374–375.

Spitzer, R. L., Williams, J. B. W., Gibbon, M., & First, M. B. (1992). The Structured Clinical Interview for DSM-III-R (SCID). *Archives of General Psychiatry, 49,* 624–629.

Spranger, E. (1928). *Types of men.* Berlin, Germany: Max Niemeyer Verlag.

Stephenson, W. (1953). *The study of behavior: Q-technique and its methodology.* Chicago: University of Chicago Press.

Stevens, S. S. (1951). Mathematics, measurement, and psychophysics. In S. S. Stevens (Ed.), *Handbook of experimental psychology* (pp. 1–49). New York: Wiley.

Stoloff, M. L., & Couch, J. V. (Eds.). (1992). *Computer use in psychology: A directory of software* (3rd ed.). Washington, DC: American Psychological Association.

Stouffer, S. A., et al. (1950). *Measurement and prediction: Vol. 4. Studies in social psychology in World War II.* Princeton, NJ: Princeton University Press.

Sundberg, N. D. (1992). Review of the Beck Depression Inventory. In J. J. Kramer & J. C. Conoley (Eds.), *The eleventh mental measurements yearbook* (pp. 79–80). Lincoln: The University of Nebraska and Buros Institute of Mental Measurements.

Super, D. E. (1973). The Work Values Inventory. In D. G. Zytowski (Ed.), *Contemporary approaches to interest measurement.* Minneapolis, MN: University of Minnesota Press.

Sweetland, R. C., & Keyser, D. J. (Eds.). (1991). *Tests* (3rd ed.). Austin, TX: Pro-Ed.

Swiercinsky, D. P. (Ed.). (1985). *Testing adults.* Kansas City, MO: Test Corporation of America.

Taylor, H. C., & Russell, J. T. (1939). The relationship of validity coefficients to the practical effectiveness of tests in selection: Discussion and tables. *Journal of Applied Psychology, 23,* 565–578.

Teeter, P. A. (1985). Review of Adjective Check List. In J. V. Mitchell, Jr. (Ed.), *The ninth mental measurements yearbook* (Vol. 1, pp. 50–52). Lincoln: University of Nebraska and Buros Institute of Mental Measurements.

Templer, D. I. (1985). Multiple Affect Adjective Check List—Revised. In D. J. Keyser & R. C. Sweetland (Eds.), *Test critiques* (Vol. 4, pp. 449–452). Kansas City, MO: Test Corporation of America.

Thissen, D., & Steinberg, L. (1986). A taxonomy of item response models. *Psychometrika, 51,* 567–577.

Thorndike, E. L. (1918). *The seventeenth yearbook of the National Society for the Study of Education,* (Pt. 2). Bloomington, IL: Public School Publishing Co.

Thurstone, L. L., & Chave, E. J. (1929). *The measurement of attitude.* Chicago: University of Chicago Press.

Tziner, A. E., & Cheatham, T. (1977). Attitude measurement through use of computer-constructed questionnaires. *Educational and Psychological Measurement, 37,* 241–243.

Vale, C. D., & Gialluca, K. A. (1985, November). *ASCAL: A microcomputer program for estimating logistic IRT item parameters* (Research Report ONR-85-4). St. Paul, MN: Assessment Systems Corporation.

Walsh, J. A. (1984). Tennessee Self Concept Scale. In D. J. Keyser & R. C. Sweetland (Eds.), *Test critiques* (Vol. 1, pp. 663–672). Kansas City, MO: Test Corporation of American.

Weaver, S. J. (Ed.). (1984). *Testing children.* Kansas City, MO: Test Corporation of America.

Weinberg, S. L. (1991). An introduction to multidimensional scaling. *Measurement and Evaluation in Counseling and Development, 24,* 12–36.

Wewers, M. E., & Lowe, N. K. (1990). A critical review of visual analogue scales in the measurement of clinical phenomena. *Research in Nursing & Health, 13*(4), 227–236.

Wexley, K. N., & Klimoski, R. (1984). Performance appraisal: An update. In K. M. Rowland & G. R. Ferris (Eds.), *Research in personnel and human resources management* (Vol. 2, pp. 35–79). Greenwich, CT: JAI Press.

Wheeler, K. G. (1985). Review of Temperament and Values Inventory. In J. V. Mitchell, Jr. (Ed.), *The ninth mental measurements yearbook* (Vol. 2, pp. 1535–1536). Lincoln: University of Nebraska and Buros Institute of Mental Measurements.

Wheeler, P. (1992). Review of the Teacher Evaluation Rating Scales. In J. J. Kramer & J. C. Conoley (Eds.), *The eleventh mental measurements yearbook* (pp. 916–917). Lincoln: University of Nebraska and Buros Institute of Mental Measurements.

Wiersma, U., & Latham, G. P. (1986). The practicality of behavioral observation scales, behavioral expectation scales, and trait scales. *Personnel Psychology, 39,* 619–628.

Wiggins, J. S. (1973). *Personality and prediction: Principles of personality assessment.* Reading, MA: Addison-Wesley.

Winer, B. J., Brown, D. R., & Michels, K. M. (1991). *Statistical principles in experimental design* (3rd ed.). New York: McGraw-Hill.

Wingersky, M. S., Barton, M. A., & Lord, F. M. (1982, February). *LOGIST user's guide.* Princeton, NJ: Educational Testing Service.

Witt, J. C., Heffer, R. W., & Pfeiffer, J. (1990). Structured rating scales: A review of self-report and informant rating processes, procedures, and issues. In C. R. Reynolds & R. W. Kamphaus (Eds.), *Handbook of psychological & educational assessment of children: Personality, behavior, & context* (pp. 364–394). New York: Guilford.

Wolfe, R. N. (1993). A commonsense approach to personality measurement. In K. H. Craik, R. Hogan, & R. N. Wolfe (Eds.), *Fifty years of personality psychology* (pp. 269–290). New York: Plenum.

Wolins, L., & Dickinson, T. T. (1973). Transformations to improve reliability and/or validity for affective scales. *Educational and Psychological Measurement, 33,* 711–713.

Wortham, S. C. (1990). *Tests and measurements in early childhood education.* New York: Merrill/Macmillan.

Worthen, B. R., Borg, W. R., & White, K. R. (1993). *Measurement and evaluation in the schools.* New York: Longman.

Wright, B. D., & Masters, G. N. (1982). *Rating scale analysis.* Chicago: MESA.

Wright, B. D., Mead, R. J., & Bell, S. R. (1979). *BICAL: Calibrating items with the Rasch model* (Research Memorandum No. 23B). Chicago: University of Chicago, Department of Education, Statistical Laboratory.

Yudofsky, S. C., Silver, J. M., Jackson, W., et al. (1986). The Overt Aggression Scale for the objective rating of verbal and physical aggression. *American Journal of Psychiatry, 143,* 35–39.

Zarske, J. A. (1985). Review of Adjective Check List. In J. V. Mitchell, Jr. (Ed.), *The ninth mental measurements yearbook* (Vol. 1, pp. 52–53). Lincoln: University of Nebraska and Buros Institute of Mental Measurements.

Zeltzer, L. K., Richie, D. M., LeBaron, S., & Reed, D. (1988). Can children understand and use a rating scale to quantify somatic symptoms? Assessment of nausea and vomiting as a model. *Journal of Consulting and Clinical Psychology, 56,* 567–572.

Zuckerman, M. (1985). Review of Temperament and Values Inventory. In J. V. Mitchell, Jr. (Ed.), *The ninth mental measurements yearbook* (Vol. 2, pp. 1536–1537). Lincoln: University of Nebraska and Buros Institute of Mental Measurements.

Zuckerman, M., & Lubin, B. (1985). *Manual for the Multiple Affect Adjective Check List—Revised.* San Diego, CA: EdITS.

Author Index

Hills, D., 242
Hoag, W. J., 240
Hoepner, R., 242
Holland, J. L., 242
Holmes, T. H., 203
Holtzman, W. H., 243
Honigfeld, G., 200
Hulin, C. L., 38, 141

Impara, J. C., 25

Jablon, J. R., 173
Jackson, W., 211, 215
Jamison, K. R., 211, 212
Joachimsthaler, E. A., 146
Johannson, C. B., 246, 250
Johnson, O. G., 25
Jordan, J. E., 237

Kane, J. S., 41
Kane, M. T., 163
Kanungo, B. N., 142
Kehoe, P. T., 141
Kendall, L. M., 141
Kendall, M. G., 65
Kendall, P. C., 200
Kerlinger, F. N., 236
Keyser, D. J., 25
Kicklighter, R. H., 180
Kilpatrick, F. P., 236
King, D. W., 243
King, L. A., 243
Kinicki, A. J., 39
Klein, S. P., 242
Kleinmuntz, B., 45
Klett, C., 200
Klimoski, R., 41
Knapp, L. F., 246
Knapp, R. R., 246
Kohn, J., 204
Korgeski, G. P., 200
Kramer, J. J., 25
Krug, S. E., 26
Kubiszyn, T., 159
Kulik, J. A., 163

Lahey, B. B., 183
Lake, D. G., 26

Lambert, N., 180
Landy, F. J., 12
Langeheine, R., 237
Lastovicka, J. L., 146
Latham, G. P., 39
Lawler, E. E., III, 41
Lazersfeld, P. F., 237
LeBaron, S., 214
LeBuffe, P. A., 183
Lee, S., 46, 47
Leigh, J. E., 180
Leland, H., 180
Lessac, M. S., 244
Levin, S., 180
Levy, P., 26
Lewis, J. F., 180
Liberman, R. P., 212
Likert, R., 231
Lindzey, G., 247
Litwin, G. H., 141
London, M., 42
Lord, F. M., 66
Lowe, N. K., 212
Lubin, B., 204, 208
Lyerly, S. B., 26

Magid, S., 231
Marsden, D. B., 173
Marsh, H. W., 163
Martin, D. V., 243
Martin, E., 240
Martin, M., 243
Martin, R. P., 32, 33
Martin, W. T., 243
Maslow, A., 195
Masters, G. N., 65
Masters, J. R., 239
Mattis, S., 215
McCall, W. A., 9
McCarney, S. B., 180
McCrae, R. R., 195
McCutcheon, A. L., 237
McDuffee, D., 240
McEvoy, G. M., 41
McGee, W. H., III, 240
McGurine, J., 183
McKeachie, W. J., 163
McReynolds, P., 15

Subject Index

Instruments Index